OSCE and VIVA VOCE in Obstetrics and Gynaecology

Calvin Chama

OSCE and VIVA VOCE in Obstetrics and Gynaecology

Evaluating the knowledge, clinical skills, and competency of medical students and residents

Springer

Calvin Chama
Obstetrics and Gynaecology
Abubakar Tafawa Balewa University
Bauchi, Nigeria

ISBN 978-3-031-77261-0 ISBN 978-3-031-77262-7 (eBook)
https://doi.org/10.1007/978-3-031-77262-7

This Springer imprint is published by the registered company Springer Nature Switzerland AG
The registered company address is: Gewerbestrasse 11, 6330 Cham, Switzerland

To Dr. Rejoice Chama, Melody Chama,
and Chinapi Chama

Foreword

Since the last decade, attention has dramatically shifted from the traditional examination to the objective structured clinical examination (OSCE) type of examination. This shift has however, not been followed by an equivalent increase in the number of quality resource materials available to both the candidates and examiners alike in the field of obstetrics and gynaecology.

OSCE Stations and VIVA VOCE in Obstetrics and Gynaecology is an excellent companion for both the candidate and examiner preparing for the OSCE examination in Obstetrics and Gynaecology.

The book is organized in a way that one can quickly glance through to the topic of interest: from the basic principles of OSCE, examination construction including blue printing, to real stations with marking schemes, and quality picture tests among others, in the various subspecialities of Obstetrics and Gynaecology.

This book will be found useful to those preparing for the postgraduate examinations in Obstetrics and Gynaecology of the West African College of Surgeons or its equivalents, and with some modifications for undergraduate examination in Obstetrics and Gynaecology.

Department of Obstetrics and Gynaecology
College of Health Sciences, University of Jos
Jos, Nigeria

Patrick H. Daru

Preface

Objective structured clinical examination (OSCE) is an approach to assessment of clinical competence in which the components of competence are assessed in a planned or structured way. Compared to the traditional clinical examination, OSCE has been shown to have higher level of validity and reliability. It is objective and equitable with minimal extraneous interference. It is globally the preferred method of clinical examination at both undergraduate and postgraduate levels.

Since the decision of the Faculty of Obstetrics and Gynaecology of the West African College of Surgeons to introduce the OSCE into the gynaecology aspect of the clinical examination in October 2017, it has successfully phased out the traditional clinical examination in both the gynaecology and obstetrics components of the membership examinations. Because most training institutions in West Africa use the traditional method of clinical examination for assessing candidates at undergraduate and postgraduate levels, there are few resource materials for conducting the OSCE examinations at all levels.

This book is intended to help consultants/lecturers to organize stations for regular assessment of their residents preparing for the membership examinations of the WACS and similar institutions in the African sub-region. It is also a useful reference material for the candidates preparing for the membership examination in obstetrics and gynaecology to understand the scope and expectations for the examination. It is not a replacement for regular training of the candidates and teachers should ensure that their students experience OSCE before the actual membership examination.

The book has been structured to touch on various topics in obstetrics and gynaecology but is by no means exhaustive. Each chapter has at least a station on communication and counselling, physical examination, diagnostic and/or therapeutic procedure, identification of abnormal test finding, and virtual sign identification or picture test. The question in any station can be modified and the checklist altered accordingly to suit the alteration. I believe this is a useful addition to the few resource materials we have for OSCE. The oral questions include those suitable for both the membership and fellowship examinations and the structured viva voce format has been followed rather than the traditional viva voce. The various subspecialities of obstetrics and gynaecology have also been touched and the questions can be *twisted* and the answer outline edited accordingly. A checklist is also provided to aide in analytic rather global scoring according to the preference of the examiner.

Calvin Chama
Bauchi, Nigeria

Acknowledgement

Although the proposed table of contents and indeed some chapters of this book had been written before contacting Springer Nature for possible publication, the reviewers made valuable contributions to make this book what it is today. I am grateful for their contributions. I wish to thank Alessandra Born and Pinky Sathishkumar who have been coordinating my work with the publishers.

The lecturers/consultants as well as residents in my department have immensely contributed in test-running the OSCE stations and the viva voce. Some have contributed useful clinical pictures and made useful contributions during our regular reviews. I wish to thank Dr Dauda Suleiman of Pathology Department of Abubakar Tafawa Balewa University Teaching Hospital, Bauchi, for the pictures of cytology and other pathology specimens from our patients.

Professor Patrick Daru, the Faculty Secretary of the Faculty of Obstetrics and Gynaecology, West African College of Surgeons, reviewed this book and wrote the foreword. May God replenish his energy and grant him more wisdom.

Contents

About the Author

Calvin Chama obtained his MBBS degree from the University of Maiduguri in June 1988. After the mandatory national youth service, he returned to his Alma-Mata as a resident in Obstetrics and Gynaecology in September 1990. He obtained the fellowship of the West African College of Surgeons in October 1997. He took up appointment with the University of Maiduguri, Nigeria, as lecturer 1 in April 2002 and rose through the ranks to become Professor of feto-maternal medicine in October 2009. Professor Chama has mentored several graduate and postgraduate medical doctors in various universities in Nigeria. He was a member of the pioneer OSCE committee of the faculty of Obstetrics and Gynaecology, West African College of Surgeons, from 2017 to 2022. He has remained a script writer for the faculty up to date.

Introduction to OSCE 1

1.1 Basic Principles of OSCE

The Objective Structured Clinical Examination (OSCE) is a way of making valid assessment of the clinical performance of medical students and resident doctors. Since its introduction by Dr. Harden and colleagues in 1975, it has gained widespread acceptance across the globe [1]. When one reviews the wide spectrum of clinical tests that can be incorporated into the OSCE, its advantages are apparent. Its major drawbacks are that it is cumbersome and expensive to set and requires a great deal of personnel for its implementation [2].

An assessment of clinical competence must ensure that the graduates who pass the examination meet the minimum standard for safe practice of obstetrics and gynaecology. A resident obstetrician and gynaecologist is expected to have an in-depth knowledge of obstetrics and gynaecology including unusual conditions. As much as possible, the examination should cover the entire syllabus for the membership and fellowship of the West African College of Surgeons, Faculty of Obstetrics and Gynaecology or its equivalent.

The Webster's dictionary defines competence as "the quality of having sufficient knowledge, judgement skill or experience for some purpose" [3]. From this, the elements of competence are knowledge, skill, attitude, and experience. Competence is a prerequisite for performance in the real clinical setting where it would be expected that a doctor operates at a higher level in most areas and demonstrates mastery in some. In medical examination, the term competence means the ability to apply clinical skills in a standardized setting, the examination setting [4]. For the purpose of assessing clinical competence, the following domains are usually examined:

- Communication and counselling skills
- Physical examination skills
- Procedural (diagnostic and therapeutic) skills
- Cognitive (knowledge) skills

C. Chama, *OSCE and VIVA VOCE in Obstetrics and Gynaecology*,
https://doi.org/10.1007/978-3-031-77262-7_1

1.1.1 Communication Skills

Doctors come across varied number of patients and circumstances, and they must gather information in order to have insight into the patient's problem. The doctor must have the skills to establish rapport with the patient, be a good listener, empathic, and be able to steer the discussion to obtain a focused history and analyse the patient's responses.

1.1.2 Physical Examination Skills

Physical examination skills are taught at an early stage of medical education, and learners are expected to master these skills as they practice on day-to-day basis during their training. With time, learners are expected to perform physical examination (including vaginal examination) to identify, elicit, and interpret the major signs of common clinical conditions.

1.1.3 Procedural Skills

Resident obstetricians and gynaecologists are expected to learn and master common and major diagnostic and therapeutic procedures. This will include diagnostic procedures like ultrasound scanning, cardiotocography (CTG), and colposcopy. Sometimes the results of these tests are presented, and the candidates are expected to interpret them. Therapeutic procedures like suturing, insertion of contraceptive devices and implants, and manual vacuum aspiration may be required.

1.1.4 Cognitive (Knowledge Application) Skills

Following patient interview and physical examination, the resident is expected to synthesize the information gathered and make an impression of the problem (initial diagnosis) before deciding on a plan of management. Relevant investigations are requested, and the resident builds a picture of the patient's problem to arrive at a definitive diagnosis. Appropriate treatment is then given. During the examination, the candidate may be assessed on knowledge application either by decision-making (diagnosis), relevant investigations, problem solving (treatment), or any combination of these.

1.2 Characteristics of a Good Assessment Instrument

Any assessment tool should be judged on the following properties [4, 5]:

- Objectivity
- Validity
- Reliability
- Educational impact

1.2.1 Objectivity

An objective tool for assessment is one in which the examiners easily agree on what is the expected response from the candidate. The chances for the examiners to manipulate the questions and answers, the candidate's performance and judgement, are minimal. All candidates go through the same questions for the same length of time.

1.2.2 Validity

This is the extent to which a test measures what it is intended to measure. A station designed to measure the knowledge of the candidate should be able to do that. Similarly, a station designed to measure the procedural skill of the candidate should principally achieve that objective. For an examination to have content validity, the stations must be carefully selected to cover the curriculum or syllabus. The more the stations the better the coverage and the better the content validity. Generally, validity depends on five sources of evidence [6]:

- The test content represents what the curriculum needs to assess, the tasks are realistic, and the right domains are being assessed.
- The responses to the test item are accurately recorded, handled, stored, and analysed.
- The test has high reliability.
- The test results correlate with the other test results assessing the similar domains and show poor correlation with those assessing different domains (convergence and divergence).
- The consequences of assessment are sound, i.e. effect on learning is positive, the penalties for failure are justifiable, and the consequences of passing are socially and professionally acceptable.

1.2.3 Reliability

This is the ability of the test or instrument, if repeated for a similar group of candidates, which will produce the same result. A reliable test results in a similar scoring across various examiners and candidates so that it reliably differentiates a good and a bad candidate. Because competences are highly domain specific, the examination should have broad sampling of domains to be tested in order to have adequate reliability. Many factors influence the reliability of any assessment method. The main influences on the reliability of an OSCE are as follows:

- The number of stations. Testing candidates across a large sample of clinical cases maximizes reliability [7]
- Standardized checklist or scoring scheme. These ensure that examiners are marking candidates against the same criteria, thereby improving consistency of scoring between candidates and examiners [8]
- Using trained examiners. There is some evidence suggesting that examiner training reduces examiner variation in scoring and improves consistency of examiner behaviour [9]
- Standardized patient performance. Poorly standardized patients who vary their performance between candidates can reduce the reliability of the examination [10]

Objectivity and validity improve reliability.

1.2.4 Feasibility

Feasibility can be defined as the degree of practicality of the assessment intervention. Compared to other assessment methods, OSCE is more resource intensive and time-consuming to set up and run. For this reason, it is important to ensure that the best use is made of the OSCE by only developing stations that require an OSCE format, i.e. assessment of performance rather than knowledge.

1.2.5 Educational Impact

All resident doctors would like to succeed and become consultants, and success is achieved only through examinations. Examinations, therefore, drive learning and the way the examination is conducted affects the way students learn. If the examination explores only basic knowledge of the subject, students are not likely to search for in-depth knowledge. An examination that drives students to learn in depth is said to have high educational impact. The OSCE can have a positive educational impact as it can drive learning [11]. This positive educational impact is dependent on realistic recreation of assessment scenarios at the OSCE stations. If candidates find it difficult to differentiate between the assessment tasks and real-life practice, then the OSCE can drive learning.

1.3 Examination Construction

1.3.1 The Blueprint

Blueprinting is the process of formally determining the content of any examination. In the case of an OSCE, this involves choosing the spread of stations to include all areas of the subject (subspecialties) and the frequency with which each appears within an examination. Each blueprint for an OSCE should take into account the context of the examination, the content which needs to be assessed mapped to the curriculum and the need for triangulation, e.g. if any domains of clinical competence should be examined with the use of more than one assessment tool [12].

The OSCE is primarily a competency-based assessment of performance in a simulated environment [13], and therefore principally tests the skill-based learning outcomes. The blueprinting process should ensure that an appropriate sample of the skill-based curriculum is examined and it is mapped to the curriculum, i.e. the examination has adequate content validity.

In order to develop an examination blueprint, the examination length needs to be determined beforehand. This will depend on the number of stations within each OSCE and the length of each station. An OSCE station typically refers to one-time limited task given to the candidates generally lasting between 5 and 10 min. The reliability (reproducibility of test results) and validity (the extent to which the test's content is representative of the actual skills learned or to be assessed) are both influenced by the number of stations and total length of the examination [14]. An appropriate and realistic time allocation for tasks at individual stations will improve the test validity. The number of stations needed to generate a reliable score is calculated using either the Cronbach's α or Generalizability (G) coefficient [15]. For practical purposes, decisions around test length generally need to balance reliability coefficients with feasibility and resource issues. As a general recommendation, with well-constructed OSCE stations, an adequate reliability could be achieved with 14–18 stations each lasting 5–10 min [16].

A blueprint normally consists of a two-dimensional matrix with one axis representing the generic competencies to be tested—communication and counselling, physical examination, and diagnostic or therapeutic procedures—and the other axis representing the problems or conditions upon which the competences will be demonstrated. An example is shown below (Table 1.1):

1.3.2 Converting the Blueprint into a Test Map

After the blueprint has been produced, the OSCE committee next agrees on the conditions (or problems) from the different sections of the subject to be examined; like VVF from urogynaecology and imperforate hymen from adolescent gynaecology. The committee then agrees on the weight given to each problem whether one or more competences should be tested for any specific problem. The problems or disease conditions are then inserted into appropriate rows according to their related section of gynaecology as shown in Tables 1.2, 1.3, and 1.4.

Table 1.1 Blueprint for gynaecological OSCE

			Domains of clinical competence						
			Communication		Examination		Procedures		
	Program		HS	CL	PE	VE	DP	TP	PT/IIR
S. no.	component	No. of stations	A	B	C	D	E	F	G
1	General gynaecology	3	1			1			1
2	Urogynaecology	2	1						1
3	Infertility/ endocrinology	3		1	1		1		
4	Gynaecological Oncology	2		1		1			
5	Adolescent gynaecology	2	1						1
6	Reproductive health	2		1				1	
	Total	14							

HS history taking, *CL* counselling, *PE* physical examination, *VE* vaginal examination, *DP* diagnostic procedure, *TP* therapeutic procedure, *PT* picture test, *IIR* interpretation of investigation result

Table 1.2 Test map for gynaecological OSCE

Blueprint cell		Disease condition or problem	Competence tested	Proposed test item
A	1	Uterine fibroid	History taking	Standardized patient
D	1	Pelvic inflammatory disease	Vaginal examination	Mannequin
G	1	Post encounter to VE	Interpretation of abnormal HVS result	Prepared microbiology report of HVS
A	2	Uterovaginal prolapse	History taking	Standardized patient
G	2	Post encounter to history of UV prolapse	Recognition of uterine procidentia	Picture of uterine procidentia with decubitus ulcer
B	3	Primary infertility	Counselling a couple for semen collection	Standardized couple
C	3	Primary infertility	General physical examination of an infertile woman	Real patient
E	3	Primary infertility	Describing laparoscopy procedure	Veress needle, trocar and cannula, laparoscopic telescope
B	4	Cervical cancer	Breaking bad news	Histology report of cervical biopsy
D	4	Cervical lesion	Vaginal examination to identify a cervical lesion	Mannequin
A	5	Imperforate hymen	History taking for primary amenorrhoea	Standardized patient
G	5	Imperforate hymen	Identify imperforate hymen	Laminated picture of imperforate hymen
B	6	Completed family size	Counselling a couple for BTL	Standardized couple
F	6	Family planning	Insertion of Jadelle implants	Model of upper arm, Jadelle and insertion trocar

Table 1.3 Blueprint for obstetric OSCE

S. no.	Program component	No of stations	Domains of clinical competence						
			Communication		Examination		Procedures		
			HT	CL	PE	VE	DP	TP	PT/IIR
			A	B	C	D	E	F	G
1	Preconception care	3		1	1		1		
2	Antenatal care	3	1			1			1
3	Medical disorders	3	1		1		1		
4	Labour and delivery	3		1		1		1	
5	The puerperium	2	1						1
	Total	14							

HT history taking, *CL* counselling, *PE* physical examination, *VE* vaginal examination, *DP* diagnostic procedure, *TP* therapeutic procedure, *PT* picture test, *IIR* interpretation of investigation result

Table 1.4 Test map for obstetric OSCE

Blueprint cell		Problem/disease condition	Competence tested	Proposed item
B	1	Intending couple	Premarital counselling and testing for HIV	Standardized couple
C	1	Woman seeking preconception care	Breast examination	Mannequin
E	1	Woman seeking preconception care	Papanicolaou smear	Mannequin
A	2	Primigravida	History taking in ANC	Standardized patient
D	2	Primigravida	Vaginal examination for dating	Mannequin
G	2	Dating pregnancy	Ultrasound picture at 14 weeks	Laminated picture of ultrasound scan
A	3	Diabetes mellitus in pregnancy	History taking	Standardized
C	3	Third trimester pregnancy	Obstetric examination of the abdomen	Real patient
E	3	Diabetes mellitus in pregnancy	Urinalysis for glycosuria	Prepared glucose solution as urine
B	4	Grand multigravida	Counselling for postpartum BTL	Standardized patient
D	4	Established labour	Vaginal examination in labour	Mannequin
F	4	Retained placenta	Manual removal of the placenta	Mannequin
A	5	Puerperal sepsis	Focused history of delivery	Standardized patient
G	5	Puerperal sepsis	Interpretation of HVS result	Microbiology report of HVS

1.3.3 Constructing Stations

In the faculty of obstetrics and gynaecology of the West African College of Surgeons (WACS), some selected group of consultants are assigned to develop OSCE scripts for storage in the data bank of the faculty. Each group is assigned a subspecialty of obstetrics and gynaecology from which the group selects clinical conditions on which to construct a station. As much as possible, a station tests only one domain of clinical competence but rarely more than one. The process is started in a meeting where the participating consultants agree on what needs to be prepared and then decide a time for the review meeting of all the drafted stations. The faculty appoints an OSCE committee which has tenure and is responsible for preparing the blueprint and the test map for the faculty examinations. The stations are then pulled out from the data bank. In preparing a station, the following are taken into consideration:

- Station's profile
- Instructions to the patient
- Instructions to the candidate
- Instructions to the examiner
- Checklist

1.3.3.1 Station's Profile

The station's profile is the characteristic of the station which includes the condition to be examined (like uterine fibroid), the time allocated, and the domain of clinical competence to be tested (like physical examination skill). It also includes whether a standardized or real patient will be used. Specially constructed plastic models or simulations may be used where repetitive or intimate nature of the task makes the use of real patients inappropriate [8]. A chaperon is needed to keep the patients comfortable and direct the candidates as may be necessary.

A dressed bed or comfortable chair for the patient, a table and chairs for the examiners and candidate, materials to be used like latex gloves, specula, laminated pictures, pencils, and erasers, and adequate checklist for examiners are needed.

1.3.3.2 Instructions to the Patient

All patients, whether real or standardized, should be told about what will happen at the station during the examination. They should also be told the appropriate clothing to wear when coming for the examination especially those that will be examined by the candidates. If a history is to be taken, it should be given in detail in writing to the patient to study if she is literate. Training of the standardized patient may be required before the examination day. If she is going to be examined, details of the examination should be given so that she is not taken by surprise. A real patient needs to be changed after a few candidates have examined her to reduce discomfort and loss of cooperation.

1.3.3.3 Instructions to the Candidate

An opening statement providing the scenario of the station to the candidate is needed. A clear instruction as to the task or skill to be demonstrated is then given. It is preferable that only one task is required per station. Rarely, the station may be integrated in which case more than one competency task is required; in such cases clear instructions for both tasks must be provided. Instructions may also include cognitive components like interacting with the examiner. For example, the candidate may be instructed to run a commentary of his findings as he performs vaginal examination. The instructions to the candidate are usually laminated on an A4 paper to prevent squeezing and staining during the examination.

1.3.4 Instructions to the Examiner

The station profile should be given to the examiner with a clear statement of the domain of clinical competence being measured. The instructions to the candidate will also be given so that the examiner knows what is expected of the candidate. If promptings are included, the examiner should know what and when the prompting will come. A checklist or marking scheme is provided for the examiner to use for scoring the candidate. The checklist should be detailed to contain specific items the candidate is expected to perform or say. Each item is rated as to whether the candidate did it well, fairly, poorly, or not done at all.

1.4 OSCE Examination Logistics

The success of an OSCE examination largely depends on comprehensive planning and organization. The organizational structure may depend on local circumstances, but the majority of the components are common to all settings.

1.4.1 OSCE Coordinator

The coordinator is responsible for overseeing the development, organization, administration, and grading of the examination. In the teaching hospitals and other accredited tertiary hospitals, the head of department of obstetrics and gynaecology or his delegate should be the coordinator. He receives input from the OSCE committee which he is a member. He must have had previous experience in organizing an OSCE examination. The coordinator must be well motivated to function effectively.

1.4.2 OSCE Committee

This consists of the coordinator and a small number of senior consultants in the department who are familiar with the training curriculum. Whether appointed or volunteered, the members of the OSCE committee must be committed to the evaluative and educational process. The number of members who make up this committee is not as important as the intensity of the investment of each member [6, 8]. Tasks should be assigned to each member like standardized patient trainer, support staff supervisor, etc. The OSCE committee develops the blueprint, selects station developers, and appoints examiners. They set the criteria for passing or failing the examination. Therefore, the committee must have the capacity and personnel to address decisions related to reliability and validity.

1.4.3 Station Developers or Script Writers

Once the blueprint has been approved by the OSCE committee, specific stations are assigned to station developers according to the test blueprint. These consist of consultants familiar with the training curriculum and with good clinical experience. All stations developed will be submitted to the OSCE committee for technical review and transforming into a uniform format. If OSCE is going to hold for the first time in the institution, it is necessary to hold a training workshop to help consultants and residents develop sound and valid stations in the prescribed format and understand the logistics of running OSCE examination.

1.4.4 Choice of Station Types

The OSCE coordinator should advise the script writers about the type of new stations needed. An understanding of the different types of OSCE station formats is essential in the choice of appropriate station types for various assessment outcomes. Once the type of station has been chosen, an appropriate template for station writing should be developed and used. A template helps authors to develop stations in a similar format to others within the bank. Such standardization prevents disadvantaging the candidates by posing questions in unfamiliar formats and helps to maintain the reliability of the scores. Below is a typical format for submission of OSCE stations:

Station number and information. e.g. station 1: Gynaecological history taking
Subject. e.g. Gynaecology
Subspecialty. e.g. Urogynaecology
Domain of clinical competence. e.g. History taking
Station objective. e.g. To assess the candidate's ability to take a focused history of a patient with urinary incontinence.
Requirements. e.g. standardized patient (SP), chaperon, table and chairs for examiners, checklist, etc.
Instructions to the standardized patient. i.e. detailed instructions about her presumed condition and how to act.
Instruction to the candidate. i.e. the task the candidate is to carry out, e.g. take a history of the patient.

Instruction to the examiners. i.e. information about the patient and the task of the candidate. A checklist is provided
A checklist complete with the scores allocated

In institutions where an OSCE is being set up for the first time, the examination blueprint governed by the curriculum outcomes would act as a good starting point to identify the topics for writing new OSCE stations. In places where an OSCE station bank already exists the OSCE coordinator or subject experts could review this to identify gaps in the assessment of certain skills or domains. The need for new stations could also arise if the curriculum is modified or the learning objectives of the module are changed. The assessment of competence should always be aligned to the teaching and learning that has taken place as specified by the course curriculum.

1.4.5 Support Staff

This should comprise at least one secretary, a consultant experienced in logistic and support services to resolve the physical issues. It has been estimated that about 80 h of secretarial time is needed to organize a large scale OSCE for the first time in an institution [9]. Resident doctors not participating in the examination, or medical students where available, can be used as support staff. Their functions include:

- Secretarial—printing and photocopying
- Setting up individual stations
- Setting up the bell system for timing and movement of candidates
- Attending the needs of standardized and real patients, candidates, and examiners
- Quarantine candidates for the examination
- Entering scores on a spreadsheet

1.4.6 Trainer

Standardized patients and sometimes real patients need to be trained on how to respond to candidates during the interviews or physical examination. This may require sessions of training. The trainer must understand the roles of standardized patients and must have good teaching skills and be capable of providing a constructive feedback. The trainer needs to liaise with station developers to understand the details of the problem to be presented.

1.4.7 Examiners

All consultant staff should be trained to be examiners. Examiners are required at stations where clinical skills are tested like history stations, counselling stations, and physical examination stations. The examiners should be clear about the objectives and standards of the station and should not interfere as much as possible. The examiner must be conversant with the checklist and be attentive during the examination so that the candidate is scored appropriately.

1.4.8 Timekeeper

This is a support staff that maintains the OSCE schedule using bell rings at precise intervals. The timekeeper must remain focused and not be distracted. A standby support is always necessary because the examination cannot go without a time keeper.

1.4.9 Monitor

A senior member of the OSCE team should be available to monitor the conduct of the examination to ensure things are going on well. The monitor directs the flow of candidates and identifies and solves any problem arising from examiners, patients, and candidates. The monitor can stop the examination to solve a particular issue at any point the need arises.

1.4.10 Standardized Patients

Standardized patients are volunteers, chronic stable patients, professional actors, students, friends, and hospital staff who have agreed and trained to simulate clinical conditions for the purpose of the OSCE examination. The reward for participating in the examination should be agreed upon and payment given promptly to motivate them. Multiple standardized patients should be trained per station depending on the number of candidates to be examined because it can be tiring to be interviewed or examined physically several times. Standardized patients who are well trained offer reliability and consistency in the quality of their presentation [10]. Real patients may also be used but it's difficult to get sufficient number of real patients with the same condition.

1.4.11 Choosing the Venue and Preparing Examination Materials

A custom-built skills laboratory or a dedicated OSCE centre is preferred but, where there is no such facility as is the case in most training facilities in West Africa, an outpatient clinic or an empty ward can be prepared to serve the purpose. In such circumstance, a long-term plan is necessary as clinical settings will need to be re-arranged to provide a functional venue for the examination.

The layout should be planned to allow smooth flow of candidates from one station to the other. Station areas should be mapped and the flow pattern shown. The layout should be such that the bell is heard throughout the examination area. Where possible, videotapes should be provided to improve the quality of training of standardized patients and in the control room to monitor each station real time.

At the venue, arrangement of furniture, equipping the stations, labelling the stations, posting signage and arrows, and identifying the quarantine room for candidates should be done at least a day before the examination.

The examination coordinator and support staff should arrive the venue early on the day of the examination. Examiners should arrive the venue at least an hour to starting time and be briefed by the coordinator. The candidates should also arrive at least 30 min before commencement of the examination and be briefed on quarantine arrangement, starting positions, and direction of flow in the circuit as well as some words of encouragement. Both the examiners and the candidates will be informed of the bell signal formula—start, stop, re-start, move, and so on. Maintaining security is important.

1.4.12 Marking Scheme and Collation of Results

The scored checklist from each station, together with the summary sheet on which each candidate's score has been recorded, is collected immediately after the examination. The scores are entered into a data sheet on Microsoft excel spread sheet (or a similar statistical package) for analysis. The marks are processed according to a predetermined format for that examination. An innovative addition, the "early feedback OSCE" first introduced by the Medical College of Ohio, USA, used the computer to compute the students score throughout the examination so that at the completion of the last station, the candidate receives a computer-generated print out of his result [6].

Various marking schemes are used to mark different types of assessment. There are two main types of marking schemes: analytical and holistic.

1.4.12.1 Analytical Scoring

This is also called the checklist, and it is a list of statements describing the actions expected of the candidates at the station. It is prepared in advance, following consultation with the OSCE committee, and in line with the content and outcomes being assessed. Checklist could be binary, with yes/No options only, or have 3 or more point ratings scale which allows examiners to mark candidates based upon the quality of the actions. The faculty of obstetrics and gynaecology of the West African College of Surgeons (WACS) uses 4-point rating scales—well done, fairly done, poorly done, and not done.

1.4.12.2 Holistic Scoring

Also called global rating, this allows the assessor to rate the whole process. Consider the performance of an expert who may not follow a predetermined sequence of steps as outlined by a checklist, yet still performs the task to a high standard with fluidity and ease. In this situation, an overall (global) assessment of the performance is required in order to accurately reflect the skill of the candidate. Global scales allow examiners to determine not only whether an action was performed, but also how well it was performed. This tool is therefore better for assessing skills where the quality with which it is performed is as important as performing it at all. It takes a more holistic view of the overall performance at a station compared to a rating scale looking at one aspect alone. Global ratings are being increasingly used over checklists for marking at OSCE stations as there is now evidence to suggest that they show greater interstation reliability, better construct validity, and better concurrent validity compared to the checklist [17].

1.5 Planning an OSCE

1.5.1 Prior to OSCE

Suitable Venue

- Book venue well in advance
- Depending on number of stations and students
- May require more than one circuit running at the same time
- Need adjacent quarantine room for students
- Adjacent resting area for standardized patients and real patients

Recruitment of Examiners

- Give advance notice
- Supply them grid of times and dates of the examination
- Invite examiners in excess in case some do not turn up

Recruitment of Standardized Patients (SPs)

- Using the blueprint, recruit sufficient number of SPs
- Inform them well ahead of time
- Train and retrain them a day before the OSCE

Running Order of the OSCE

- Number and label the stations
- Provide rest stations; usually one every 40 min of examination

List of All the Equipment

- To be checked a day before the examination
- Detailed by station, with some spare in case of breakages and tear
- Liaise with technicians of skill laboratory if available

1.5.2 On the Day of OSCE

Signs

- Indicating examination venue, rooms for students, and resting area for SPs
- Stations per room or cubicles

Briefing

- Students briefed in the quarantine room as well as when starting the circuit
- Examiners reminded of the conduct of the exam; no interference, use of checklist, switch off phones, etc.

Timing

- Electronic timing program or manual bell
- Positioned so that all students and examiners hear the bell

Chaperons

- To direct students, SPs, and examiners
- To look after the welfare of the people involved in the exam
- Refreshment for all participants including examiners

1.5.3 After the OSCE

Collection of Marking Sheets

- Members of OSCE committee usually assigned to do this
- Can be done after each bell or at the end of running the circuit
- Ensure checklists are properly filled and signed

Care of Patients and SPs

- At least reimburse transport money
- Thank them for coming

Thank You Letters

- To all examiners, patients, SPs, and chaperons

References

1. Haden RM, Stevenson M, Dawnie WW. Assessment of clinical competence using the objective structured clinical examination. BMJ. 1975;1:447–9.
2. Carpenter JL. Cost analysis of the objective structured clinical examination. Acad Med. 1995;70:828–33.
3. Webster dictionary, 10th ed. Merriam Webster Incorporated; 2020.
4. Ware J, El-Mardi A, Abdulghani H, Saddiqui I. Examination construction. In: OSCE manual. Saudi Commission for Health Specialties; 2014. pp. 24–31.
5. McCoy JA, Merrick HW. The role of the OSCE in the assessment of students' performance. In: OSCE manual. ASE Educational Clearinghouse; 2001. pp. 18–26.
6. American Educational Research Association. Standards for educational and psychological testing. Washington, DC; 1999.
7. Khan KZ, Ramachandran S, Gaunt K, Pushkar P. The objective structured clinical examination (OSCE). AMEE guide no 81. Part I: an historical and theoretical perspective. Med Teach. 2013;35(9):e1437–46.
8. Smee S. ABC of learning and teaching in medicine, "skill-based assessment". BMJ. 2003;326:707–6.
9. Van Der Vleutin CPM, Van Luyk SJ, Van Ballengooijen AMJ, Swansons DB. Training and experience of examiners. Med Educ. 1989;23:290–6.
10. Waren J, El-Mardi A. Relevant principles of assessment. In: OSCE manual. Saudi Commission for Health Specialties; 2014. pp. 1–9.
11. Boursicot K. Structured assessment of clinical competence. Br J Hosp Med. 2010;71:342–4.
12. Vargas AL, Boulet JR, Errichetti A, Zanten MV, Lopez MI, Reta AM. Developing performance-based medical school assessment programs in resource-limited environments. Med Teach. 2007;29:192–8.
13. Khan KZ, Ramachandran S, Gaunt K, Pushkar P. The objective structured clinical examination (OSCE). AMEE guide no 81. Part II: organization and administration. Med Teach. 2013;35(9):e1447–63.
14. Newble D. Techniques for measuring clinical competence. Objective structured clinical examination. Med Educ. 2004;38:199–203.
15. Pell G, Fuller R, Homer M, Roberts T. How to measure the quality of the OSCE: a review of metrics. AMEE guide no 49. Med Teach. 2010;32:802–11.
16. Epstein RM. Assessment in medical education. N Engl J Med. 2007;356:387–96.
17. Turner JL, Dankoski ME. Objective structured clinical examination: a critical review. Fam Med. 2008;40:574–8.

General Gynaecology OSCE Stations

2

2.1 Station 2.1 Focused History of Hypomenorrhea

Subject: Gynaecology.
Subspecialty: General gynaecology.
Domain of clinical competence: Focused history taking.
Station: Focused history of hypomenorrhea.
Station objective: To assess the candidate's ability to take a focused history of a patient with reduced menstrual flow.
Requirements: Standardized patient (SP), instructions to the standardized patient, instructions to the candidate, instructions to the examiner with sufficient checklist for the number of candidates, a table and 3 chairs for the examiners and the candidate, plain papers to be used by the candidates as a jotter, dressed bed or an office chair for the standardized patient, and a chaperon (Fig. 2.1).

2.1.1 Instructions to the Standardized Patient (SP)

Biodata

Name: Mrs, JH	Religion: Christianity
Age: 25 years	Tribe: Kilba
Address: Flat 4, Block C5, APDC Estate, Abuja	Marital status: Married
Occupation: Seamstress	Parity: P1 + 1 A1
Educational level: University graduate	LMP: 2 days ago

Presenting Complaints

- Scanty menstrual flow
- Duration—for 3 months

C. Chama, *OSCE and VIVA VOCE in Obstetrics and Gynaecology*,
https://doi.org/10.1007/978-3-031-77262-7_2

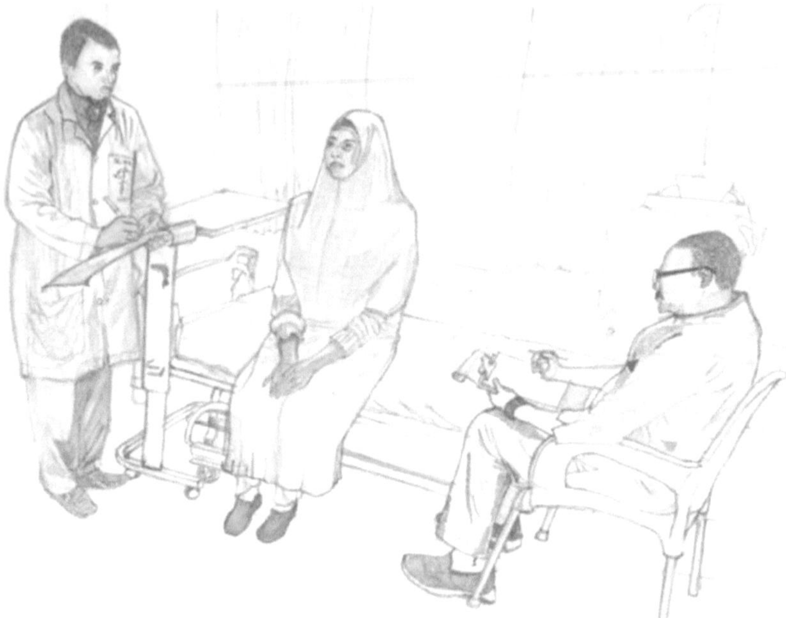

Fig. 2.1 History taking during OSCE examination. (Courtesy of Jonathan Edache Otache)

History of Presenting Complaints

I have been apparently well until 3 months ago when I noticed my menses had reduced flow. Since then, it has gradually reduced to mere one day of spotting of blood. I used to see my menses for 4 days and had to use 2–3 sanitary pads a day. I also experience severe lower abdominal pains when the menses comes, and I use feldene (Piroxicam) capsules to relief the pain. Earlier on I had a miscarriage of a 3-month pregnancy for which I was seen in a private hospital and my womb was washed. I was discharged home on some tablets but had to return after 3 days with fever, lower abdominal pain, and foul-smelling vaginal discharge. I was taken to the theatre again, and my womb was washed because they did a scan which showed some parts of the pregnancy remaining inside my womb. The first procedure was done using a big syringe, and I was awake even though they gave me an injection. The second procedure was done after I was put to sleep. I was given some drip (IVF) and injections with some relief and was discharged home after 2 days on some capsules and tablets for one week. The pain and discharge subsided but my first menses after that was scanty, and it lasted 3 days.

I do not have any other complaints (if asked whether you have milky breast discharge, undue feeling of cold or heat or neck swelling, just answer NO). If asked whether you want to have more children, answer YES.

Gynaecological History
I started seeing my menses when I was 14 years of age, and I menstruate for 4 days every 26–28 days. The flow was moderate, and there were no associated lower abdominal cramps until after the miscarriage. I have never contracted sexually transmitted infection, and my husband is my only sexual partner. I am aware of methods of preventing pregnancy but have not used any so far. I had Pap smear done 2 years ago which was normal.

Obstetrics History
My only child is 3 years old. He was conceived 6 months after my marriage, and I had antenatal care in the same private hospital. The pregnancy was carried to term, and I delivered normally in the same hospital. The child was breastfed for 6 months exclusively and is fully immunized for age. He is doing well in nursery school.

Past Medical and Surgical History
If asked whether you have been diagnosed or admitted for any medical or surgical condition, answer NO

Family and Social History
I am the only wife of my husband who is a Director with the Federal Ministry of Works and Housing. I run a designer shop for women, and I have 6 workers in my employment. We live in a 4-bedroom flat in the APDC Estate Abuja. I don't know of any close relative with hypertension, diabetes, sickle cell disease, or twining. I do not smoke or take alcoholic beverages.

Systemic Review
If asked of any other abnormal feeling today like headache, dizziness, etc.; answer NO

2.1.2 Instructions to the Candidate

The patient in front of you was referred from a private clinic to the gynaecological clinic in your hospital. Your task is to take her history.

2.1.3 Instructions to the Examiner

The candidate has been instructed to take a focused history of this patient who presents with hypomenorrhea of 3 months duration following repeated evacuation for incomplete miscarriage. Use the checklist provided to score the candidate.

Checklist for history taking on hypomenorrhea

Tasks;	**Well done**	**Fairly done**	**Poorly done**	**Not done**
Greets patient, introduces self, obtains consent		2	1	0
Biodata – Name, age, address, religion, level of education, occupation, marital status		2	1	0
Asks for Parity, LMP		2	1	0
Asks for presenting complaint and duration		2	1	0
History of presenting complaint				
Confirms last normal menstrual period		2	1	0
Obtains pattern of normal cycle before present problems and compares with current state	4	2	1	0
Associated dysmenorrhoea		2	1	0
Associated fertility concerns		2	1	0
Identifies precipitating factor - miscarriage		2	1	0
Details of uterine evacuation	4	2	1	0
Details of post uterine evacuation complications - fever, abdominal pain, offensive vaginal discharge	4	2	1	0
Details of second uterine evacuation		2	1	0
Rules out symptoms suggestive of thyroid disorders	4	2	1	0
Rules out any discharge from breast	4	2	1	0
No care received yet for the complaint		2	1	0
Gynaecology history Menarche, Duration and frequency of menstruation, any menstrual abnormality, Contraceptive history, TOPs? Cervical smear?		2	1	0
Past Obstetrics History Year of pregnancy and delivery, mode of delivery, child alive and well.		2	1	0
PMSHx - Nil of note			1	0
Family and Social History Family setting, fertility desires, social habits			1	0
Systemic Review			1	0
Summarises history and tells patient of probable diagnosis and next steps			1	0
Thanks patient			1	0
PENALTY(IES) Disorderliness/Disorganization, poor clarity of spoken English	-4	-2	-1	0
Total Marks	49			
Candidate's score …/49				

Examiner's Name____________________________Signature________________________

2.2 Station 2.2 Post Encounter to History Station

Station objective: To assess the candidate's ability to manage a patient who presents with hypomenorrhea following an abortion.

Requirements: Clearly written and numbered management questions regarding the patient clerked on the last station, plain papers for the candidate to write his answers (he may be asked to answer the questions verbally also), comfortable chairs and a table for candidate and examiners, marking scheme or checklist for examiners to score the candidate, pencils and erasers, a chaperon to attend to examiners and candidates.

2.2.1 Instruction to the Candidate

Clearly written tasks, pasted to the table so that it is not blown away or mishandled:

1. Give a summary of the history of the patient you clerked on the last station.
2. List 4 differential diagnoses?
3. List 5 relevant investigations you would request and why.
4. What is the most likely diagnosis and what is the treatment of choice?

2.2.2 Instructions to the Examiners

The candidate took the history of a patient with hypomenorrhea following repeated uterine curettage on the last station. He is supposed to answer the questions provided regarding the patient he clerked on the last station. Use the answer guide (or checklist) to score the candidate.

Answers

1. Mrs. JH is a 25-year-old P1 + 1, one alive **(2 marks),** who presented with scanty menstrual flow of 3 months duration (2 **marks**), following repeated uterine curettage for incomplete miscarriage **(2 marks).** She has no galactorrhea or heat or cold intolerance **(2 marks).**
2. The differential diagnoses are: **(2 marks each)**
   (a) Intrauterine adhesion (Asherman's syndrome)
   (b) Pituitary necrosis (Sheehan's syndrome)
   (c) Hyperprolactinemia
   (d) Thyroid disease (hyper-/hypothyroidism)
3. Five relevant investigations include:
   (a) Full blood count **(2 marks)** to rule out anaemia and on-going sepsis **(2 marks)**
   (b) Renal function tests (EUCr) **(2 marks)** to rule out renal injury following sepsis and possible haemorrhage (**2 marks**)

(c) High vaginal swab for MCS **(2 marks)** to rule out any genital tract infections **(2 marks)**
(d) Pelvic ultrasound scan (TVS) **(2 marks)** to rule out other pelvic pathologies and possibly saline sonohysterogram to diagnose intrauterine adhesions **(2 marks)**
(e) HSG or hysteroscopy **(2 marks)** for diagnosis and treatment of intrauterine adhesions **(2 marks)**

4. The most likely diagnosis is intrauterine adhesions **(4 marks)** due to repeated uterine curettage following incomplete miscarriage complicated by sepsis **(4 marks).**

Checklist for post encounter station to hypomenorrhea

Tasks	Well done	Fairly done	Poorly done	Not done
Summary of history - Identity and parity of patient - Presenting complaints - Most probable cause of the problem - Important negatives		 2 2 2 2		 0 0 0 0
Differential diagnoses - Intrauterine adhesions - Pituitary necrosis - Hyperprolactinemia - Thyroid disease		 2 2 2 2		 0 0 0 0
Relevant investigations (2 marks) and reasons for the test (2 marks):				
FBC to rule out anaemia and sepsis	4	2		0
EUCr to rule out renal injury	4	2		0
HVS for MCS to rule out genital sepsis	4	2		0
Pelvic USS (TVS) to rule out other pelvic pathologies	4	2		0
HSG or Hysteroscopy for diagnosis and treatm3ent	4	2		0
The most likely diagnosis is intrauterine adhesions (2) due to repeated uterine curettage and sepsis (2)	4	2		0
Total marks	40			
Candidate's score .../40				

Examiner's signature Date

2.3 Station 2.3 Performing Vaginal Examination

Subject: Gynaecology.
Subspecialty: General gynaecology.
Domain of clinical competence: Diagnostic procedure.
Station objective: To assess the candidate's ability to perform vaginal examination in a patient presenting with lower abdominal pain and vaginal discharge for the purpose of diagnosing the disease condition.
Requirements: A mannequin of the female pelvis fitted with uterus and cervix of various sizes, a table or dressed bed on which to place the mannequin, a table and 2 chairs for examiners, Cusco's speculum, a packet of latex hand gloves, swab sticks, a Galli pot containing wet swab, sterile water as vaginal lubricant, enough checklist, pencils and erasers for the examiners, a chaperon, a light source, litter bin and drapes for the mannequin (Fig. 2.2).

2.3.1 Instruction to the Candidate

Mrs. JH is a 24-year-old P2 + 0 A2 whose LCB was 4 years ago. She has been having chronic pelvic pain with vaginal discharge for the past one year. She received several drugs from the police clinic where her husband works. She has come to the gynaecological clinic of your hospital on referral.

Use the pelvic model provided (Fig. 2.2) to demonstrate, with running commentary how you would perform a pelvic examination on her.

2.3.2 Instruction to the Examiners

Provided is a pelvic model fitted with uterus and cervix. The candidate is supposed to demonstrate how to perform a pelvic examination on a patient complaining of lower abdominal pain and vaginal discharge. Use the checklist provided to score the candidate.

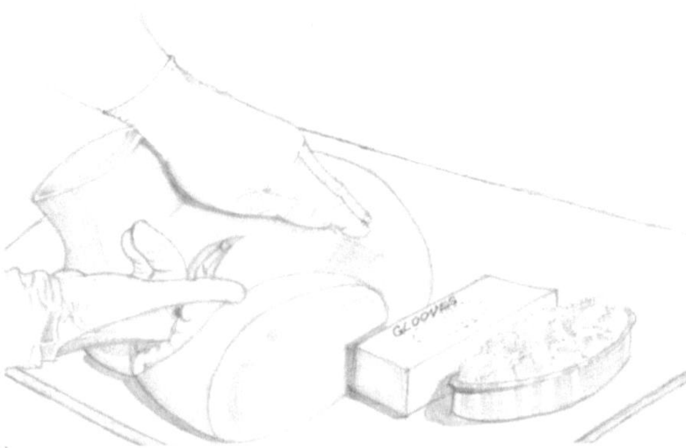

Fig. 2.2 Performing vaginal examination on a mannequin. (Courtesy of Jonathan Edache Otache)

Checklist for vaginal examination

Tasks	**Well done**	**Fairly done**	**Poorly done**	**Not done**
Greets patient and introduces self		2	1	0
Explains the procedure and obtains permission from patient		2	1	0
Requests the chaperon to screen the patient, positions patient		2	1	0
Examination part 1				
- Scrubs and wears sterile gloves.		2	1	0
- Parts the labia and inspects the vulva.		2	1	0
- Asks patient to strain or cough		2	1	0
Examination part 2				
- Lubricates Cusco's speculum with sterile water and inserts correctly.		2	1	0
- Opens the valves of the speculum and takes HVS swab correctly.		2	1	0
- Closes the valves of the speculum and withdraws the speculum gently from the vagina		2	1	0
Examination part 3				
- Parts the labia and inserts middle and index fingers of the dominant hand.		2	1	0
- Performs bimanual examination with comment on uterine size and position.		2	1	0
- Examines the adnexa in sequence.		2	1	0
- Examines the Pouch of Doughlas with comment.		2	1	0
- Performs cervical excitation tenderness with comment.		2	1	0
- Withdraws fingers and checks for vaginal discharge and odor.		2	1	0
Thanks the patient and positions her supine		2	1	0
Says he will document findings and fill the form for HVS for MCS	4	2	1	0
Penalties – examination not in sequence, rough, does not engage chaperon	-4	-2	-1	0
Total marks	36			
Candidate's score ..../36				

Examiner's signature Date

2.4 Station 2.4 Examination of Abdominal Mass

Subject: Gynaecology
Subspecialty: General gynaecology
Domain of clinical competence: Physical examination
Station: Abdominal examination of a patient with uterine fibroids
Station objective: To assess the candidate's ability to examine the abdomen for the purpose of characterizing the nature of an abdominal mass to arrive at the diagnosis of uterine fibroids.
Requirements: Patients with large uterine fibroids are common in our environment and such patients can be booked for OSCE examinations. An office table and 2 office chairs for examiners, a dressed bed and covering for the patient, and enough checklists for the examiners are required. A chaperone is required to keep the patient comfortable and attend to her when necessary. A mannequin with various sizes of uterine models can be used but hardly brings out the features of uterine fibroids (Fig. 2.3).

2.4.1 Instruction to the Candidate

Your task is to examine her abdomen. The patient on this station is a 35-year-old nullipara who was referred from the General Outpatient Department (GOPD) to the gynaecological clinic.

2.4.2 Instruction to the Examiners

The patient is a 35-year-old nullipara with multiple uterine fibroids of about 22 weeks size. The candidate is to examine her abdomen while running commentary on his findings. Use the check list provided to score the candidate.

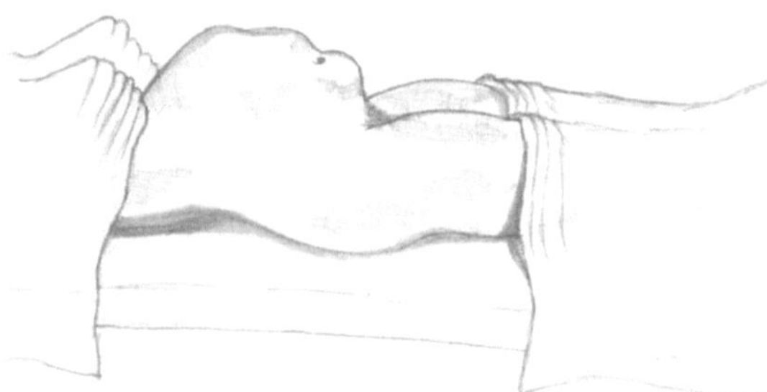

Fig. 2.3 Appropriate exposure for abdominal examination. (Courtesy of Jonathan Edache Otache)

Checklist for abdominal examination with uterine fibroids

Task	Well done	Fairly done	Poorly done	Not done
Greets the patient and introduces self		2	1	0
Explains the procedure and takes permission from patient		2	1	0
Asks patient to expose her abdomen as he helps her appropriately		2	1	0
Inspection with comment				
-abdominal contour		2		0
-any scarifications		2		0
-hair distribution		2		0
Palpation with comment				
-asks patient for any area of tenderness		2	1	0
-light palpation for masses and tenderness		2	1	0
-palpates for liver, spleen, and kidneys		2	1	0
-palpates for abdomino-pelvic mass				
* Lower abdominal mass 22 weeks size		2	1	0
* Firm and nodular		2	1	0
* Mobile in both planes		2	1	0
* Tenderness		2	1	0
* Can get below it		2	1	0
Percussion with comment				
-from center to the flanks		2	1	0
-no shifting dullness		2	1	0
Auscultation for bowel sounds or bruit		2	1	0
Thanks the patient and helps to cover her		2	1	0
Gives summary of findings	4	2	1	0
Penalties: not sequential, rough, no eye contact	**-4**	**-2**	**-1**	**0**
Total score	40			
Candidate's score .../40				

Examiner's name Date

2.5 Station 2.5 Interpreting Laparoscopic Findings of Endometriosis

Subject: Gynaecology.
Subspecialty: General gynaecology.
Domain of clinical competence: Interpretation of abnormal test finding (IATF).
Station: Interpreting laparoscopy finding in endometriosis.
Station objective: To assess the candidate's ability to interpret the findings at laparoscopy which was diagnostic of endometriosis and counsel the patient for plan of management.
Requirements: Standardized or real patient, photographs or video of laparoscopic clips if available, a copy of the report of laparoscopic findings, an office table and 2 chairs for examiners, a dressed bed or chair for the patient, a chair for the candidate, pencils and erasers for examiners, plain papers for rough use by candidates.

2.5.1 Instruction to Standardized Patient

You have been coming to the gynaecology clinic of this hospital for the past 2 years because of pelvic pain that is worse just before menses. You have received some medications but obtained little or no relieve of the pain. Recently when you travelled to Saudi Arabia for the Hajj, you visited King Faad Hospital and had laparoscopy done. You were told you had endometriosis. You have come for your regular follow-up and want to share the result of the laparoscopy with your doctor. You are the only wife of your husband whom you married one year ago and for the past 3 months you experience pain when having sexual intercourse with your husband. You have never conceived but the pelvic pain is your major concern.

2.5.2 Instruction to the Candidate

Mrs. RY is a known patient of chronic pelvic pain. She has come for her regular follow-up. She is a nullipara and has received analgesics for the pelvic pain in the past. Attend to her and address her current issues. She was last seen 6 weeks ago.

2.5.3 Instruction to the Examiner

The patient is a known case of chronic pelvic pain who has been on analgesics. Recently she travelled to Saudi Arabia on Hajj and visited a hospital there with the same complaint. She had a laparoscopy and was told she had endometriosis. She has come with the laparoscopy report to share with the doctor and obtain more insight into her problem. The candidate is supposed to ask her for any new complaints before the patient discloses that she had laparoscopy recently.

Checklist for endometriosis

Task	Well done	Fairly done	Poorly done	Not done
Greets patient and introduces self		2	1	0
Welcomes patient and asks how she has been doing since last visit	4	2	1	0
Asks patient if she has any new complaint		2		0
Collects the laparoscopy report from patient, reads it and begins to explain to her what endometriosis is:				
- Presence of lining of the uterine cavity outside the uterus		2	1	0
- During menses the tissue also sheds but cannot come out like normal menses		2	1	0
- Your body reacts to the shedding endometriotic tissue causing pain.		2	1	0
- It may also be responsible for your inability to conceive.		2	1	0
- It can only be visualized by laparoscopy as was done		2	1	0
Asks patient what she understands by what he said		2		0
Makes further clarification on the nature of endometriosis		2	1	0
Asks patient if she knows any way of treating endometriosis		2		0
Explains the options of treatment of endometriosis.				
- Can be treated with analgesics, COCP, progestogens, GnRH analogues.		2	1	0
- In complicated cases, surgery may be required.		2	1	0
- Where pregnancy is desired, ART is helpful		2	1	0
Allows her to ask for any clarification		2		0
Further explains the options of treatment and asks for her preference	4	2	1	0
Thanks her for listening and feedback and gives her appointment	4	2	1	0
Communication skills: empathic, eye contact, allows feedback	4	2	1	0
Total marks	42			
Candidate's score .../42				

Examiner's name Date

2.6 Station 2.6 Understanding Parts and Functions of Karman's Syringe and Cannula

Subject: Gynaecology.
Subspecialty: General gynaecology.
Domain of clinical competence: Instrumentation.
Station: Understanding the Karman's syringe for manual vacuum aspiration.
Station objective: To test the candidate's understanding of the parts and functions of the Karman's syringe and cannula for the purpose of manual vacuum aspiration.
Requirements: IPAS plus Karman's syringe and cannulas (or any other model of Karman's syringe) can be assembled or disassembled, written instructions to the candidates, sufficient checklist for examiners, a table and chairs for examiners and candidates, a chaperon (Fig. 2.4).

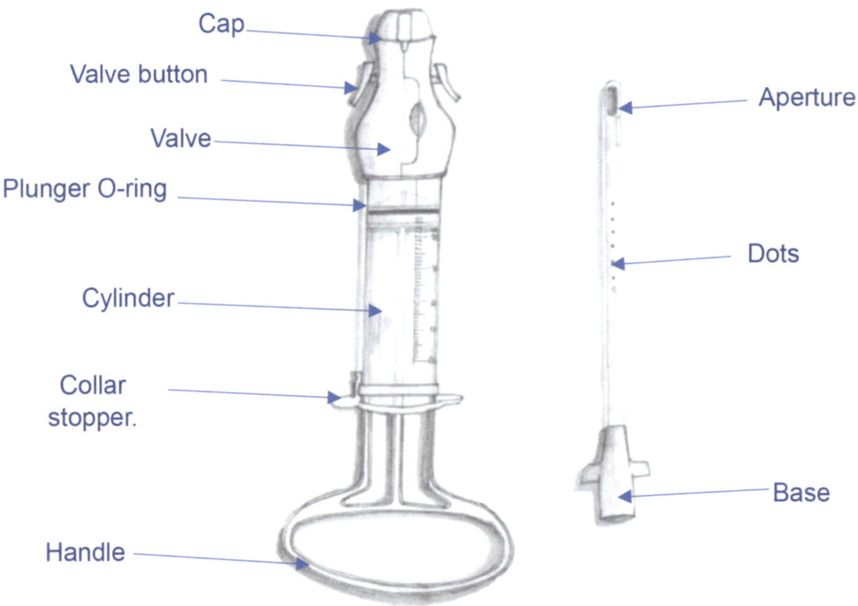

Fig. 2.4 Parts of Karman's syringe and cannula. (Courtesy of Jonathan Edache Otache)

2.6.1 Instruction to the Candidate

Provided are IPAS MVA plus syringe and cannula (or any other model of Karman's syringe). Your task is to describe the parts of the syringe and cannula, giving the function of each part you describe to the hearing of the examiners. Lastly, list the steps in processing this instrument.

2.6.2 Instructions to the Examiners

The candidate is expected to first describe the various parts of the Karman's syringe and cannulas provided, giving the function of each part and secondly, mention the steps in processing this instrument. Use the checklist provided to score the candidate.

Checklist for parts and functions of Karman's syringe

Task	Well done	Fairly done	Poorly done	Not done
Parts and functions of Karman's syringe:				
Cap (2), holds the cannula (2)	4	2		0
Latch (2), opens the valve (2)	4	2		0
Valve buttons (2), control release of vacuum (2)	4	2		0
Valve (2), maintains vacuum (2)	4	2		0
O-ring (2), eases movement of the plunger (2)	4	2		0
Cylinder (2), holds the aspirated products of conception (2)	4	2		0
Clip (2), holds the collar stop in place (2)	4	2		0
Colar stop (2), prevents plunger from slipping out (2)	4	2		0
Plunger with handle (2), creates the vacuum (2)	4	2		0
Parts and functions of Karman's cannula:				
Aperture (2), curette, passage of uterine contents (2)	4	2		0
Dots (2), uterine sound in cm (2)	4	2		0
Wing (2), for easy grip of cannula (2)	4	2		0
Base (2), fits into the cap of the syringe (2)	4	2		0
Steps in processing Karman's syringe and cannula:				
decontamination		2		0
Cleaning		2		0
Disinfection/sterilization		2		0
Storage		2		0
Total marks	60			
Candidate's score .../60				

Examiner's name Date

2.7 Station 2.7 Picture Test on Unruptured Interstitial Pregnancy

Subject: Gynaecology.
Subspecialty: General gynaecology.
Domain of clinical competence: Virtual sign identification (VSI) or picture test.
Station: Picture test on unruptured interstitial pregnancy.
Station objective: To test the candidate's ability to identify interstitial pregnancy based on laparotomy finding of an abnormal uterine swelling following 16 weeks of amenorrhoea.
Requirements: A picture of unruptured interstitial pregnancy with questions for the candidate, preferably on the same page. Plain papers for the candidate to write his answers on, an office table and 2 chairs for the examiners, a chair for the candidate, pencils and erasers, marking scheme or checklist for examiners, a chaperon.

2.7.1 Instruction to the Candidate

Mrs. FU is a 26-year-old G3P2 + 0 A2 who presented with 16 weeks of amenorrhoea and a dull lower abdominal pain for 2 weeks. A pregnancy test done at 8 weeks of amenorrhoea was positive. She was evaluated and eventually had laparotomy. The picture below shows the finding at laparotomy. Carefully study the picture and answer the questions that follow (Fig. 2.5).

1. What is the diagnosis?
2. Give 2 differences between this condition and ampullary ectopic pregnancy
3. List 3 modes of treatment of this condition
4. What special test needs to be done postoperatively?
5. Give one important information she needs to know concerning her future reproductive career.

Answers

1. Unruptured interstitial pregnancy (**4 marks**)
2. Differences between interstitial and ampullary ectopic pregnancies (**4 marks each**)
   (a) Interstitial pregnancy attains greater size (14–16 weeks) than ampullary ectopic pregnancy.
   (b) Ruptured interstitial pregnancy leads to more severe haemorrhage than ruptured ampullary ectopic pregnancy.
3. Three modes of treatment (**4 marks each**)
   (a) Cornual wedge resection and salpingectomy
   (b) Cornuostomy—analogous to linear salpingostomy
   (c) Medical treatment in selected cases

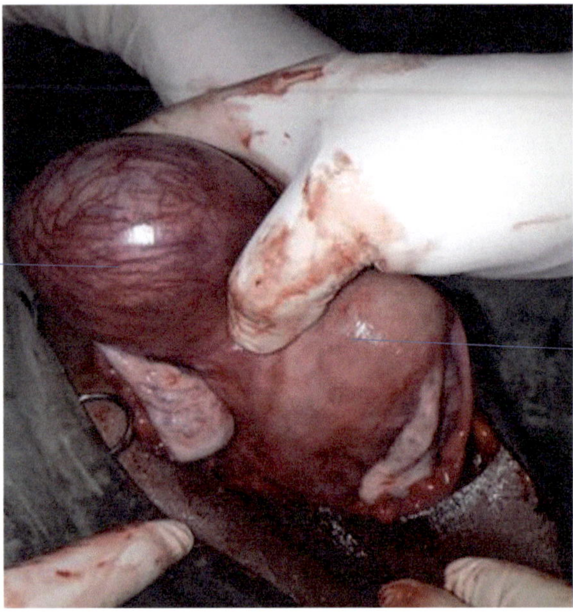

Fig. 2.5 Picture of unruptured interstitial pregnancy

4. Serial beta-HCG needs to be done postoperatively **(4 marks)**
5. Concerning future pregnancy (**4 marks**)
   (a) Rate of future ectopic pregnancy in the remaining tube is higher than after other ectopic pregnancies.
   (b) Rate of uterine rupture in subsequent pregnancy is as high as following classical caesarean section.

Checklist for unruptured interstitial pregnancy

Task	**Well done**	**Fairly done**	**Poorly done**	**Not done**
Diagnosis: Unruptured (2), interstitial pregnancy (2)	4	2		0
Differences between interstitial and ampullary pregnancy (2)				
- Interstitial pregnancy usually grows into second trimester		2		0
- Rupture of interstitial pregnancy usually leads to catastrophic haemorrhage		2		0
Methods of treatment of unruptured cornual pregnancy				
- Cornual wedge resection		2		0
- Cornuostomy, similar to linear salpingostomy		2		0
- Medical treatment in selected cases		2		0
Special postoperative test: serial (2) β-hCG (2)	4	2		0
Important information to patient concerning future pregnancy				
- Rate of ectopic pregnancy in the remaining tube is higher than following other types of ectopic pregnancy.		2		0
- Rate of uterine rupture in subsequent pregnancy is as high as following classical CS.		2		0
Total marks	22			
Candidate's score .../22				

Examiner's signature Date

Paediatric and Adolescent Gynaecology OSCE Stations

3

3.1 Station 3.1 History Taking of Acute Abdomen in an Adolescent

Subject: Gynaecology.
Subspecialty: Adolescent gynaecology.
Domain of clinical competence: Focused history taking.
Station: History of acute abdominal pain in an adolescent.
Station objective: To assess the candidate's ability to take a focused history of an adolescent presenting with acute abdominal pain with the aim of arriving at a diagnosis.
Requirements: Standardized patient (Role player), a table and 2 chairs for examiners, a dressed bed for standardized patient, a chaperone to attend to patient, a chair for candidate, enough copies of checklist for examiners, plain papers for use by candidates, pencils and erasers for examiners.

3.1.1 Instructions to the Standardized Patient

Biodata

Name: AD	Religion: Moslem
Age: 16 years	Tribe: Hausa
Address: Federal Government Girls College, Bauchi	Education: SS 2 student
Parity: P0 + 0	LMP: 2 weeks ago

C. Chama, *OSCE and VIVA VOCE in Obstetrics and Gynaecology*,
https://doi.org/10.1007/978-3-031-77262-7_3

Presenting Complaint

Lower abdominal pain

Duration: one day

History of Presenting Complaint

I was apparently well until yesterday evening when I had sudden lower abdominal pain which was gripping and severe. The pain is more on the right side and moves down my right thigh. I vomited once when the pain started but there was no fever. I had no dizziness or fainting attack, and I don't have problem with passing urine or moving my bowels. My roommate contacted the hostel matron who took me to the school clinic where I was given an injection which relieved the pain but the pain came back a couple of hours after the injection. The school nurse then brought me to this hospital.

I noticed a lower abdominal swelling on the right side about 3 months ago and has been gradually increasing in size. The swelling has been painless until this episode. (If asked whether you have vaginal discharge or bleeding, answer NO)

Gynaecological History

I started menses at the age of 13 years and menstruate for 3 days every 20–30 days. The flow is moderate and associated with mild lower abdominal pain the first day. (If asked whether you are sexually active, or uses contraceptives, or has had a Pap smear, say NO)

Obstetric History

I have never known a man

Medical and Surgical History

I have never been admitted to hospital for any illness or operation. I have been treated for malaria fever a few times as outpatient. I am not allergic to any of the drugs I have taken.

Family and Social History

I am the second of four children in my family. My father is a secondary school teacher while my mother is a trader with a provision store. We live in our own house in Sabon Kaura ward of Bauchi. I do not smoke or take alcoholic beverages. I do not know of any of my relations with diabetes, hypertension, or sickle cell disease.

Systemic Review

If asked whether you any other complaints like headache, fever, diarrhoea, etc.; say NO.

3.1.2 Instruction to the Candidate

The patient in front of you has been referred from the school clinic of Federal Government Girls College, Bauchi to the gynaecological emergency of your hospital. Take her history.

3.1.3 Instruction to the Examiners

The patient is a 16-year-old SS 2 pupil from Federal Government Girls College, Bauchi who was referred with acute abdominal pain. The candidate is supposed to take her history. Use the checklist provided to score the candidate.

Checklist for history of acute abdomen

Task	Well done	Fairly done	Poorly done	Not done
Greets patient and introduces self		2	1	0
Biodata; name, age, address, occupation, tribe, religion, education	4	2	1	0
Parity, LMP		2	1	0
Presenting complaints: lower abdominal pain (2), duration (2)	4	2		0
History of presenting complaint				
- Site		2		0
- Nature		2		0
- Radiation		2		0
- Aggravating and relieving factors		2		0
- Associated lower abdominal swelling (2), increasing in size (2)	4	2		0
- Any associated fever, urinary symptoms, nausea, vomiting, dizziness	4	2		0
GH: menarche, LMP, periods, cycle, flow, contraception, sex	4	2	1	0
OH: parity, abortions		2		0
PMH: admissions, drug allergy, surgery		2		0
FSH: siblings, parents, HT, DM, SCD, alcohol, smoking	4	2	1	0
Systemic review; headache, anorexia,		2		0
Summary of history		2	1	0
Total marks	44			
Candidate' score .../44				

Examiner Date

3.2 Station 3.2 Post Encounter to History of Acute Abdomen

Domain of clinical competence: Virtual sign identification.

Station objective: To test the candidate's ability to investigate and diagnose adnexal torsion at laparotomy and offer appropriate treatment.

Requirements: A picture of finding at laparotomy (adnexal torsion), clearly written questions for candidate, preferably on the same page with the picture, a table and 2 chairs for examiners, a chair for the candidate, plain papers for answering the questions by the candidate, a marking scheme for examiners, a chaperon.

3.2.1 Instruction to the Candidate

The patient you clerked on the last station was evaluated and eventually had emergency laparotomy. The picture below shows the findings at laparotomy. Answer the questions that follow (Fig. 3.1).

Questions

- From the history, what were your differential diagnoses?
- What specific investigations would you have requested to establish the diagnosis?
- Based on the finding at laparotomy, what was the diagnosis?
- Which adnexum is more commonly affected in this condition?
- What proportion of such cases occur in pregnancy?
- What does the pedicle look like on ultrasound scan?
- What does it suggest if fever were present at presentation?
- What procedures are done at laparotomy for the treatment of this condition?
- What additional treatment is required after surgery if she were 14 weeks pregnant?

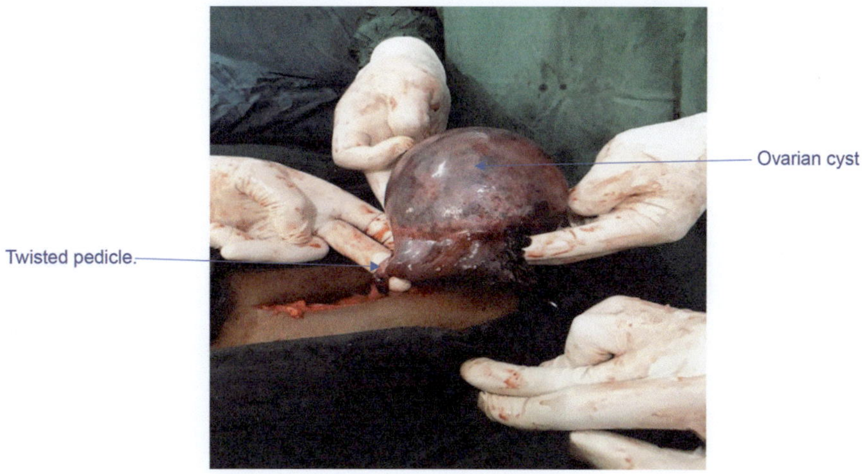

Fig. 3.1 Laparotomy finding of adnexal torsion (Chama et al. 2019)

Answer

Differential Diagnoses (2 Marks Each; Maximum of 5)

- Adnexal torsion (twisted ovarian cyst)
- Acute pelvic inflammatory disease
- Acute appendicitis
- Acute cystitis
- Ureteric colic
- Ruptured ectopic gestation.

Specific Investigations (2 Marks Each; Maximum of 5)

- Abdominopelvic ultrasound scan
- MRI where available
- IVU to rule out renal tract pathologies Acute pelvic inflammatory disease
- FBC to rule out sepsis
- Serum B-hCG to rule out pregnancy
- Urine MCS

Diagnosis at Laparotomy—Adnexal Torsion (4 Marks)

The right adnexum is commonly involved; rectosigmoid colon probably limits torsion on the left (2 marks).

20–25% adnexal torsions occur in pregnancy **(2 marks)**.

The pedicle appears like "snail shell" or "Bull eye" on ultrasound scan **(2 marks).**

The presence of fever suggests necrosis **(2 marks)**.

The procedure involves: **(2 marks each)**

- Detorsion (untwisting)
- Cystectomy with or without
- Oophoropexy

No additional treatment is needed; she would require progesterone support if she were <12 weeks pregnant **(4 marks).**

Checklist for management of adnexal torsion

Tasks	**Well done**	**Fairly done**	**Poorly done**	**Not done**
Differenal diagnoses: (Max.of 5)				
- Adnexal torsion		2		0
- Acute pelvic inflammatory disease		2		0
- Acute appendicis		2		0
- Ureteric colic		2		0
- Acute cyss		2		0
- Ectopic pregnancy		2		0
Specific invesgaons:				
- Abdominopelvic ultrasound		2		0
- MRI if available		2		0
- FBC to tule out sepsis		2		0
- Urine MCS		2		0
- Serum B-hCG		2		0
Diagnosis – Adnexal torsion (twisted ovarian acceptable)	4			0
Right adnexum commonly involved		2		0
20-25% adnexal torsion occurs in pregnancy		2		0
The pedicle appears like "snail shell"or "Bull eye"on USS		2		0
The presence of fever suggests necrosis		2		0
The procedure involves"				
- Detorsion (untwisting)		2		0
- Cystectomy and		2		0
- Oophooropexy (optional)			1	0
No additional treatment needed; she would require progesterone support if she were less than 12 weeks pregnant	4	2	1	0
Total marks	41			
Candidate's score .../41				

Examiner's signature Date

3.3 Station 3.3 History Taking of a Patient with Primary Amenorrhoea

Subject: Gynaecology.
Subspecialty: Adolescent gynaecology.
Domain of clinical competence: Focused history taking.
Station: History of primary amenorrhoea complicated by acute urinary retention.
Station objective: To test the candidate's ability to take a focused history of primary amenorrhoea complicated by acute urinary retention with the purpose of arriving at a diagnosis.
Requirements: Standardized or real patient, a table and 2 chairs for examiners, enough copies of checklist, pencils and erasers, dressed bed or chair for patient or Role player, a chair for the candidate, plain papers for use by candidates, a clearly written task for the candidate.

3.3.1 Instructions to the Standardized Patient

Biodata

Name: JJ	Religion: Christianity
Age: 16 years	Tribe: Bura
Parity: P0 + 0	Educational status: SS 3 pupil
Address: Old GRA Maiduguri	Marital status: A child (unmarried)

Presenting Complaints

Lack of menses since birth
Inability to pass urine for 24 h

History of Presenting Complaints

I am a 16-year-old SS 3 student of Government Girls College, Maiduguri, who has never seen her menses. I first noticed breast development at the age of 13 years followed by appearance of pubic and axillary hair at the age of 14 (if asked). Although

I started experiencing monthly lower abdominal pains last year, I did not seek medical advice until now because I was unable to pass urine last night and I informed my mother who decided to bring me to see a gynaecologist. There is associated lower abdominal swelling which is gradually increasing in size (if asked). I had no preceding problem with passing urine or moving my bowels.

Past Medical and Surgical History
I have never been admitted in hospital for any reason. I have been treated for malaria fever several times on outpatient basis both at home and in school. I am not allergic to any of the drugs I have taken. I received childhood immunizations.

Family and Social History
I live with my parents in a 4-bedroom flat in Old GRA Maiduguri, I am the last of 5 children: 3 boys and 2 girls. My sister has no similar problem. There is no family history of hypertension and sickle cell disease, but my father is diabetic on treatment. I am not sexually active, never known a man.

Systemic Review
I have no other complaint.

3.3.2 Instruction to the Candidate

The patient before you is a senior secondary school student (SS 3) who was brought to the hospital by her mother to see a gynaecologist. Your task is to take her history.

3.3.3 Instruction to the Examiners

Ms. JJ is a 16-year-old SS 3 student who was brought to the gynaecological clinic by her mother on account of primary amenorrhoea and acute urinary retention of about 24 h duration. The candidate is expected to take her history. Use the checklist provided to score the candidate.

Checklist for history of primary amenorrhoea

Task	Well done	Fairly done	Poorly done	Not done
Greets paent and introduces self and obtains permission to talk to her	4	2	1	0
Obtains Biodata: name, age, address, occupaon, tribe, religion, etc.	4	2	1	0
Asks for LMP		2		0
Presenng complaints: - Lower abdominal pain (1) for 1 year (1) - Inability to pass urine (1) for 24 hours (1)		 2 2	 1 1	 0 0
History of presenng complaints: - Characterize the abdominal pain; cyclical, aching, radiaon - Is there associated lower abdominal swelling? - When did she noce breast development? - When did she noce appearance of pubic/axillary hair? - Was there difficulty in passing urine before the retenon? - Any other urinary symptom; frequency, dysuria, urgency? - Any bowel symptoms		 2 2 2 2 2 2 2		 0 0 0 0 0 0 0
Past medical and surgical history; previous illness, surgery, drug allergies, regular medicaon	4	2	1	0
FSH: siblings, similar problem in siblings, sexual history, HT, DM, SCD	4	2	1	0
Systemic review: Nil of note		2		0
Summary of history	4	2	1	0
Total score	42			
Candidate's score......../42				

Examiners name and signature Date

3.4 Station 3.4 Post Encounter to History of Acute Urinary Retention

Domain of clinical competence: Virtual sign identification (Picture test).

Station object: To test the candidate's ability to recognize imperforate hymen and explain the pathogenesis and treatment of the condition.

Requirements: A laminated picture of the vulva of a patient showing imperforate hymen, questions to the candidate on imperforate hymen preferably on the same page with the picture, a table and 3 chairs for the examiners and the candidate, pencils and erasers for the examines, plain papers on which to answer the questions, a chaperon.

3.4.1 Instruction to Candidate

Below is the picture of the exposed vulvar of the 16-year old SS3 student you clerked on the last station with acute urinary retention. Carefully study it and answer the questions that follow (Fig. 3.2).

Questions

1. What is the diagnosis?
2. List 2 differential diagnosis
3. From which embryonal tissue is the structure causing this problem derived from?
4. List 4 symptoms she might present with
5. List 3 complications of this problem in the neonate
6. What is the treatment of the condition?

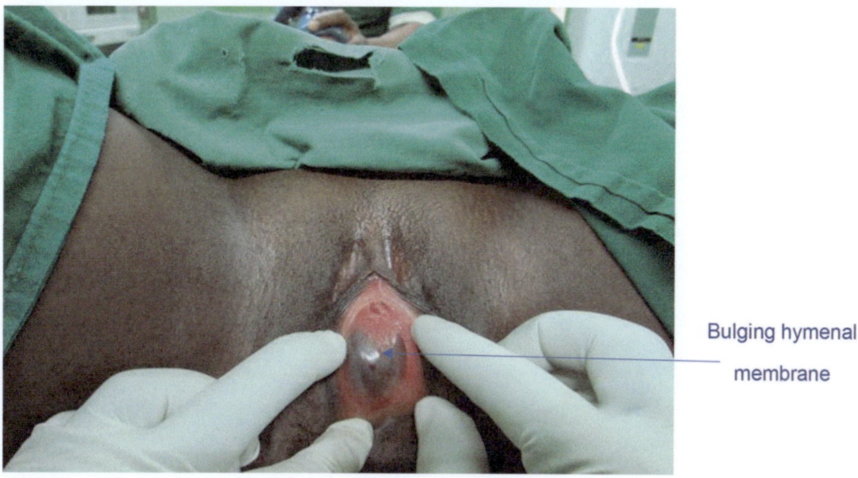

Fig. 3.2 Imperforate hymen on vulvar exposure (Chama 2014)

Answers

1. Imperforate hymen (**4 marks**)
2. Differentials (**maximum of 4 marks**)
   (a) hymeneal cyst = 2 marks
   (b) transverse vaginal septum = 2 marks
   (c) labial agglutination = 2 marks
3. The hymen is derived from the ***urogenital membrane (4 marks)***
4. Possible symptoms in a 14-year-old girl (**maximum of 8 marks**)
   (a) cyclic lower abdominal pain = 2 marks
   (b) primary amenorrhoea = 2 marks
   (c) acute abdominal pain = 2 marks
   (d) difficulty with urination = 2 marks
   (e) difficulty with defaecation = 2 marks
5. Possible complications in the neonate (**maximum of 6 marks**)
   (a) hydro/mucocolpos = 2 marks
   (b) hydronephrosis = 2 marks
   (c) acute renal failure = 2 marks
   (d) respiratory failure = 2 marks
6. The treatment for this condition is **hymenectomy (4 marks)**

Maximum marks for the station = 30

Checklist for imperforate hymen

Task	**Well done**	**Fairly done**	**Poorly done**	**Not done**
Diagnosis: Imperforate hymen	4			0
Differenal diagnosis:				
- Hymeneal cyst		2		0
- Transverse vaginal septum		2		0
- Labial agglunaon		2		0
The hymen is derived from the urogenital membrane	4			0
Possible symptoms in a 14 year old girl:				
- Cyclical lower abdominal pain		2		0
- Primary amenorrhea		2		0
- Acute lower abdominal pain		2		0
- Acute urinary retenon		2		0
- Difficulty with defaecaon		2		0
Possible complicaons in the neonate:				
- Hydro/mucocolpos		2		0
- Hydronephrosis		2		0
- Acute renal failure		2		0
- Respiratory failure		2		0
The definive treatment of this condion is Hymenectomy (give 2 points for hymenotomy or I&D)	4	2		0
Total score	34			
Candidate's scor.../34				

Examiner's signature Date

3.5 Station 3.5 Vaginal Examination in a Paediatric Patient

Subject: Gynaecology.
Subspecialty: Paediatric and adolescent gynaecology.
Domain of clinical competence: Physical examination.
Station: Vaginal examination in a child presenting with vaginal discharge.
Station objective: To assess the candidate's ability to examine a paediatric patient for the purpose of establishing a diagnosis.
Requirements: Standardized mother, a female doll or mannikin, dressed bed for standardized mother and mannikin, latex gloves, kidney dish with wet swabs, swab stick, non-toothed dissecting forceps, a table and chairs for examiners, sufficient checklists, pencils and erasers, a chaperon (Fig. 3.3).

3.5.1 Instruction to the Standardized Mother

I have listened to your complaints concerning your 6-year-old daughter who is experiencing serous vaginal discharge with some blood stain. I want to thank you also for answering the questions I have asked you concerning her condition. Now I would like to examine her to further assess her condition, and I need your

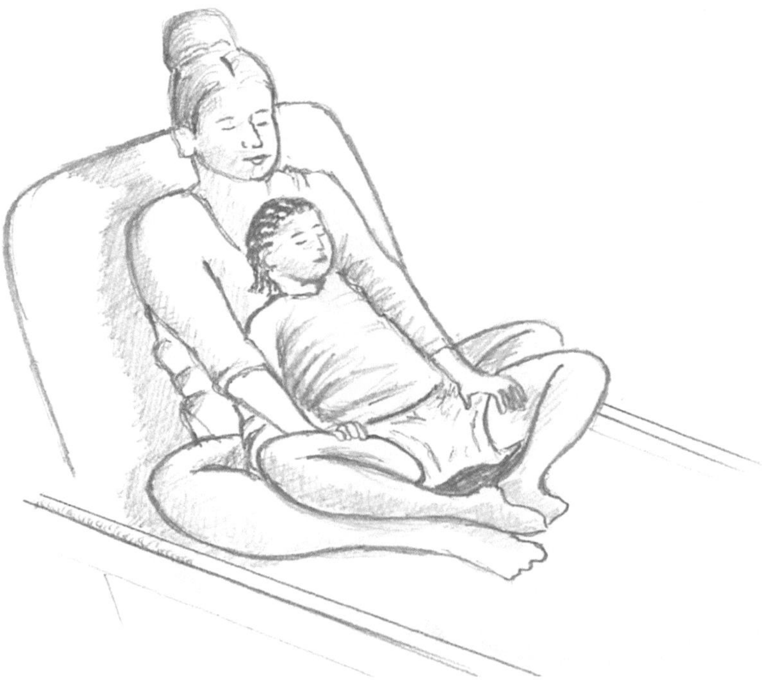

Fig. 3.3 Frog-leg position. (Courtesy of Jonathan Edache Otache)

participation in the procedure to obtain her cooperation. I will use this mannikin to demonstrate how your daughter will be examined.

You will lie on this bed with the head raised while your daughter sits on your lap with her legs straddling your thighs like this (demonstrate to her). You would have undressed her so that I can examine her thoroughly including her private part. Thank you for your cooperation.

3.5.2 Instructions to the Candidate

The girl on the bed is a 6-year-old nursery school pupil sitting beside her mother. Her mother complained that she has noticed a blood-stained serous discharge from the private part of her daughter. Using the mannikin provided, demonstrate step by step how you would examine the child.

3.5.3 Instructions to the Examiner

Mrs. FD has brought her 6 years old daughter to the clinic, having noticed blood-stained serous discharge on her pants for the past one week. Using the mannikin provided, the candidate is supposed to examine the child with the aim of establishing a diagnosis. Use the checklist provided to score the candidate.

Checklist for paediatric vaginal examination

Task	Well done	Fairly done	Poorly done	Not done
Greets the SP, introduces self and obtains permission		2	1	0
Explains the procedure and seeks her parcipaon		2	1	0
Speaks to the child nicely, offers her an object (doll), or chocolate		2	1	0
Requests the mother to sit comfortably on the bed and put her daughter on her lap, assuming the frog-leg posion	4	2	1	0
Starts with less inmate examinaon: eyes, ears, mouth, auscultate her chest for heart sounds and breath sounds	4	2	1	0
Vaginal exam (with mother keeping child in frog-leg posion) - Inspects the external genitalia for discharge, lesions etc. - Takes a swab of the discharge		 2 2	 1 1	 0 0
Holds each labia between thumb and forefinger and pull forward and laterally to inspect: - Introitus for discharge, inflammaon, foreign body - Hymen for tears or laceraons - Lower vagina for foreign body, tumors		 2 2 2	 1 1 1	 0 0 0
If foreign body seen, irrigate with normal saline in 50ml syringe to expel foreign body behind the hymen	4	2	1	0
If there is tumor or persistent foreign body, schedule for EUA and vaginoscopy	4	2	1	0
Clean paent, thank the mother and reposion child		2	1	0
Penales – rough, non-sequenal, child irritated	-4	-2	-1	0
Total marks				
Candidate's score …/				

Examiner's signature Date

3.6 Station 3.6 Breast Examination in an Adolescent

Subject: Gynaecology.
Subspecialty: Paediatric and adolescent gynaecology.
Domain of clinical competence: Physical examination (PE).
Station: Breast examination in an adolescent with lack of development of one breast.
Station objective: Breast examination of an adolescent with lack of development of one breast with the aim of establishing a diagnosis and developing management plan.
Requirements: Mannikin of an adolescent chest with asymmetric breast development, latex gloves, dressed bed for the mannikin, a table and chairs for the examiners, sufficient checklist for use by the examiners, pencils and erasers, a chaperon to take care of the mannikin and attend to the examiners (Fig. 3.4).

3.6.1 Instruction to the Candidate

Ms. JA is a 16-year-old Senior Secondary School class 3 pupil who was brought to the gynaecology clinic by her mother because her left breast is not developing like the right breast. Your task is to use the mannequin to demonstrate how you would examine her breasts. Run a commentary on your findings to the hearing of the examiners as you perform the breast examination.

3.6.2 Instructions to the Examiners

Ms. Joy is a 16-year-old SSS 3 pupil who came with her mother to the gynaecology clinic because her left breast is not developing. The candidate is supposed to use the mannequin to demonstrate how he would examine Joy's breasts. Use the checklist provided to score the candidate.

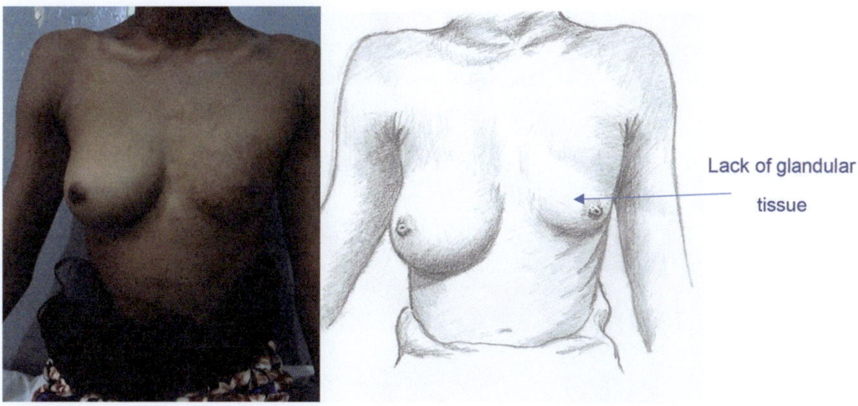

Fig. 3.4 Lack of glandular tissue in one breast (Chama 2022) (Drawing on the right, Courtesy of Jonathan Edache Otache)

Checklist for breast examination

Tasks	Well done	Fairly done	Poorly done	Not done
Greets the patient and introduces self		2	1	0
Explains the procedure and obtains permission		2	1	0
Requests the chaperon to screen the patient and be present		2	1	0
Requests the patient to sit straight with hands by her side		2	1	0
Inspection:				
- Symmetry of breasts; left obviously smaller		2		0
- Nipples; flat, retracted, everted		2		0
- Any scar, particularly over smaller breast?		2		0
- Skin coloration; areola, any others		2		0
Requests patient to sit akimbo or hold hands over her head		2	1	0
Palpation:				
- Hands previously washed and wore latex gloves		2	1	0
- Stabilize breast with one hand and palpate with the other		2	1	0
- Examines all quadrants and the areola for masses		2	1	0
- Gently squeezes the base of the nipple for secretions		2	1	0
- Reports on normal glandular masses		2	1	0
- Presence or absence of any abnormal masses		2	1	0
- Palpates axillary lymph nodes		2	1	0
Additional palpation of small breast				
- Palpates infraclavicular area (attachment of pectoralis-major)		2		0
- Palpates intercostal spaces for deficiency of pectoral muscles		2		0
- Palpates bulk of latissimus dorsi muscle		2		0
Thanks patient and repositions		2		0
Reassures patient that her condition will be investigated and treated accordingly	4	2	1	0
Summarizes findings to the examiners	4	2	1	0
Total score	48			
Candidate's score .../48				

Examiner's signature Date

3.7 Station 3.7 Excision of Urethral Prolapse

Subject: Gynaecology.
Subspecialty: Paediatric gynaecology.
Domain of clinical competence: Therapeutic procedure.
Station: Excision of urethral prolapse in a child.
Station objective: To assess the ability of the candidate to correctly excise a symptomatic urethral prolapse in a 4-year-old girl.
Requirements: Picture of the vulva of a girl child with urethral prolapse (a mannequin may also be used if available), latex gloves, kidney dish with sterile gauze, Gali pot with wet swab, needle holder, non-toothed dissecting forceps, vicryl 3-0 sutures, paediatric Foley's catheter, 5 mL syringe and needles, dressed bed or trolley for the mannequin, a table and chairs for examiners, sufficient checklist, pencils and erasers, a chaperon (Fig. 3.5).

3.7.1 Instruction to the Candidate

A 3-year-old girl was seen in the gynaecology clinic with bloodstaining of her pants for 2 weeks. She was evaluated and found to have urethral prolapse. She was placed on oestrogen cream for 6 weeks without improvement of her symptoms. She is scheduled for excision of the urethral prolapse. Using the mannequin provided, describe step by step how you would perform the procedure. Run a commentary as you perform the procedure to the hearing of the examiners.

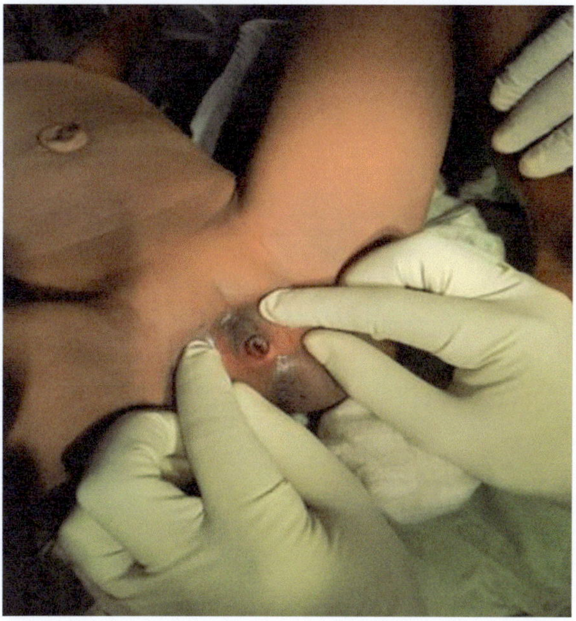

Fig. 3.5 Urethral prolapse in a female child (Chama 2017)

3.7.2 Instruction to the Examiners

The candidate has been provided with a mannequin of a female child with urethral prolapse scheduled for excision. He is supposed to demonstrate step by step how he would perform the procedure. Use the checklist provided to score the candidate.

Checklist for excision of urethral prolapse

Tasks	Well done	Fairly done	Poorly done	Not done
Preoperative preparation: PCV, renal function tests, urine MCS, any abnormality treated, and written consent obtained from parents/guardians	4	2	1	0
Patient under GA, positioned in frog-leg position to expose vulva		2	1	0
I will clean and gown, then clean and drape the patient		2	1	0
I will pass paediatric foley's catheter, inflate balloon with 3ml savlon or normal saline		2	1	0
With non-toothed dissecting forceps to hold the prolapsed tissue, I will excise it circumferentially using blade number 15	4	2	1	0
The cut edges will be approximated with vicryl 3-0 sutures at 12, 3, 6, and 9 O'clock positions	4	2	1	0
The vulva is cleaned, and the catheter left in-situ for 2-3 days		2	1	0
The patient is positioned supine and transferred to recovery room		2	1	0
I will document the procedure and prescribe postoperative management	4	2	1	0
The patient can be discharged home after removing the foley's catheter and given appoint to the clinic		2	1	0
Total score	36			
Candidate's score .../36				

Examiner's signature Date

Infertility and Assisted Reproductive Technology OSCE Stations

4

4.1 Station 4.1 History Taking in Primary Infertility

Subject: Gynaecology.
Subspecialty: Infertility and assisted reproductive technology.
Domain of clinical competence: History taking.
Station: Focused history of primary infertility.
Station objective: To assess the candidate's ability to take a focused history of a patient with primary infertility with the aim of eliciting the possible cause of the problem.
Requirements: Standardized patient (role player), a dressed bed for the patient, a table and 2 chairs for the examiners, pencils and erasers, enough copies of checklist, a chair for the candidate, some plain papers for use by the candidate, a chaperon.

4.1.1 Instruction to Standardized Patient

Biodata

Name: TA	Tribe: Tsayawa
Age: 25 years	Religion: Christianity
Address: Federal Low Cost, Bauchi	Parity: P0 + 0
Occupation: Secondary school Teacher	LMP: 2 weeks ago

Presenting Complaint
Inability to conceive.
Duration of 3 years

C. Chama, *OSCE and VIVA VOCE in Obstetrics and Gynaecology*,
https://doi.org/10.1007/978-3-031-77262-7_4

History of Presenting Complaint
I am 25 years old and married for the past 3 years. I have not been able to conceive and that is why I came to the hospital to seek for solution. I stay with my husband in a 3 bedroom flat at Federal Low Cost estate, Bauchi and we meet (sexual intercourse) about 3 times a week except during menses. My husband achieves good erection and ejaculates during sexual intercourse. I don't experience undue pains during sexual intercourse.

I have noticed some milky discharge from both my nipples when I press my breasts; this has been on-going for about one year now. There is no headache except when I have malaria fever which is not often. I have never been admitted in hospital for any illness. My husband is the first and only person I have had sexual intercourse with. However, my husband confessed to me that he was treated for gonorrhoea once when he was a student in the university. He is a graduate of Building Engineering. I have never been treated for any sexually transmitted infection. I have never had any neck swelling and do not have undue feeling of cold or heat.

Past Medical and Surgical History
I have never been treated or operated for any major illness.

Family and Social History
I am the only wife of my husband and neither of us drink alcohol or smoke cigarettes. None of my immediate relations have diabetes, hypertension, or sickle cell disease. My husband had no groin surgery or any surgery for that matter.

Systemic Review
I have no other complaint.

4.1.2 Instruction to the Candidate

The patient in front of you has come to the gynaecological clinic. Take her history.

4.1.3 Instructions to the Examiners

The candidate has been instructed to take the history of a married nulligravida who has come to the gynaecological clinic with primary infertility. Use the checklist provided to score the candidate.

Checklist for history of infertility candidate's number………

Tasks	Well done	Fairly done	Poorly done	Not done
Greets patient, introduces self and obtains permission to discuss her problem with her	4	2	1	0
Biodata: name, age, occupation, address, tribe etc.	4	2	1	0
Presenting complaints:				
- Inability to conceive(1) for 3 years (1)		2	1	0
- Milky discharge from the breasts (1) for 1 year (1)		2	1	0
History of presenting complaints				
- Duration of marriage		2		0
- Coital frequency		2		0
- Whether husband achieves erection and ejaculation		2		0
- Knowledge of fertile period		2		0
- History of PID/neck swelling		2		0
- Any abnormal hair growth pattern		2		0
- Milky breast discharge		2		0
- History of STI in husband	4	2		0
- Any child outside marriage	4	2		0
		2		0
GH: menarche, LMP, periods, cycle, dysmenorrhea, contraception	4	2	1	0
Obstetric history: P0+0		2		0
PMH: nil of note		2		0
FSH: only wife of husband, does not smoke or take alcohol		2	1	0
Systemic review: headache, lower abdominal pain, vaginal discharge		2		0
Give a summary of the history to the examiners	4	2	1	0
Communication skill	4	2	1	0
Total score	56			
Candidate's score………/56				

Examiner's signature Date

4.2 Station 4.2 Counselling a Couple for Semen Analysis

Subject: Gynaecology.
Subspecialty: Infertility and ART.
Domain of clinical competence: Communication and Counselling .
Station: Counselling a couple for collection of semen for analysis.
Station objective: To test the candidate's ability to counsel a couple on how to collect semen for analysis for the purpose of identifying possible male factor infertility.
Requirements: Standardized or real couple, samples of semen collection bottles, a table and 2 chairs for examiners, 2 chairs or dressed bed for the couple, a chair for the candidate, enough copies of the checklist, pencils and erasers, and a chaperon (Fig. 4.1).

4.2.1 Instructions to the Role Couple

You have been married for 3 years now without achieving pregnancy. You have seen a gynaecologist who has discussed your concern with you and examined you and your wife. The gynaecologist has requested that your wife carry out some investigations and you are also requested to bring your semen for analysis. The gynaecologist is going to give you further instructions on obtaining your semen for analysis.

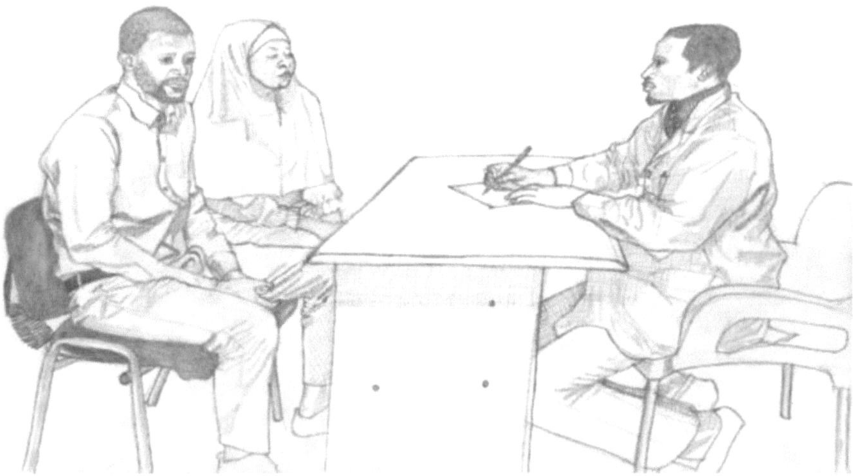

Fig. 4.1 Couple counselling session. (Courtesy of Jonathan Edache Otache)

4.2.2 Instructions to the Candidate

The couple before you have seen a gynaecologist for primary infertility. The husband has been requested to produce his semen for analysis as one of the investigations they have to carry out. Your task is to counsel the couple on obtaining semen for analysis.

4.2.3 Instructions to the Examiners

The candidate is supposed to counsel the couple on how to obtain semen for analysis. Use the checklist provided to score the candidate.

Checklist for counselling for semen collection

Task	Well done	Fairly done	Poorly done	Not done
Greets couple and introduces self		2	1	0
Introduces the topic; like I understand you are expected to provide your semen for laboratory analysis….	4	2	1	0
Asks the husband if he achieves ejaculation during sexual intercourse		2	1	0
Informs the couple they must abstain from sexual intercourse for at least 2 days but not more than one week before the test in order not to produce premature or aging sperm cells for analysis	4	2	1	0
Allows couple to ask questions or seek clarifications		2	1	0
Explains how to collect semen by masturbation:				
- Couple can use a special room within the laboratory or their home if living nearby.		2	1	0
- They should romance without penetrative intercourse using the most sensitive parts of their bodies.		2	1	0
- When the husband is about to ejaculate, he puts the semen into the bottle provided		2	1	0
- The specimen should be taken to the laboratory immediately		2	1	0
Asks the couple if they can collect semen this way		2		0
Explains alternative methods:				
- Electrical stimulators from the laboratory can be used.		2	1	0
- Coitus interruptus can be used but the specimen may be contaminated.		2	1	0
- Silicon condom can be used but removing the semen from the condom is incomplete		2	1	0
Inform the couple whichever method they want to use, the specimen must reach the laboratory within 30 minutes		2	1	0
Asks the couple which method they prefer to use		2		0
Thanks the couple for listening and gives them appointment		2		0
Communication skills	4	2	1	0
Maximum score	36			
Candidate's score …/36				

Examiner's signature Date

4.3 Station 4.3 Interpreting Semen Analysis Result

Subject: Gynaecology.
Subspecialty: Infertility and ART.
Domain of clinical competence: Interpretation of abnormal test finding (IATF).
Station: Interpreting the result of semen analysis.
Station objective: To test the candidate's ability to correctly identify the abnormalities in the result of semen analysis and the possible causes and proffer appropriate treatment.
Requirements: Standardized couple, result sheet of the semen analysis, comfortable chairs or dressed bed for the couple, a table and 2 chairs for examiners, a chair for the candidate, pencils and erasers, enough copies of the checklist, and a chaperon.

4.3.1 Instruction to the Candidate

The couple you counselled on the last station had the semen analysis done and they have come with the result to the follow-up clinic. Study the result as shown below and answer the questions, which follow.

4.4 XX, Bauchi

4.4.1 Microbiology Report Form

Name	HA	**Consultant** Dr. CC
Age	40 years	
Address	Yelwa ward, Bauchi	
Date	20/11/2023	
Specimen: Semen for analysis		**Macroscopy**
Time produced: 9:00 a.m.		Volume: 3.5 mL
Time received: 9:20 a.m.		Colour: pale yellow
Time analysed: 9:30 a.m.		Viscosity: viscous
		pH: 7.4
Microscopy		**Culture**
Count	10 million/mL	Gardnerella vaginalis isolated
Motility 10% progressively active		15% sluggish
		75% immotile
WBC 10–15/hpf; *clue cells present.*		
		Signature of microbiologist

Questions

1. What is your diagnosis in the male partner?
2. List 2 possible causes of the abnormality in this result in your environment
3. What treatment would you offer him immediately?
4. When would you like to repeat the semen analysis?
5. What is the likely diagnosis in the female partner?
6. How would you confirm the likely diagnosis in the female partner?
7. If left untreated, what would be the possible complications if she gets pregnant?

Answers

1. Oligoasthenozoospermia (4 marks)
2. Possible causes of oligoasthenozoospermia (2 marks each; maximum 4 marks)
   (a) STI
   (b) Alcohol consumption
   (c) Cigarette smoking
3. Oral metronidazole 400 mg 8 hourly for one week (tinidazole, secnidazole acceptable; drug 2 marks, dosage 2 marks)
4. Repeat the semen analysis 3 weeks after treatment (2 marks)
5. The likely diagnosis in his wife is bacterial vaginosis because of the presence of clue cells in the semen; Gardnerella vaginalis can be harboured in the male urethra (4 marks).
6. Gram stain of HVS would show Gardnerella vaginalis and few or absent lactobacilli (4 marks)
7. If left untreated and the woman conceives, possible complications of bacterial vaginosis in pregnancy include: (2 marks each, maximum 6 marks)
   (a) Second trimester miscarriage followed by PID
   (b) Premature rupture of membranes
   (c) Preterm birth
   (d) Postpartum endometritis

Checklist for interpretation of semen analysis result

Task	Well done	Fairly done	Poorly done	Not done
Diagnosis: Oligo-(2)asthenozoospermia (2)	4	2		0
Possible causes of Oligoasthenozoospermia:				
- STI		2		0
- Alcohol consumption		2		0
- Smoking		2		0
Tabs metronidazole (2) 800mg 8 hourly for one week (2)	4	2		0
Repeat semen analysis (2) 3 weeks after treatment (2)	4	2		0
Likely diagnosis in his wife is bacterial vaginosis (2) because of the presence of Gardnerella vaginalis in the semen (2)	4	2		0
Gram statin of HVS would show Gardnerella vaginalis (2) and few or no lactobacilli (2)	4	2		0
If left untreated and the woman conceives, possible complications:				
- Second trimester miscarriage		2		0
- Premature rupture of membranes		2		0
- Preterm birth		2		0
- Postpartum endometritis		2		0
Total score	30			
Candidate's score .../30				

Examiner's signature Date

4.5 Station 4.4 Counselling a Couple for Invitro Fertilization (IVF)

Subject: Gynaecology.
Subspecialty: Infertility and ART.
Domain of clinical competence: Communication and counselling.
Station: Counselling a couple for IVF-ET.
Station objective: To test the candidate's ability to counsel a couple to take up IVF and embryo transfer (ET) for the purpose of achieving pregnancy using their own gametes.
Requirements: Standardized or real patient, a table and 2 chairs for examiners, enough copies of the checklist, pencils and erasers, a chair for the candidate, plain papers for rough use by the candidate, and a chaperon.

4.5.1 Instruction to Standardized Couple

I am a 25-year-old housewife who has been coming to the hospital for the past 3 months because I am not able to conceive after 3 years of marriage. I and my husband have gone through several tests and received treatment for the problems identified by the doctor. I was treated for a sexually transmitted infection and abnormal flow of milk from my breasts. My husband has also been treated for the same infection, but his sperm count has remained low after three repeated tests over the past 3 months. Both of us were requested to come today for further interaction on the way forward concerning our inability to conceive. We have no new complaints.

4.5.2 Instructions to the Candidate

Mrs. TA and her husband have been evaluated for primary infertility in this facility. Her husband has oligospermia on three consecutive specimens over the last 3 months. They were both treated for Gardnerella vaginalis infection with metronidazole with good effect. They were requested to come to the clinic today to receive counselling for in vitro fertilization and embryo transfer. Your task is to counsel them for this purpose.

4.5.3 Instructions to the Examiners

The couple present are known patients of this hospital who have been evaluated for primary infertility following 3 years of marriage. The husband has oligospermia, and they have been requested to come for counselling for in vitro fertilization and embryo transfer. The candidate is supposed to counsel the couple for this purpose. Use the checklist provided to score the candidate.

Checklist for counselling for IVF

Task	Well done	Fairly done	Poorly done	Not done
Greets couple and introduces self		2	1	0
Empathizes with the couple and assure them the situation is not hopeless	4	2	1	0
Biodata: name, age, address, occupation, education, religion	4	2	1	0
Parity, LMP, cycle, periods		2	1	0
Asks the couple what they know about IVF		2		0
Explains about IVF-ET				
- She will be screened and treated if need be for conditions that will interfere with the IVF process like fibroids, medical diseases etc.		2	1	0
- Ovulation induction will make her produce many eggs in a cycle.		2	1	0
- Development of the eggs will be monitored and harvested when sufficiently mature.		2	1	0
- The eggs will be fertilized using her husband's sperm and growth of embryo monitored in the laboratory.		2	1	0
- 2 embryos (babies) will be transferred into your womb for further growth.		2	1	0
- Drugs will be given to her to support the pregnancy in the early stages		2	1	0
Ask couple to give feedback on what they understand by the explanation so far		2		0
Further explanation				
- Pregnancy test will be done 2 weeks after the ET		2	1	0
- Pregnancy will be confirmed 4 weeks after embryo transfer.		2	1	0
- The chances of successfully getting pregnant is about 25%		2	1	0
Ask couple if they want further clarifications		2		0
If successful she will book for ANC early; possible complications include ectopic pregnancy, OHSS and needs prompt treatment	4	2	1	0
Thanks the couple for the discussion and gives them appointment		2		0
Communication skills	4	2	1	0
Total scores	46			
Candidate's score .../46				

Examiner's signature Date

4.6 Station 4.5 Transvaginal Ultrasound for Follicle Tracking

Subject: Gynaecology.
Subspecialty: Infertility and ART.
Domain of clinical competence: Diagnostic procedure.
Station: Transvaginal ultrasound for follicle tracking.
Station objective: To assess the candidate's ability to correctly perform a transvaginal ultrasound scan with the purpose of monitoring follicular growth in a patient on gonadotrophin stimulation.
Requirements: Mannequin of female pelvis, transvaginal ultrasound probe, male condoms, ultrasound jelly, latex gloves, a table or dressed bed for the mannequin, table and chairs for the examiners, checklists, pencils and erasers, tissue paper, antiseptic swipes, and a chaperon (Fig. 4.2).

4.6.1 Instructions to the Candidate

The patient on the bed is a nullipara who is being treated for secondary infertility. She is being prepared for IVF-ET indicated by bilateral tubal blockage. She has been on 75 mg FSH IM daily for the past 5 days and is scheduled to have TVS today for follicle tracking. Using the mannequin and the transvaginal probe provided, demonstrate step by step how you would perform transvaginal ultrasound on her and report your findings to the hearing of the examiners as you perform the procedure.

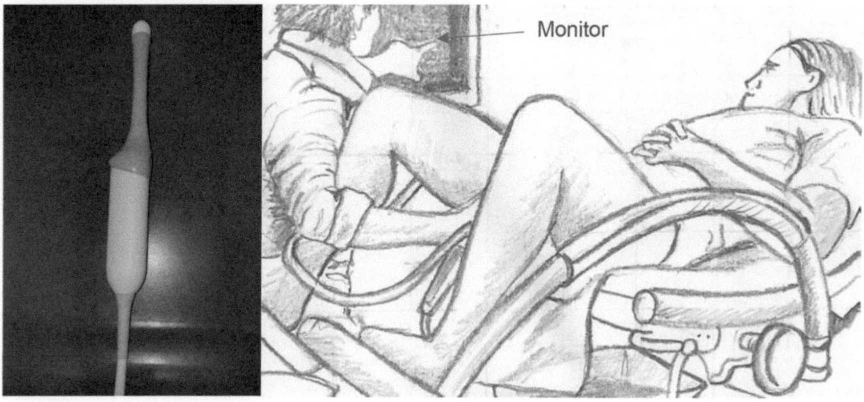

Transvaginal probe *Transvaginal scan procedure*

Fig. 4.2 Performing transvaginal ultrasound. (Drawing in the right—Courtesy of Jonathan Edache Otache)

4.6.2 Instructions to the Examiners

The patient is a known case of secondary infertility on ovarian stimulation using FSH for the purpose of IVF-ET. The candidate is supposed to use the pelvic model and the transvaginal probe to demonstrate how he would perform TVS for the purpose of monitoring follicular growth. Use the checklist provided to score the candidate.

Checklist for TVS for follicular tracking

Tasks	Well done	Fairly done	Poorly done	Not done
Greets the patient and introduces self		2	1	0
Explains the procedure and obtains permission		2	1	0
Requests the presence of chaperon and asks patient to go and empty her bladder		2	1	0
Wears latex gloves, positions patient supine, thighs abducted, and knees flexed	4	2	1	0
Introduces jelly into the tip of a male condom (or sheath) and covers the transvaginal probe, adds sufficient jelly to tip of probe	4	2	1	0
Holds the probe in the dominant hand with the knob pointing upwards		2	1	0
Parts the labia with the non-dominant hand and introduces the tip of the probe into the vagina	4	2	1	0
With pushing and pulling, rotational, rocking, and panning movements: - A longitudinal view of the uterus is obtained. - Locate each ovary turn by turn, count developing follicles. - Measure the ovary in 3 diameters and calculate volume. - Measure each developing follicle in 3 diameters and obtain the volume. - Use doppler to assess stromal vascularity. - Use 3D to differentiate follicles from cysts; also, more accurate in assessing volume. - Follicles with mean diameter of 16-20mm are mature		2 2 2 2 2 2 2	1 1 1 1 1 1 1	0 0 0 0 0 0 0
Withdraw the probe and provide the patient with tissue paper to clean herself		2		0
Remove the condom and clean the probe with antiseptic swipe		2		0
Thank the patient, explain the findings, and give her appointment	4	2	1	0
Document your findings		2		0
Total marks	44			
Candidate's score .../44				

Examiner's signature Date

4.7 Station 4.6 Electroejaculation for Semen Analysis in a Paraplegic

Subject: Gynaecology.
Subspeciality: Infertility and ART.
Domain of clinical competence: Therapeutic procedure.
Station: Electroejaculation in a paraplegic for the purpose of semen analysis.
Station objective: To test the candidate's ability to collect semen by electrical stimulation in a paraplegic who is unable to ejaculate and presents with primary infertility.
Requirements: Male mannequin, electroejaculator, latex gloves, liquid paraffin, Gali pot with wet swab, sterile bottle for collecting semen, a dressed bed for the mannequin, a table and chairs for the examiners, sufficient checklist, pencils and erasers, and a chaperon (Fig. 4.3).

4.7.1 Instruction to the Candidate

Mr. SB and his wife have been evaluated for primary infertility. Mr. Suleiman who became paraplegic 5 years ago following road traffic accident is unable to ejaculate during sexual intercourse. He is scheduled for electro-ejaculation for semen analysis and possible intrauterine insemination. Use the mannequin provided to demonstrate step by step how you would obtain semen from Mr. Suleiman using electro-ejaculation.

4.7.2 Instruction to the Examiners

The candidate has been instructed to use the mannequin provided to demonstrate how to obtain semen by electro-ejaculation for the purpose of semen analysis. He is supposed to report each step verbally to your hearing. Use the checklist provided to score the candidate.

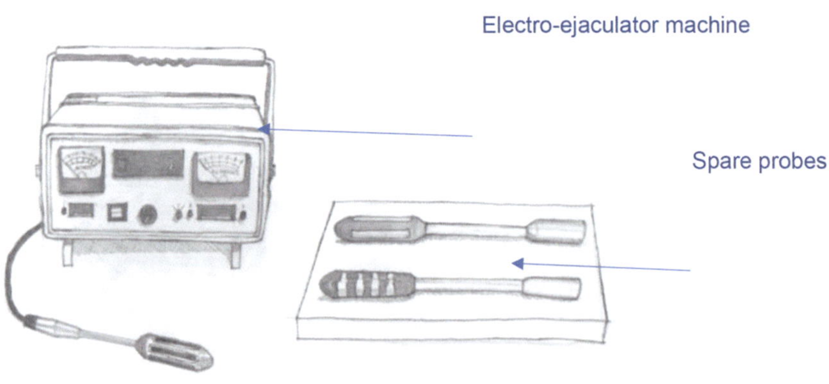

Fig. 4.3 Typical electroejaculator machine with spare probes. (Courtesy of Jonathan Edache Otache)

Checklist for electro-ejaculation

Tasks	Well done	Fairly done	Poorly done	Not done
Greets patient and introduces self		2	1	0
Explains the procedure and obtains permission		2	1	0
Instructs the assistant on how to collect the semen	4	2	1	0
Request chaperon to screen the patient		2	1	0
Checks the functionality of equipment		2	1	0
Scrubs and gowns, asks assistant to position patient in left lateral position	4	2	1	0
Mount electrodes on a cylindrical rod and lubricated with liquid paraffin.		2	1	0
With non-dominant hand exposing the anal verge, the rod is held with the dominant hand and the electrodes gently introduced into the anus with the electrodes facing the prostate	4	2	1	0
The assistant holds the penile shaft, pointing into a wide-mouthed bottle		2	1	0
Using the non-dominant hand, turn the voltage of the electro-ejaculator from 0-5volts, immediately return to 0 volts		2	1	0
If there is no ejaculation, repeat and increase voltage to 6 volts, progressively increase the voltage till ejaculation is seen.		2	1	0
Continue stimulation at this level until ejaculation stops	4	2	1	0
Cover specimen, label bottle and send to lab for analysis	4	2	1	0
Remove the rod, cover the patient, and debrief him, then give him appointment	4	2	1	0
Document the procedure and findings		2	1	0
Total marks	42			
Candidate's score .../42				

Examiner's signature Date

4.8 Station 4.7 The Diagnosis of PCOS

Subject: Gynaecology.
Subspecialty: Infertility and ART.
Domain of clinical competence: Identification of abnormal test finding (IATF).
Station: Investigation of a suspected polycystic ovarian syndrome.
Station objective: To test the candidate's ability to establish the diagnosis of polycystic ovarian syndrome and outline its management.
Requirements: The result of the hormonal profile of a patient presenting with clinical features of polycystic ovarian syndrome, clearly written tasks to the candidate, answer guideline or checklists for the examiners, plain papers for use by the candidate, pencils and erasers for examiners, a table and chairs for examiners and candidate, and a chaperon (Fig. 4.4).

4.8.1 Instruction to the Candidate

Mrs. MS is a 26-year-old P1 + 0 A1 whose last childbirth was 4 years ago. She was referred from a primary health centre to your facility with secondary infertility of 2 years duration. She was evaluated, and a transvaginal scan done showed the feature above. Her hormonal profile was also requested, and the result is shown below. Carefully study the result of her hormonal profile and answer the questions which follow:

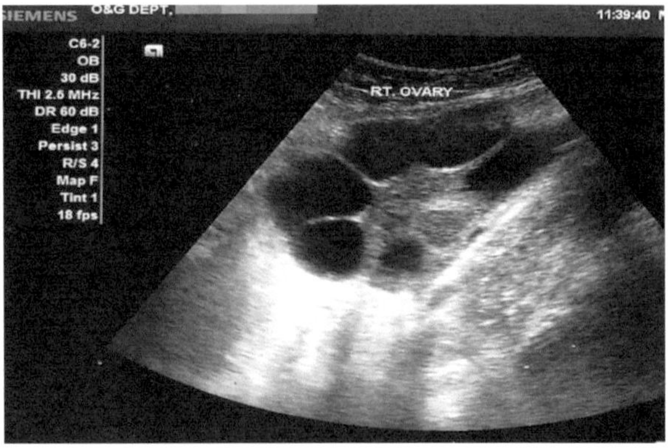

Fig. 4.4 Polycystic ovary on transvaginal scan (Chama 2014)

Chemical pathology

Test	Parameters			
	Name	Value	Unit	Reference value
Follicle Stimulating Hormone	FSH	8.2	mIU/ml	2 – 12
Luteinizing Hormone	LH	19.2	mIU/ml	0.5 – 10.5
Prolactin	PrL	16	ng/ml	1.2 – 19.5
Estrogen	Estrogen	60	pg/ml	30 - 100
Progesterone	Progesterone	5.8	ng/ml	2 - 25

1. What is the most likely diagnosis?
2. What additional clinical information would you request to strengthen your diagnosis?
3. What other investigations are necessary for her management?
4. Mention 2 classes of drug and an example each, that used for the treatment of this condition.

4.8.2 Instruction to the Examiners

The candidate is presented the hormonal profile of a patient presenting with secondary infertility and oligomenorrhea. Based on the result of the hormonal profile and the history of the patient, the candidate is supposed to answer the questions provided. Use the answer guide (if answers are to be written) or the checklist (if candidate is to say the answers) to score the candidate.

Answers

1. Polycystic ovarian syndrome is the likely diagnosis (5 marks)
2. Additional clinical information required to establish the diagnosis are (any 2 of the following features):
   (a) History of oligoamenorrhoea (2 marks)
   (b) Clinical hyperandrogenism; abnormal hair distribution, voice changes, baldness (2 marks)
   (c) Polycystic ovaries on transvaginal scan (2 marks)
3. Other necessary investigations include (2 marks each; maximum of 5):
   (a) TSH to rule hypo- or hyperthyroidism
   (b) Serum prolactin can cause oligoamenorrhoea
   (c) LH/FSH ratio ≥ 2
   (d) 17-alpha progesterone to rule out late congenital adrenal hyperplasia
   (e) Testosterone is elevated in androgen secreting tumors
   (f) DHEAS is elevated in adrenal adenoma
4. Two classes of drugs used for treating infertility in PCOS are (4 marks each):
   (a) Insulin sensitizing agents, for example metformin
   (b) Ovulation induction drugs, for example clomiphene citrate

Checklist for diagnosis and management of PCOS

Tasks	Well done	Fairly done	Poorly done	Not done
The most likely diagnosis is PCOS	4			0
Additional information required(any 4):				
- History of oligo-amenorrhea		2		0
- Clinical hyperandrogenism (abnormal hair distribution)		2		0
- Polycystic ovaries on TVS		2		0
- Obesity		2		0
- Premature adrenarche		2		0
Other necessary investigations (maximum of 5):				
- TSH to rule out hypo-/hyperthyroidism.		2		0
- Serum prolactin – elevated levels can cause amenorrhea.		2		0
- LH/FSH ratio ≥2		2		0
- 17a-progesterone in late adrenal hyperplasia		2		0
- Testosterone elevated in androgen secreting tumors.		2		0
- DHEAS elevated in adrenal adenoma		2		0
Two classes of drugs for treating PCOS:				
- Insulin sensitizing agents (2) like metformin (2)	4	2		0
- Ovulation induction drugs (2) like clomiphene (2)	4	2		0
Total marks	30			
Candidate's score .../30				

Examiner's signature Date

5 Gynaecological Oncology OSCE Stations

5.1 Station 5.1 History of Postcoital Bleeding

Subject: Gynaecology.
Subspecialty: Gynaecological oncology.
Domain of clinical competence: History taking.
Station: Focused history taking in a patient with postcoital vaginal bleeding.
Station objective: To assess the candidate's ability to obtain a focused history in a patient presenting with postcoital vaginal bleeding with the aim of establishing a diagnosis.
Requirements: A standardized patient, a chair or dressed bed for the patient, a table and chairs for the examiners, plain papers for use by the candidate, script for the standardized patient, clearly written tasks for the candidate, sufficient checklists, pencils and erasers, a chaperon to take care of the SP and attend to the examiners.

5.1.1 Instructions to the SP

Biodata

Name: ZM	Tribe: Hausa
Age: 36 years	Religion: Islam
Address: Sabon kaura, Bauchi	Parity: P8 + 0 A7
Occupation: House wife	LCB: 2 years ago
LMP: one week ago	

Presenting Complaints
Vaginal bleeding following sexual intercourse.
Duration (when asked) of one year
Vaginal discharge (if asked of any other complain) of 6 months duration.

C. Chama, *OSCE and VIVA VOCE in Obstetrics and Gynaecology*,
https://doi.org/10.1007/978-3-031-77262-7_5

History of Presenting Complaints

I was apparently well until about a year now when I noticed vaginal bleeding whenever I meet my husband. The bleeding is scanty and stops in a day or two. There is no undue pain during sexual intercourse, and I have not noticed any growth on my private part or coming out of my private part. There is no lower abdominal swelling. I urinate normally without pain or any difficulty. My urine is clear in colour.

About 6 months ago, I started having mucoid vaginal discharge which has offensive smell. It stains my underwear which I have to change twice a day. The smell is relieved by taking flagyl (metronidazole) I procure from a chemist, but the discharge does not stop. It is sometimes stained with blood. I have not noticed any weight loss, and my appetite is good. However, I have been worried over the discharge and went to see the doctor in the general hospital where I delivered all my children. The doctor examined me and referred me to see a specialist in this hospital.

Gynaecological History

I started seeing my menses when I was about 14 years old. The menses was irregular the first year but after that I bleed for 4 days every 28–30 days. I experience mild lower abdominal pains during menses and use 2 sanitary pads per day for the first 2 days. My first sexual intercourse was at the age of 15 years. I got married at the age of 18 and since then have sex only with my husband. I have had a total of 3 sexual partners in my life. I have heard about family planning during antennal clinics but have never used any method.

Obstetric History

All my pregnancies were supervised at Bayara General Hospital, Bauchi, and I delivered them in the same hospital. I have never had any surgery. I breastfed all my children for about a year before weaning them off breastmilk. I lost the second child due to a febrile illness with convulsion at the age of 3 years. I have 3 boys and 4 girls alive and doing well.

Family and Social History

I am the first daughter of my mother who had 8 children: 4 boys and 4 girls. My mother died of vaginal bleeding 5 years ago. She had lost a lot of weight then and was told she had cancer in the mouth of the womb. My father had 4 wives and 20 children. He was a trader. There is no family history of hypertension or diabetes.

I am the first of 2 wives of my husband who is a trader. He sells textile material, and we live in our own house at Sabon kaura, Bauchi. I do not smoke cigarette or drink alcohol.

Systemic Review

I have no cough or difficulty in breathing, I can do my household chores normally, I have not noticed any weight loss.

5.1.2 Instruction to the Candidate

The patient on the bed was referred to this hospital from Bayara General Hospital for expert management. Your task is to take her history.

5.1.3 Instruction to the Examiners

The candidate is supposed to take a focused history of this patient who was referred to this facility with postcoital bleeding. Use the checklist provided to score the candidate.

Checklist for history of postcoital bleeding

Tasks	Well done	Fairly done	Poorly done	Not done
Greets the patient and introduces self		2	1	0
Explains the purpose of coming and obtains permission		2	1	0
Obtains patient's biodata: Name, age, address, occupation, etc.	4	2	1	0
Parity, LMP		2	1	0
Presenting complaints:				
- Postcoital bleeding (2) for one year (2)	4	2		0
- Vaginal discharge (2) for 6 months (2)	4	2		0
History of presenting complaints:				
- Severity of bleeding		2		0
- Any associated dyspareunia		2		0
- Any relation of menses?		2		0
- Nature/color of discharge		2		0
- Odor of discharge		2		0
- Quantity of discharge		2		0
- Any relieving or aggravating factor		2		0
Gynaecological history: menarche, periods, cycle, LMP	4	2	1	0
Sexual history: coitarche, No of sexual partners, contraception	4	2	1	0
Obstetric history: parity, ANC, SVDs, breastfeeding		2	1	0
FSH: polygamous, mother died of cervical cancer	4	2	1	0
Systemic review: No weight loss, no weakness, no anorexia		2	1	0
Summary of history	4	2	1	0
Penalty: none sequential, judgmental, vulgar	-4	-2	-1	0
Total marks	52			
Candidate's score .../52				

Examiner's signature Date

5.2 Station 5.2 Examination of Abdominal Mass

Subject: Gynaecology.
Subspecialty: Gynaecological oncology.
Domain of clinical competence: Physical examination.
Station: Abdominal examination of a patient with suspected ovarian tumor.
Station objective: To assess the candidate's ability to systematically examine the abdomen in a patient suspected to have ovarian tumor with the aim of arriving at a diagnosis.
Requirements: A real patient or mannequin with abdominal mass, a dressed bed for the mannequin, a table and chairs for the examiners, sufficient checklist, pencils and erasers, and a chaperon (Fig. 5.1).

5.2.1 Instructions to the Candidate

The patient is a 50-year-old nullipara who presented with abdominal swelling of 6 months duration. The swelling has rapidly increased in size over the past one month. Her menses has been regular, and the LMP was last week. Your task is to examine her abdomen and report your findings to the hearing of the examiners as you proceed.

5.2.2 Instructions to the Examiners

The candidate is supposed to examine the abdomen of a 50-year-old nullipara suspected to have ovarian tumor. Use the checklist provided to score the candidate.

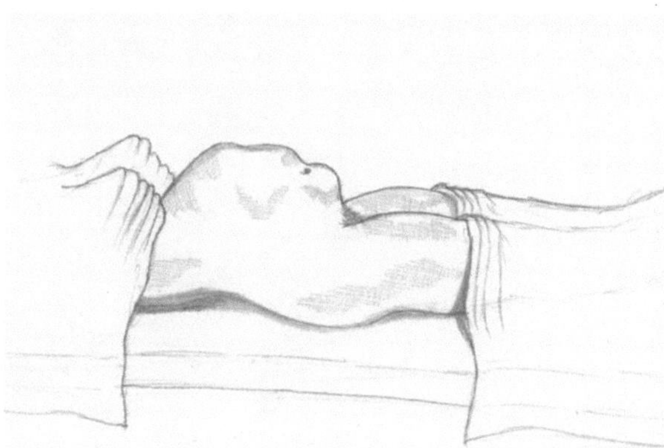

Fig. 5.1 Exposure for examination of abdominal mass. (Courtesy of Jonathan Edache Otache)

Checklist for examination of abdominal mass

Tasks	Well done	Fairly done	Poorly done	Not done
Greets the patient and introduces self		2	1	0
Explains the procedure and obtains permission to proceed		2	1	0
Helps patient to expose the abdomen adequately		2	1	0
Inspection:				
- Contour		2		0
- Scarification marks		2		0
- Umbilicus		2		0
- Striae		2		0
Palpation:				
- Asks patient for any area of tenderness.		2	1	0
- Light palpation of 4 quadrants for masses and tenderness		2	1	0
- Deep palpation for liver, spleen, and kidneys		2	1	0
Examines for inguinal hernias and lymph nodes		2	1	0
Palpating the abdominal mass:				
- Size and position		2	1	0
- Surface		2	1	0
- Consistency		2	1	0
- Mobility		2	1	0
- Attempt getting below it		2	1	0
Percussion:				
- Dullness and its extent		2	1	0
- Shifting dullness/fluid thrill		2	1	0
Thanks patient, covers her, helps to reposition her comfortably	4	2	1	0
Summarizes the findings to the examiners	4	2	1	0
Total marks	44			
Candidate's score .../44				

Examiner's signature Date

5.3 Station 5.3 Performing a Papanicolaou Smear

Subject: Gynaecology.
Subspecialty: Gynaecological oncology.
Domain of clinical competence: Diagnostic procedure.
Station objective: To assess the candidate's ability to identify instruments used for Pap smear and demonstrate how to perform the procedure.
Requirements: Ayre's or plastic spatula (A), endocervical brush (B), plastic broom (C), glass slides, alcohol container, pelvic model fitted with cervix, latex gloves, Cusco's speculum, a table, office chairs, checklists, pencils and erasers, and a chaperon (Fig. 5.2).

5.3.1 Instructions to the Candidate

- Identify the objects A, B, and C
- Demonstrate, using the pelvic model provided how to use object A
- What is the advantage of using C over the others?

5.3.2 Instructions to the Examiners

The candidate is supposed to identify Ayre's spatula (A), endocervical brush (B), and plastic broom (C). Using the pelvic model provided, the candidate is supposed to demonstrate how to take a Pap smear. Use the checklist provided to score the candidate.

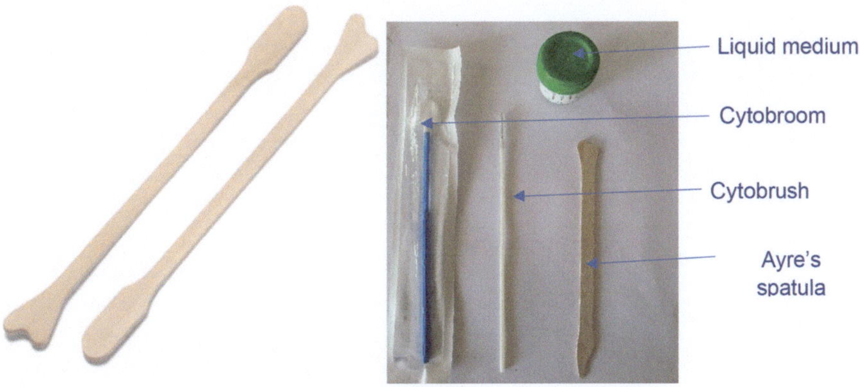

Fig. 5.2 Materials needed for taking Pap smear

Checklist for taking Pap smear

Task	Well done	Fairly done	Poorly done	Not done
Identification of objects - A = Ayres's spatula - B = Endocervical brush - C = Plastic broom		 2 2 2		 0 0 0
Says all objects are used for obtaining Pap smear		2		0
Demonstrating how to take a Pap smear:				
Says he will greet the patient and introduce himself		2	1	0
Request for a chaperone and ensure patient is comfortable		2	1	0
Says he will explain the procedure to the patient		2	1	0
Will allow patient to ask questions		2		0
Will obtain permission to proceed with the procedure		2		0
Checks the equipment tray to ensure all requirements are available		2		0
Will ask the patient to empty her bladder if she feels like passing urine before lying in the dorsal position		2		0
Washes his hands and wears sterile gloves		2		0
Helps patient to flex her hips and knees with slight abduction		2	1	0
Inspects the vulva for any abnormality and then parts the labia	4	2	1	0
Correctly inserts the Cusco's speculum, opens the blades and inspects the cervix for gross pathology	4	2	1	0
A cotton wool soaked in normal saline is used to clean mucus from the cervical os		2		0
The long arm of the Ayres's spatula is inserted into the cervical os and rotated 360 degrees	4	2	1	0
The specimen is spread on 2 labelled glass slides in a circular form and placed immediately in 95% alcohol	4	2	1	0
Unscrews and removes the speculum and drops it into a decontaminant container		2		0
Thanks the patient as he offers her a tissue paper to clean herself		2	1	0
Removes the gloves and discard them, washes hands and fill the requisition form and sends along with specimen to the laboratory	4	2	1	0
Explains the findings to the patient and gives appointment to see her with the result	4	2	1	0
Advantages of using C over the others: - Debris, mucus and blood are eliminated - Cell overlap are eliminated		 2 2		 0 0
- Cells distributed over a small area on the glass slide		2		0
Total score	60			
Candidates score.../60				

Examiner's signature Date

5.4 Station 5.4 Interpreting a Pap Smear Result

Subject: Gynaecology.
Subspecialty: Oncology.
Domain of clinical competence: Identification of abnormal test finding (IATF).
Station: Interpretation of a picture of Pap smear.
Station objective: To test the candidate's ability to correctly interpret the findings on Pap smear and use it to plan for patient management.
Requirements: A picture of ×10 magnification of a normal Pap smear, preferably laminated to prevent squeezing and staining, a clearly written set of questions for the candidate preferably on same page with the picture for easy cross checking by the candidate, a table and 2 chairs for examiners, a marking scheme for the examiners, a chair for the candidate and plain answer sheets and a chaperon.

5.4.1 Instruction to the Candidate

The patient you took Pap smear for on the last station brought the result to the gynaecological clinic after one week. A picture clip of the result was given to her and is shown below (Fig. 5.3). Study the picture carefully and answer the questions which follow:

1. Name 3 types of cell you can identify on the picture.
2. What is the diagnosis.
3. List 2 other uses of the Pap smear
4. List 4 conditions to be avoided before performing this test.
5. List 4 important information that should be provided on the request form.

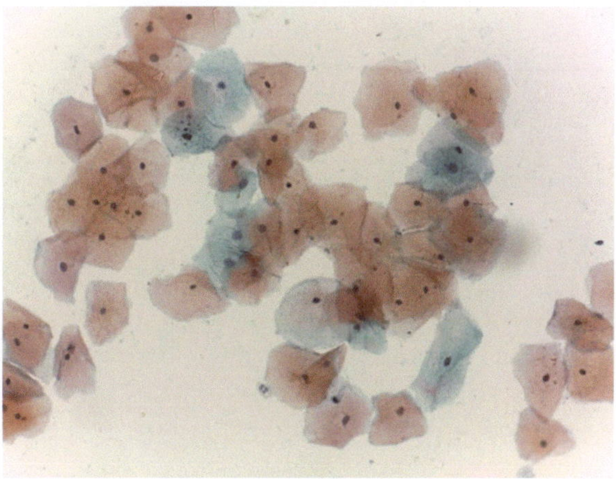

Fig. 5.3 Appearance of normal Pap smear (courtesy of Dr. Dauda Suleiman 2023)

5.4.2 Instruction to the Examiner

The candidate has been provided with a snap shot of the slide of a normal Pap smear. He is supposed to study the picture and answer the questions which follow. Use the checklist provided to score the candidate.

Checklist for interpretation of Pap smear

Task	Well done	Fairly done	Poorly done	Not done
Types of cells on the slide				
- Pinkish flat ectocervical cells		2	1	0
- Bluish flat endocervical cells		2	1	0
- Dark bluish dots of lactobacilli		2	1	0
The diagnosis is normal pap smear	4			0
Other uses of the pap smear include:				
- Diagnosis of bacterial vaginosis		2		0
- Diagnosis of cervicitis		2		0
- Diagnosis of endometrial carcinoma		2		0
Conditions to be avoided before performing pap smear				
- Menses; should stop at least 24-48 hours before pap smear		2		0
- Vaginal intercourse at least 24 hours before pap smear		2		0
- Douching		2		0
- Contraceptive creams		2		0
- Vaginal medications like pessaries and suppositories		2		0
Important information on the request form to the Pathologist				
- LMP of the patient		2		0
- Pregnancy or menopause		2		0
- Exogenous hormone use		2		0
- Result of previous pap smear if applicable		2		0
- Abnormal vaginal bleeding		2		0
- Use of IUCD (if in-situ)		2		0
Total score	32			
Candidate's score.../32				

Examiner's signature Date

5.5 Station 5.5 EUA, Biopsy, and Staging of Cervical Cancer

Subject: Gynaecology.
Subspecialty: Gynaecological oncology.
Domain of clinical competence: Diagnostic procedure.
Station: Examination under anaesthesia, biopsy, and staging of suspected cancer of the cervix.
Station objective: To assess the candidate's ability to perform EUA in correct sequence for the purpose of biopsy and staging of cancer of the cervix. This is important in planning further management of the condition.
Requirements: Mannequin of the pelvis fitted with uterus and cervix with a lesion, a table or dressed bed for the mannequin, Cusco's speculum, latex hand gloves, angle poise lamp, a cystoscope, proctoscope, and a chaperon to attend to the mannequin after each examination, a table and 2 chairs for examiners, enough copies of checklist, a chair for the chaperon, and boldly written instructions to the candidate (Fig. 5.4).

5.5.1 Instruction to Candidate

Mrs. AH is a 42-year-old P7 + 0 A7 whose last childbirth was 2 years ago. She presented with postcoital bleeding of 3 months duration. A cervical mass was demonstrated on pelvic examination with contact bleeding. A diagnosis of cancer of the cervix was made. Using the pelvic model, demonstrate how you would perform examination under anaesthesia, biopsy, and staging of the tumor.

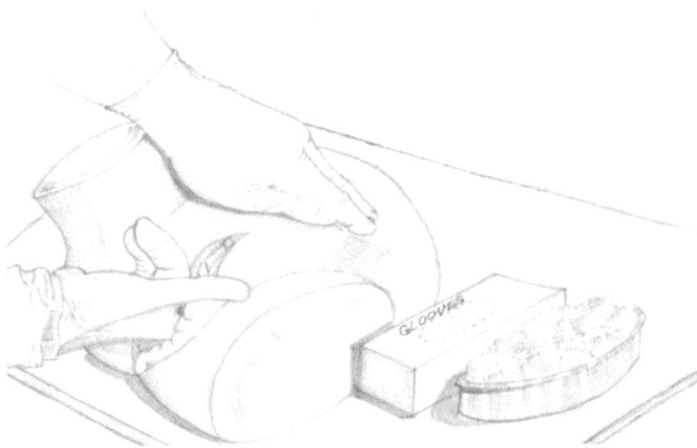

Fig. 5.4 Vaginal examination using mannequin. (Courtesy of Jonathan Edache Otache)

5.5.2 Instruction to the Examiners

The candidate has been given a scenario in which a grand multipara who presented with postcoital bleeding was examined and found to have a cervical mass suspected to be cancer of the cervix. He is supposed to use the mannequin provided to demonstrate how he would perform examination under anaesthesia for the purpose of biopsy and staging of cancer of the cervix in the patient. Use the checklist provided to score the candidate.

Checklist for EUA, biopsy, and staging

Task	Well done	Fairly done	Poorly done	Not done
Patient in lithotomy position under regional or general anaesthesia		2	1	0
Will scrub, gown and clean and drape patient, exposing operation field		2	1	0
Empty bladder with metal catheter, examine urine for blood or debris		2	1	0
Do cystoscopy to rule out bladder lesion or growth	4	2	1	0
Do proctoscopy to rule out rectal involvement	4	2	1	0
Change gloves (remove and wear new ones)		2		0
Gently insert a bivalve speculum to expose the cervix and: - Inspect the nature and extent of the lesion		2		0
- Take biopsy involving both healthy and diseased tissue - Preserve tissue in formalin		2 2		0 0
Bimanual examination: - Reassess nature and extent of lesion; friable, contact bleeding - Uterine size, fixity - Adnexa; thickening of broad ligament - Feel vaginal mucosa for induration		2 2 2 2		0 0 0 0
Rectal examination - Thickening of broad ligament better appreciated PR - Uterine size - Rectal mucosa for thickening or induration		2 2 2		0 0 0
Clean patient and pack the vagina if there is active bleeding		2	1	0
Reposition patient supine, reverse anaesthesia and transfuse if needed	4	2	1	0
Document findings and fill requisition forms and prescribe postoperative management	4	2	1	0
Total score				
Candidate's score				

Examiner's signature Date

5.6 Station 5.6 Breaking Bad News

Subject: Gynaecology.
Subspecialty: Gynaecological oncology.
Domain of clinical competence: Communication and counselling.
Station: Breaking bad news to a patient.
Station objective: To test the candidate's ability to compassionately break the bad news to a patient in order not to cause unnecessary anxiety and wrong decisions in management of the condition.
Requirements: Standardized patient, a copy of the histology report, a comfortable chair or dressed bed for the patient, a table and 2 chairs for the examiners, enough copies of the checklist, a chair for the candidate, pencils and erasers, and plain papers for rough use by the candidate.

5.6.1 Instruction to the Standardized Role Player

I am a 42-year-old housewife who has delivered 7 children. The youngest is 3 years old, and my last menses started one week ago. The bleeding lasted 4 days which is normal. I presented to this hospital 3 weeks ago complaining of bleeding from my private part each time I meet my husband. This has been going on for about 3 months now. I was examined and the need to further examine me in the theatre was explained to me. This was done 2 weeks ago, and a portion of the disease seen on the mouth of my womb was taken and sent to the laboratory for analysis. I was given an appointment today to come and discuss the result with my doctor. I have come along with my husband.

5.6.2 Instruction to the Candidate

The patient in front of you had examination under anaesthesia for the purpose of biopsy and staging of suspected cervical cancer. The tumor was staged as 4A as the bladder mucosa was involved on cystoscopy. She has come to the clinic with the histology result that confirms squamous cell carcinoma of the cervix with urinary bladder involvement. Your task is to disclose the bad news to the patient.

5.6.3 Instruction to the Examiner

Mrs. HT had EUA, biopsy, and staging for suspected cancer of the cervix. She has come for follow-up, and the histology report confirms squamous cell carcinoma of the cervix with urinary bladder involvement. The candidate is supposed to break the bad news to the patient. Use the checklist provided to score the candidate.

Checklist for disclosing advanced cervical cancer

Task	Well done	Fairly done	Poorly done	Not done
Greets the patient and introduces self		2	1	0
Confirm patients' identity and demand the presence of spouse or relative	4	2	1	0
Inform the patient you are about to break the bad news; like 'I'm sorry but I have some bad news for you'	4	2	1	0
Ask patient how much she knows about her condition		2	1	0
With compassion, frankly, explain the condition.				
- The test result confirms you have cancer.		2	1	0
- This cancer has no cure as it is extensive at this stage.		2	1	0
- It has spread beyond the mouth of the womb to involve the urinary bladder.		2	1	0
- However, radiotherapy and anti-cancer drugs will check its spread.		2	1	0
- With treatment you will be able to live a reasonably good quality of life		2	1	0
Allow some time for her to absorb the shock		2	1	0
Ask her what she understands by your explanation so far, encourage her to ask questions	4	2	1	0
Repeat some important points for her understanding	4	2	1	0
Outline subsequent management plan including referral for radiotherapy if not available in your Centre	4	2	1	0
Give her appointment		2		0
Ask if she would like the services of her spiritual leader		2		0
Thank her for giving you the time to talk with her		2		0
Communication skill	4	2	1	0
Maximum score	44			
Candidate's score .../44				

Examiner's signature Date

5.7 Station 5.7 Picture Test of Vulvar Cancer

Subject: Gynaecology.
Subspecialty: Gynaecological oncology.
Domain of clinical competence: Virtual sign identification (VSI).
Station: Picture test on locally advanced vulvar cancer.
Station objective: To test the candidate's ability to identify a locally advanced vulvar cancer with the aim of planning its management.
Requirements: Picture of locally advanced vulvar cancer, written questions concerning the picture, preferably on the same page, structured answer guide or checklist, a table on which the laminated picture is plastered and a chair for the candidate, a table and chairs for the examiners, and pencils and erasers (Fig. 5.5).

Questions
1. What is your diagnosis?
2. What structures may be affected in this stage of the disease?
3. List 5 risk factors for the condition
4. How would you treat this stage of the disease?
5. List 2 preventive measures for this disease

5.7.1 Instructions to the Candidate

The patient is a 65-year-old P4 + 0 A4 who is 15 years postmenopausal. She presented with 6 months history of ulceration on her private part which is spreading

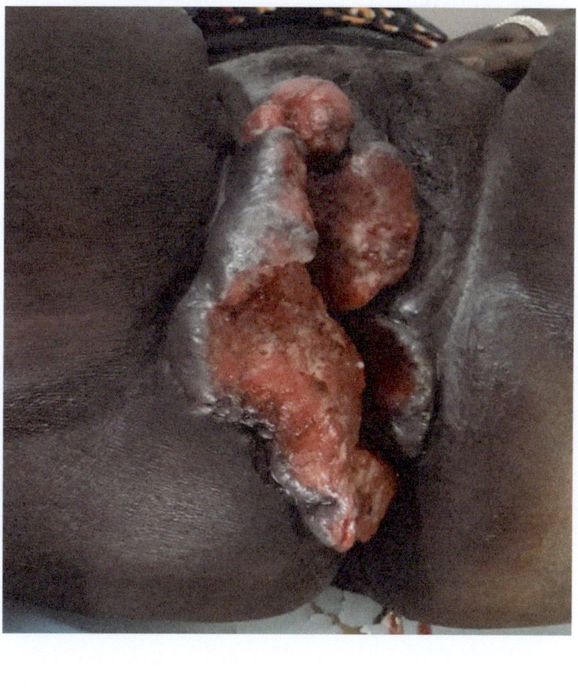

Fig. 5.5 Advanced vulvar carcinoma (Chama 2021)

toward the anal region. Recently, she has noticed involuntary leakage of soft stool through the vagina. The picture is a snap shot of her perineum. Your task is to answer the questions below the picture.

5.7.2 Instructions to the Examiners

Provided is a picture of a locally advanced vulvar cancer with faecal fistula. The candidate is supposed to answer the questions written below the picture. Use the answer guide to score the candidate.

Answers

1. The diagnosis is advanced vulvar carcinoma **(2 marks)**, probably stage IVA due to involvement of the rectum (**2 marks**).
2. The structures that may be affected in stage IVA vulva cancer are: (**2 marks each, max 5**)
   (a) Proximal (upper 2/3) urethra
   (b) Proximal (upper 2/3) vagina
   (c) Bladder mucosa
   (d) Rectal mucosa
   (e) Pelvic bone
   (f) With or without inguinal lymph node involvement
3. Risk factors for vulvar cancer are: (**2 marks each, max 5**)
   (a) Age > 60 years
   (b) High-risk HPV infection
   (c) Herpes simplex virus infection
   (d) Smoking
   (e) High-grade VIN
   (f) Immunosuppression (organ transplant, HIV infection)
   (g) Lichen sclerosis
4. Treatment of advanced vulvar cancer would involve: (**4 marks each**)
   (a) Neoadjuvant chemoradiation
   (b) Radical vulvectomy ± pelvic exenteration
5. Preventive measures for vulvar cancer include: (**2 marks each**)
   (a) Vaccination with Gardasil 9
   (b) Vulvoscopy and biopsy in high-risk patients
   (c) Early treatment of HIV infection

Checklist for vulvar cancer (To be used when the candidate is instructed to express the answers verbally to the hearing of the examiners)

Tasks	Well done	Fairly done	Poorly done	Not done
Diagnosis: advanced vulvar cancer (2) likely stage IVA (2)	4	2		0
Structures that may be affected in stage IVA vulvar cancer (max 5)				
- Proximal (upper 2/3) urethra		2		0
- Proximal (upper 2/3) vagina		2		0
- Bladder mucosa		2		0
- Rectal mucosa		2		0
- Pelvic bone		2		0
- Inguinal lymph nodes		2		0
Risk factors for vulvar cancer (max 5)				
- Age >60 years		2		0
- High risk HPV infection		2		0
- HSV infection		2		0
- Smoking		2		0
- High grade VIN		2		0
- Immunosuppression		2		0
- Lichen sclerosis		2		0
Treatment of stage IVA vulvar cancer involves:				
- Neoadjuvant chemoradiation		2	1	0
- Radical vulvectomy ± pelvic exenteration		2	1	0
Preventive measures to vulvar cancer include:				
- Vaccination with Gardasil 9		2	1	0
- Vulvoscopy and biopsy in high-risk patients		2	1	0
- Treatment of HIV		2	1	0
Total marks	34			
Candidate's score .../34				

Examiner's signature Date

6 Urogynaecology OSCE Stations

6.1 Station 6.1 History Taking for VVF Patient

Subject: Gynaecology.
Subspecialty: Urogynaecology.
Domain of clinical competence: History taking.
Station: Focused history taking of a patient with vesico-vaginal fistula.
Station objective: To assess the candidate's ability to obtain a focused history of patient presenting with involuntary leakage of urine following prolonged obstructed labour with the aim of arriving at a diagnosis.
Requirements: Standardized patient (role player), dressed bed for the patient, 2 office chairs and a simple table for examiners, enough copies of checklist, pencils and erasers, an office chair for the candidate, plain papers for use by the candidate, and a chaperon.

6.1.1 Instruction to Standardized Patient

Biodata

Name: AB	Tribe: Hausa
Age: 19 years	Religion: Islam
Address: Toro, Bauchi state	Education: Completed primary school
Occupation: Housewife	

Presenting Complaint

Leakage of urine through my private part
Duration of 3 months (if asked)

C. Chama, *OSCE and VIVA VOCE in Obstetrics and Gynaecology*,
https://doi.org/10.1007/978-3-031-77262-7_6

History of Presenting Complaint

I am a 19-year-old married woman, a Hausa Moslem and got married last year. I had a stillbirth 3 months ago following a 9 months pregnancy. I registered for antenatal care at General Hospital, Toro at about 5 months of pregnancy and had 4 antenatal visits, all of which were uneventful. The blood and urine tests carried out on me were said to be normal.

When I was getting to 9 months of pregnancy, I went to my village to deliver in my parents' house as is our custom. I was in labour for about 2 days and was attended to by a traditional birth attendant. I had a stillbirth, and on the third day of delivery, I started leaking urine through my private part.

I was then taken to the hospital where I had antenatal care and a rubber was passed through my private part but the urine leakage continued with only a small quantity entering the rubber. The rubber was removed after 3 weeks, and I was given a letter to come here after 3 months for treatment.

I am the only wife of my husband who is a farmer and is supportive to me. I have no new complaints today.

Gynaecological History

I started seeing menses at the age of 14 years and I bleed for 3 days every 26–28 days. I experience mild lower abdominal pains during menses and I use 2–3 sanitary pads per day. I have not yet resumed menses since I delivered 3 months ago.

Obstetric History

This incident occurred following my first delivery. I was never pregnant before.

6.1.2 Instruction to Candidate

Mrs. AB is a 19-year-old primipara who was referred from General Hospital Toro for expert management. Your task is to obtain her history.

6.1.3 Instruction to Examiners

The patient is a 19-year-old primipara who sustained vesico-vaginal fistula following prolonged obstructed labour about 3 months ago. There has been no attempted repair of the VVF elsewhere. She has been referred to the teaching hospital for expert management.

The candidate is expected to take her history. Use the checklist provided to score the candidate

Checklist for history of VVF

Task	Well done	Fairly done	Poorly done	Not done
Greets patient, introduces self and obtains permission to discuss her problem	4	2	1	0
Biodata: name, age, address, occupation, tribe, religion	4	2	1	0
Parity, LMP		2	1	0
Presenting complaint: leakage of urine PV (2), for 3 months (2)	4	2		0
History of presenting complaint - History of ANC - Place of labour and delivery - Duration of labour - Attendant in labour (midwife, TBA) - Type of delivery; SVD, assisted VD, CS - When did urine leakage start? - Any catheterization, for how long - Any urge to urinate - Any faecal incontinence - Any gait abnormality - Any perineal rashes		2 2 2 2 2 2 2 2 2 2 2 2 2		0 0 0 0 0 0 0 0 0 0 0 0 0
PMH: treatment received including attempted repair, perineal care	4	2	1	0
Gynae. History: menarche, periods, cycle, contraception	4	2	1	0
Obstetric history: Parity, LMP		2	1	0
FSH: husband's occupation, social support, DM, HT, SCD		2	1	0
Systemic review: fever, loin pains, bowel symptoms		2	1	0
Summary of history	4	2	1	0
Communication skill	4	2	1	0
Total score	60			
Candidate's score .../60				

Examiners name Date

6.2 Station 6.2 Postoperative Acute Urinary Retention

Subject: Gynaecology.
Subspecialty: Urogynaecology.
Domain of clinical competence: Diagnostic and therapeutic procedures.
Station: Acute urinary retention following VVF repair.
Station objective: To test the candidate's ability to recognize poor urinary output following VVF repair, find out the cause, and institute appropriate therapeutic measures.
Requirements: An office table and 2 chairs for examiners, a chair for the candidate, boldly written task for the candidate, plain papers to serve as answer sheets for the candidate, enough copies of checklist, pencils and erasers for examiners, and a chaperon.

6.2.1 Instruction to the Candidate

The patient you clerked on the last station eventually had VVF repair. Three hours postoperatively, the nurse in the postoperative ward called you to see the patient because there was no urine entering the urine bag for the past one hour.

Describe step by step how you would manage the situation.

6.2.2 Instruction to the Examiners

The candidate is expected to explain step by step, how he would manage acute urinary retention 3 h post-VVF repair on the ward. Use the checklist provided to score the candidate.

Checklist for postoperative urinary retention

Task	Well done	Fairly done	Poorly done	Not done
Greets patient and introduces self		2	1	0
Explains to the patient why he was called and obtains permission to examine her	4	2	1	0
Checks her hourly input/output chart to know whether her urinary output was satisfactory before the past one hour		2	1	0
Check the urinary catheter for positioning (over the thigh) and any kinking – correct any of these where necessary		2	1	0
Check the patient's bedsheet for wetness – which may suggest breakage of repair		2	1	0
If the bed is dry and the catheter is in correct position and no kinking, examine the patient for pain which is suggestive of obstructive uropathy		2	1	0
Examine the abdomen for loin tenderness and full bladder		2	1	0
If bladder is full, the most likely thing is blockage with blood clot		2	1	0
Use 50ml syringe to flush the catheter with normal saline; this dislodges small clots and drainage established	4	2	1	0
If bladder haemorrhage is massive – can be confirmed with ultrasound scan – suprapubic cystostomy and evacuation may be necessary in the theatre	4	2	1	0
Explain what had happened to patient and reassure her		2		0
If she is bedwetting, explain to her the repair has failed and another repair would have to be rescheduled later		2		0
Leave catheter in-situ even if bedwetting; there is a chance the VVF could heal within 6 weeks of continuous bladder drainage		2		0
Communication skill	4	2	1	0
Total score	36			
Candidate's score .../36				

Examiners name Date

6.3 Station 6.3 Vaginal Examination for Stress Incontinence

Subject: Gynaecology.
Subspecialty: Urogynaecology.
Domain of clinical competence: Physical examination.
Station: Vaginal examination in a patient with stress incontinence.
Station objective: To assess the candidate's ability to correctly demonstrate the possibility of stress incontinence in a patient who presents with involuntary loss of urine when coughing.
Requirements: A mannequin of half-body female pelvis, a dressed bed for the mannequin, latex gloves, Gali pot containing dry swabs, Sims speculum, sponge-holding forceps, office table and chairs for examiners, pencils and erasers, sufficient checklists, and a chaperon (Fig. 6.1).

6.3.1 Instructions to the Candidate

Mrs. FA is a 48-year-old P8 + 0 A8 who is 2 years postmenopausal. She presents with the complaint of wetting of her pants when she coughs or sneezes for the past one year. The symptom is gradually getting worse. Using the mannequin provided, perform vaginal examination on her and report your findings to the hearing of the examiners as you proceed.

6.3.2 Instruction to the Examiners

The patient is a 48-year-old grand multipara who is 2 years postmenopausal. She presents with worsening involuntary leakage of urine when she coughs or sneezes. The candidate is supposed to use the mannequin to perform a pelvic examination on her and report the findings to your hearing. Use the checklist provided to score the candidate.

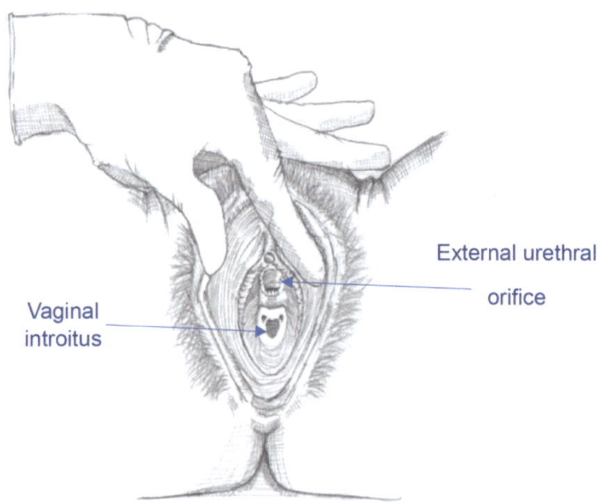

Fig. 6.1 Exposure of the vulva. (Courtesy of Jonathan Edache Otache)

Checklist for stress incontinence

Task	Well done	Fairly done	Poorly done	Not done
Greets the patient, introduces self and obtains permission		2	1	0
Explains the procedure and seeks her cooperation		2	1	0
Asks chaperon to screen the patient		2	1	0
Positions the patient in lithotomy position (dorsal position fair)		2	1	0
Washes hand and wear gloves		2	1	0
Inspection - Normal external genitalia - Evidence of atrophy of external genitalia Absent/present sub-urethral cyst or dilatation		 2 2 2		 0 0 0
Neurologic evaluation - Bulbospongiosus reflex using cotton wool or swab stick. - Anal wink reflex using cotton wool		 2 2		 0 0
Pelvic support assessment - Valsalva maneuver or cough - Observe for escape of urine per urethra. - Assess descent of cervix beyond hymenal ring - Bimanual examination for other pelvic pathologies		 2 2 2 2		 0 0 0 0
Use Sim's speculum to examine vaginal walls in Sim's position	4	2	1	0
Clean the patient, reposition, and thank her	4	2	1	0
Penalties – rudeness, clumsy, haphazard examination	-4	-2	-1	0
Total scores	36			
Candidate's score .../36				

Examiner's signature Date

6.4 Station 6.4 Simple Cystometry

Subject: Gynaecology.
Subspecialty: Urogynaecology.
Domain of clinical competence: Diagnostic procedure.
Station: Bedside cystometry.
Station objective: To assess the candidate's ability to perform a simple cystometry for the purpose of evaluating bladder function in a patient complaining of intermittent urinary incontinence.
Requirements: Half-body female mannequin with bladder, a dressed bed for the mannequin, under lay sheet, Gali pot or kidney dish containing wet swab, latex gloves, Foley's urethral catheter size (14 or 16), 60 mL plastic bladder syringe, 1000mLs of normal saline, cystometry form, pen, measuring cylinder, bed pan, 10mLs syringe and needles, 10mLs water for injection, office table and chairs for the examiners, sufficient checklist, pencils and erasers, and a chaperon.

6.4.1 Instructions to the Candidate

Mrs. KP is a 45-year-old P6 + 1, 5 children alive, last childbirth was 16 years ago. She presented with complaint of some urine escaping before she reaches the toilet of about 4 weeks duration. She first noticed that her symptoms were gradually worsening and could not hold urine before reaching the toilet anymore. She also wakes up to pass urine 3–4 times at night. Using the mannequin provided, demonstrate step by step how to perform a simple cystometry procedure on her as you report your findings to the hearing of the examiners.

6.4.2 Instructions to the Examiners

The candidate has been given a scenario of a patient presenting with intermittent urinary incontinence for a duration of about 4 weeks. Using the mannequin provided, he is supposed to demonstrate how to perform a simple cystometry on the patient for the purpose of assessing the type of incontinence the patient has. Please study the checklist provided and use it to score the candidate (Fig. 6.2).

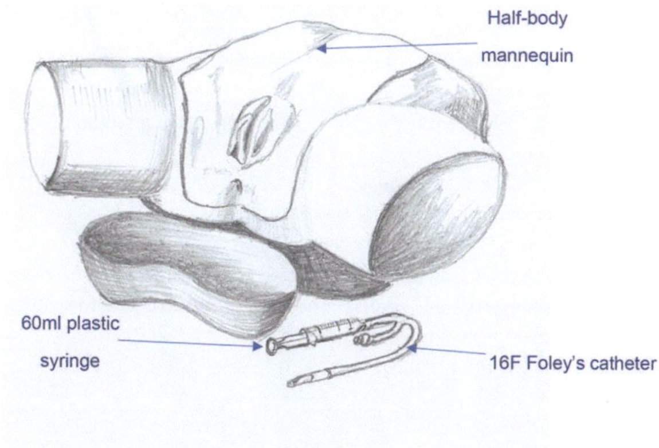

Fig. 6.2 Requirements for simple cystometry. (Courtesy of Jonathan Edache Otache)

Checklist for simple urethrocystometry

Tasks	Well done	Fairly done	Poorly done	Not done
Greets patient and introduces self		2	1	0
Explains the procedure and obtains permission for the test	4	2	1	0
Asks the patient to empty her bladder while he checks the tray for completeness of materials needed.	4	2	1	0
Asks chaperon to screen patient, she undresses and lies in supine lithotomy position		2	1	0
Scrubs and gowns, wears sterile gloves		2	1	0
Parts labia, cleans vulva and asks patient to cough; if urine leaks after emptying bladder, then patient requires more sophisticated urodynamic study	4	2	1	0
If no leakage, passes foley's catheter and measure residual volume		2	1	0
Connect 60ml syringe to catheter, remove plunger and hold vertically above the bladder (about 15cm)	4	2	1	0
Pinch the catheter and fill syringe with NS to 60ml mark.		2	1	0
Before filling the bladder, ask the patient to report when she feels pain, the desire to void, when there is an urge to void, and when there is strong desire to void (note volume of NS at each stage)	4	2	1	0
Release the pinch and allow NS to flow under gravity into the bladder		2		0
Observe the meniscus for any rise (sign of detrusor instability)		2		0
Observe for any peri-catheter leakage		2		0
At strong urge (cannot hold more NS), remove catheter and ask patient to cough.		2	1	0
If no change of meniscus and leakage of urine is positive, patient has genuine stress incontinence	4	2	1	0
Ask patient to void into bedpan, then repass catheter to measure post-test residual volume	4	2	1	0
Remove catheter, clean patient, thank and reposition her	4	2	1	0
Summarize your findings to examiners	4	2	1	0
Penalty: non-sequential, patient uncomfortable, clumsy	-4	-2	-1	0
Total marks	54			
Candidate's score .../54				

Examiner's signature Date

6.5 Station 6.5 Interpretation of Cystometry Findings

Subject: Gynaecology.
Subspecialty: Urogynaecology.
Domain of clinical competence: Interpretation of abnormal test finding.
Station: Interpretation of simple cystometry.
Station objective: To assess the candidate's ability to correctly interpret the findings at simple cystometry with the aim of arriving at a diagnosis of the type of incontinence the patient may have.
Requirements: Result of simple cystometry, questions on the findings on cystometry, answer guide (or checklist if candidate is to answer the questions verbally), a table and chairs for examiners and candidate, plain paper for candidate to use as answer sheet, pencil and erasers for examiners, and a chaperon.

6.5.1 Instruction to the Candidate

Study the result of the simple cystometry you performed on the last station and answer the following questions:

1. During the initial voiding by the patient, what another useful test could you have performed?
2. Mention 4 key parameters you could assess during the procedure to help arrive at a diagnosis of the patient's condition
3. List 3 abnormalities on simple cystometry that could suggest urge, stress, or mixed (both urge and stress) incontinence
4. Mention 3 types of incontinence that are not suitable for assessment with this procedure
5. List 5 conditions that may suggest low bladder compliance

6.5.2 Instructions to the Examiners

The candidate performed simple cystometry on a patient with urine incontinence on the last station. Provided is a set of questions on simple cystometry for the candidate to answer. Use the answer guide to score the candidate.

Answers
1. Uroflowmetry could have been assessed during the initial voiding (**2 marks**).
2. Parameters that can be assessed during simple cystometry include (**2 marks each; max 8 marks**):
   (a) Bladder compliance (bladder volume change per detrusor pressure change)
   (b) Stress incontinence
   (c) Urgency or pain

   (d) Intravesical pressure (Pves)
   (e) Bladder capacity
3. Abnormalities suggestive of urge, stress, or mixed incontinence (**2 marks each; max 6 marks**):
   (a) First desire to void at less than 100 mL (normal range 150–250 mL)
   (b) Bladder capacity of less than 400 mL or more than 650 mL (normal range 450–650 mL)
   (c) Post void residual volume of less than 50 mL (normal range 50–100 mL)
   (d) Pain or incontinence during filling
4. Incontinence that are not suitable for simple cystometry (**2 marks each; max 6 marks**):
   (a) Neurologic abnormalities
   (b) Fistulous incontinence
   (c) Previous bladder neck surgery
   (d) Voiding disorders
   (e) Bladder outlet obstruction.
5. Causes of low bladder compliance (**2 marks each; max of 10 marks**)
   (a) UTI
   (b) Detrusor instability
   (c) Stress incontinence
   (d) Fibrosis due to chronic schistosomiasis
   (e) Post radiation (pelvic malignancy)
   (f) Interstitial cystitis
   (g) Neurogenic bladder

Total marks = 32

Checklist for simple cystometry (If a candidate is to answer verbally)

Tasks	Well done	Fairly done	Poorly done	Not done
Uroflowmetry could be assessed during initial voiding		2		0
Parameters assessed during simple cystometry (Max 4):				
- Bladder compliance		2		0
- Stress incontinence		2		0
- Urgency or pain		2		0
- Intravesical pressure		2		0
- Bladder capacity		2		0
Abnormalities suggestive of urge, stress or mixed incontinence				
(Max 3)		2		0
- First desire to void at less than 100ml		2		0
- Bladder capacity of <400ml or >650ml		2		0
- Post void residual volume <50ml		2		0
- Pain or incontinence during filling				
Incontinence not suitable for assessment by simple cystometry				
(Max 3)		2		0
- Neurologic abnormalities		2		0
- Fistulous incontinence		2		0
- Previous bladder neck surgery		2		0
- Voiding disorders		2		0
- Bladder outlet obstruction				
Causes of low bladder compliance (Max 5)				
- UTI		2		0
- Detrusor instability		2		0
- Stress incontinence		2		0
- Fibrosis due to chronic schistosomiasis		2		0
- Post radiation (pelvic malignancy)		2		0
- Interstitial cystitis		2		0
- Neurogenic bladder		2		0
Total marks	32			
Candidate's score .../32				

Examiner's signature Date

6.6 Station 6.6 Picture Test on Uterine Procidentia

Subject: Gynaecology.
Subspecialty: Urogynaecology.
Domain of clinical competence: Virtual sign identification (VSI).
Station: A picture of uterine procidentia with decubitus ulcer.
Station objective: To test the candidate's ability to identify uterine procidentia complicated by decubitus ulcer.
Requirements: A laminated picture of third-degree uterovaginal prolapse, clearly written questions preferably on the same page with the picture, plain papers for the candidate to answer the questions on, marking scheme for examiners, pencils and erasers for examiners, a simple office table and 2 chairs for examiners and a chair for the candidate, and a chaperon.

6.6.1 Instruction to the Candidate

The patient you clerked on the last station was examined, and some of the features on vaginal examination are shown in the picture below. Answer the questions that follow (Fig. 6.3).

Questions
1. What is the diagnosis?
2. List 5 predisposing factors to this condition
3. What are the various modalities of treatment?
4. List 4 complications of the pathology
5. Which complication can you see in this patient?
6. What is the cause of this complication?

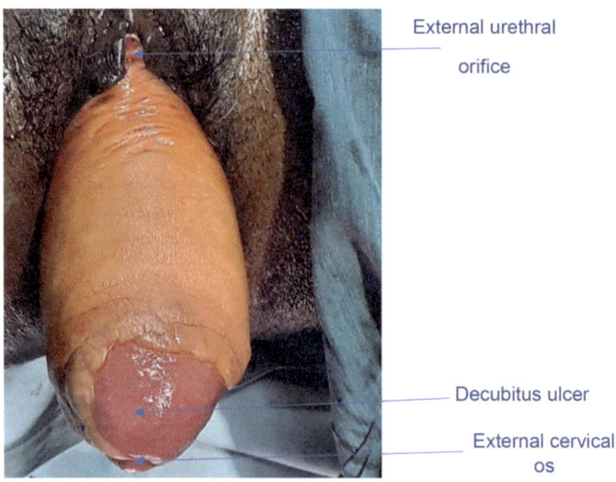

Fig. 6.3 Uterine procidentia with decubitus ulcer (courtesy of Dr. Dattijo 2023)

Answers

1. Diagnosis
   (a) Third-degree uterovaginal prolapse or uterine procidentia **(4 marks)**
2. Predisposing factors **(2 marks each, max. 10 marks)**
   (a) High parity
   (b) Postmenopausal status
   (c) Advanced age
   (d) Difficult vaginal deliveries
   (e) Medical conditions—chronic cough, constipation, abdominal mass
   (f) Occupation—lifting heavy objects, farming, pushing heavy loads
3. Methods of treatment **(4 marks each, max. 8 marks)**
   (a) Conservative with pessaries and or physiotherapy
   (b) Surgical
      - Vaginal hysterectomy
      - Colpocleisis
4. Complication of procidentia **(2 marks each, max. 10 marks)**
   (a) Urinary retention leading to UTI
   (b) Urinary incontinence
   (c) Ureteric kinking leading to renal failure
   (d) Decubitus ulcer
   (e) Chronic constipation
   (f) Psychosexual problems
5. The complication seen in this patient is "Decubitus ulcer" **(4 marks)**
6. Decubitus ulcer is caused by avascular necrosis due to kinking of the uterine arteries **(4 marks)**

Checklist for uterine procidentia with decubitus ulcer

Task	Well done	Fairly done	Poorly done	Not done
The diagnosis is 3rd degree Uterovaginal prolapse or uterine procidentia	4			0
Predisposing factors to this condition include: (max. 5)				
- High parity		2		0
- Postmenopausal condition		2		0
- Advanced age		2		0
- Difficult vaginal deliveries		2		0
- Medical disorders; chronic cough, abdominal mass, etc.		2		0
- Occupation: lifting heavy weights, pushing heavy loads, etc.		2		0
Methods of treatment				
- Conservative; pessaries, physiotherapy		2	1	0
- Surgery; hysterectomy, Colpocleisis		2	1	0
Complications of procidentia: (max. 5)				
- Urinary retention leading to UTI		2		
- Urinary incontinence		2		
- Ureteric kinking leading to renal failure		2		
- Decubitus ulcer		2		
- Psychosexual disorders		2		
- Chronic constipation		2		
The complication seen in this picture is decubitus ulcer		2		0
Decubitus ulcer is caused by avascular necrosis (1) due to kinking of uterine vessels (1)		2	1	0
Total score	32			
Candidate's score .../32				

Examiner's name/signature Date

6.7 Station 6.7 Interpreting Abnormal Test Finding

Subject: Gynaecology.
Subspecialty: Urogynaecology.
Domain of clinical competence: Interpretation of abnormal test finding (IATF).
Station: FBC and chemistry in a patient with uterine procidentia.
Station objective: To test the candidate's ability to identify abnormal FBC and blood chemistry in a patient with uterine procidentia for the purpose of optimizing her for surgery.
Requirements: Full blood count and renal function results of the patient, clearly written questions concerning the interpretation of the results, answer guideline or checklist, a table and chairs for the candidate and examiners, plain papers as answer sheets for the candidate, pencils and erasers, and a chaperon.

6.7.1 Instructions to the Candidate

The patient you examined on the last station with uterine procidentia was requested to do some investigations. Below is the result of her full blood count and renal function tests. Study the results of the tests carefully and answer the questions that follow.

6.8 XX Hospital

6.8.1 Pathology Department

FBC	Hb 9.2 g/dL	(n = 11–14 g/dL)
	WBC 4.6 × 10^9/L	(n = 4.0–11.0 × 10^9/L)
	MVC 88 fl	(n = 80–95 fl)
	MCH 20 pg	(n = 27–34 pg)
	Platelets 164 × 10^9/L	(n = 150–400 × 10^9/L)
EUCr	Na 126mmol/L	(n = 134–146 mmol/L)
	Ka 4.8 mmol/L	(n = 3.5–5.5 mmol/L)
	Cl 113mmol/L	(n = 92–106 mmol/L)
	HCO 24 mmol/L	(n = 20–30 mmol/L)
	Urea 12.5umol/L	(n = 1.7–9.0 mmol/L)
	Creatinine 280 mmol/L	(n = 72–125 umol/L)

Questions

1. What is your diagnosis based on the results?
2. Give 2 possible reasons for these findings in this patient
3. How would you manage the abnormalities detected in these tests?
4. Give 2 possible treatment modalities for the patient

Answers

1. The diagnosis is chronic renal failure with mild anaemia (**4 marks**).
2. Two possible reasons for renal failure and anaemia in this patient are (**2 marks each**):
   (a) Kinking of the ureters leading to obstructive uropathy and renal failure.
   (b) Urethral obstruction, leading to urinary stasis, hydronephrosis and renal failure.
   (c) Any of the two above can cause ureteric or renal stone formation and renal failure.
3. Management of the patient (**2 marks each**):
   (a) Admit patient into the gynaecological ward.
   (b) Reduce the procidentia.
   (c) Pack the vaginal with sterile gauze soaked in antiseptic like eusol (pessary will worsen the decubitus ulcer)
   (d) Abdominal USS or IVU to rule out bladder/renal calculi and hydronephrosis
   (e) Monitor renal function till normal
4. The 2 modalities of treatment of this patient are (**2 marks each**):
   (a) Vaginal hysterectomy and pelvic floor repair when she is stabilized.
   (b) Use of pessaries to retain the uterus in position when decubitus ulcer has healed.
   (c) Colpocleisis is also an option.

Checklist for IATF if candidate is requested to verbally answer the questions

Tasks	Well done	Fairly done	Poorly done	Not done
Diagnosis: chronic renal failure (2) with mild anaemia (2)	4	2		0
Possible reasons for renal failure (Max 2):				
- Kinking of ureters causing obstructive uropathy.		2	1	0
- Urethral obstruction causing obstructive uropathy.		2	1	0
- Calculi along urinary tract due to any of the above reasons		2	1	0
Management of patient (Max 5):				
- Admit into gynaecological ward.		2		0
- Reduce procidentia.		2		0
- Pack vagina with gauze soaked in antiseptics.		2		0
- Abdominal USS or IVU for calculi and hydronephrosis		2		0
- Monitor renal functions till normal.		2		0
- Give haematinics		2		0
Modalities of treatment (Max 2):				
- Vaginal hysterectomy and pelvic floor repair		2	1	0
- Use pessaries when decubitus ulcer has healed.		2	1	0
- Colpocleisis if unfit for major surgery		2	1	0
Total marks	22			
Candidate's score .../22				

Examiner's signature Date

Family Planning OSCE Stations 7

7.1 Station 7.1 Counselling for Use of Combined Oral Contraceptive Pills

Subject: Gynaecology.
Subspecialty: Family planning.
Domain of clinical competence: Communication and counselling.
Station: Counselling a client for use of combined oral contraceptive pills.
Station objective: To test the candidate's ability to counsel a client for correct use of the combined oral contraceptive pills for the purpose of family planning.
Requirements. Standardized client (role player), samples of the combined oral contraceptive pills, the WHO medical eligibility criteria wheel, a comfortable chair for the client, a chair for the candidate, a table and 2 chairs for the examiners, enough copies of the checklist, pencils and erasers, and a calendar chart.

C. Chama, *OSCE and VIVA VOCE in Obstetrics and Gynaecology*,
https://doi.org/10.1007/978-3-031-77262-7_7

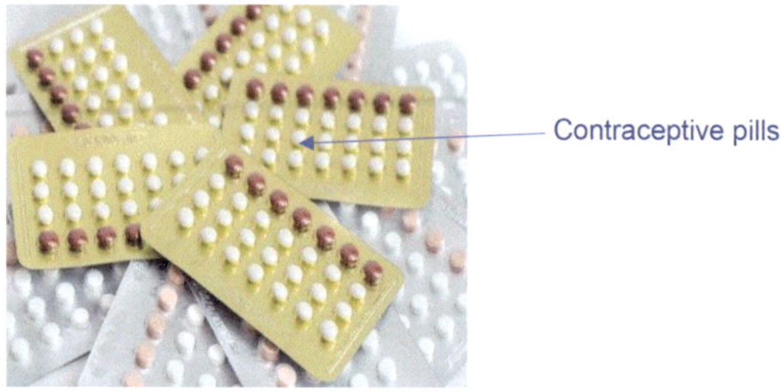

Fig. 7.1 Oral contraceptive pills

7.1.1 Instructions to the Candidate

Mrs. JJ is a 24-year-old P1 + 0 A1 whose last confinement was about 6 weeks ago. She had group counselling on family planning in the postnatal clinic, and she wants to use the combined oral contraceptive pills. Using the medical eligibility criteria wheel and samples of the combined oral contraceptive pill sachets, counsel her to favourably use the combined oral contraceptive pills (Fig. 7.1).

7.1.2 Instructions to the Examiner

The candidate is to use the tools provided to counsel Mrs. HJ who wants to use the combined oral contraceptive pills. Use the checklist below to score the candidate.

Checklist for counselling for use of COCPs

Task	Well done	Fairly done	Poorly done	Not done
Greets patient, introduces self and obtains permission to discuss the use of COCPs with her	4	2	1	0
Asks about her knowledge of the birth control pills		2		0
Uses the MEC wheel to confirm patient is suitable to use the pills		2	1	0
Explains to patient how the pill works; mentions some benefits as well as side effects	4	2	1	0
Shows a sachet and explains the active tablets and the iron placebos	4	2	1	0
Tells her to take one tablet daily, starting with the first and following the arrow daily, preferably at about the same time each day	4	2	1	0
Allows her to ask questions or seek clarifications		2		0
Explains that if she forgets to take a pill on time (delayed) or for a day (missed), she should take the pill as soon as she remembers and take the next pill at the right time even if it means taking 2 pills in the same day. No additional contraception needed	4	2	1	0
If she misses 2 or more pills, she should take the recently missed pill as soon as possible and take the next pill at the usual time even if it means taking 2 pills the same day. Use a back-up method like condoms.	4	2	1	0
Asks her to repeat what he has said about missed pills and make any corrections if any		2		0
If the pills were missed in the last week (D15-28), omit the placebo pills after completing the hormonal pills and start the new pack. A back-up method is needed until after 7 days of taking hormonal pills	4	2	1	0
Emergency contraception should also be considered if a hormonal pill is missed in the first week.		2		0
Ask if she has any questions and let her repeat the instructions so far given to check her understanding		2		0
Provide her with the pills and give her appointment for follow-up in 6 weeks to evaluate any challenges she might be facing with the pills		2		0
Thank her for her attention and hope you have been of assistance to her		2		0
Communication skills	4	2	1	0
Total score	48			
Candidate's score .../48				

Examiner's name and signature Date

7.2 Station 7.2 Demonstrating How to Use the Male condom

Subject: Gynaecology.
Subspecialty: Family planning.
Domain of clinical competence: Therapeutic procedure.
Station: Demonstrating how to use the male condom.
Station objective: To test the candidate's ability to demonstrate to a client how to use the male condom for the purpose of family planning and prevention of sexually transmitted infections.
Requirements: Samples of the male condom, a wooden or plastic model of the penis, condom lubricant, latex hand gloves, standardized couple (Role players), 2 comfortable chairs for the couple, a table and 2 chairs for the examiners, enough copies of the checklist, pencils and erasers, a chair for the candidate, and a chaperon to clear the table after each examination.

7.2.1 Instruction to Candidate

Mrs. FA is a 30-year-old P5 + 0 A5 who's last childbirth was 6 weeks ago. She and her husband were counselled in the postnatal clinic on family planning, but they have not made up their mind on a long-term contraceptive. They have decided to use the male condom in the interim.

Your task: Using the male condom sample and wooden penis model, explain to the couple, while demonstrating, how to use the male condom (Fig. 7.2).

7.2.2 Instruction to Examiners

The candidate is to use the male condom and the wooden penis model to demonstrate to the couple how to use the male condom. Use the checklist provided to score the candidate

Fig. 7.2 Wooden penis model and packs of male condoms. (Courtesy of Jonathan Edache Otache)

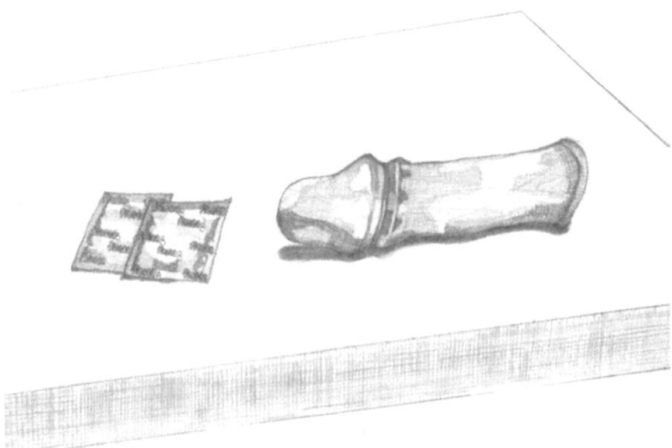

Checklist for condom use

Task	Well done	Fairly done	Poorly done	Not done
Greets the couple, introduces self and obtains permission to discuss the use of the male condom	4	2	1	0
Introduces the subject e.g. I understand you want to use the male condom in the interim before you make up your mind on ………	4	2	1	0
Asks couple what they understand about the male condom		2		0
Introductory statements - Condoms are made of thin latex rubber and hardly cause irritation. - When used correctly it is effective in preventing pregnancy. - It has the added advantage of preventing premature ejaculation. - It can also prevent STI		2 2 2 2		0 0 0 0
Demonstrates how to wear the condom: - Have a foreplay so that the penis becomes erect. - Tear open the package; do not use scissors or teeth. - Correctly places the condom on the wooden penis with the rolled side out - Unrolls the condom to the base of the wooden penis		2 2 2 2		0 0 0 0
Asks the couple to open a new condom and roll it over the wooden penis as he has done	4	2	1	0
Further explanation - The penis can now be inserted into the vagina with the condom. - After ejaculation, hold the base of the condom and withdraw the penis from the vagina. - Use a new condom after each ejaculation. - Dispose the condom properly		2 2 2 2		0 0 0 0
Ask the couple if they have any questions or clarification		2		0
Thanks the couple for listening and hope they will use the condom correctly and consistently		2		0
Communication skill	4	2	1	0
Total score	50			
Candidate's score …/50				

Examiners name and signature date

7.3 Station 7.3 Counselling for Bilateral Tubal Ligation

Subject: Gynaecology.
Subspecialty: Family planning.
Domain of clinical competence: Communication and counselling.
Station: Counselling a couple for bilateral tubal ligation (BTL).
Station objective: To test the candidate's ability to counsel a couple for BTL, making the couple understand not only its effectiveness, but also its irreversibility, so that they do not regret their decision.
Requirements: Standardized couple (role players), 2 comfortable chairs or a dressed bed for the couple, a table and 2 chairs for examiners, enough copies of the checklist, pencils and erasers, a chair for the candidate, plain papers for use by the candidate, a model of the uterus with tubes and ovaries to be used for demonstration to patients by the candidate (a chart of the female reproductive organs can also be used) (Fig. 7.3).

7.3.1 Instruction to the Role Player

I am 42 years old and carrying my seventh pregnancy, having delivered 6 times with all my children alive; 3 boys and 3 girls. I registered for antenatal care 2 weeks ago and informed my doctor that I want to stop having children after this pregnancy. I was counselled on the various available methods but I do not

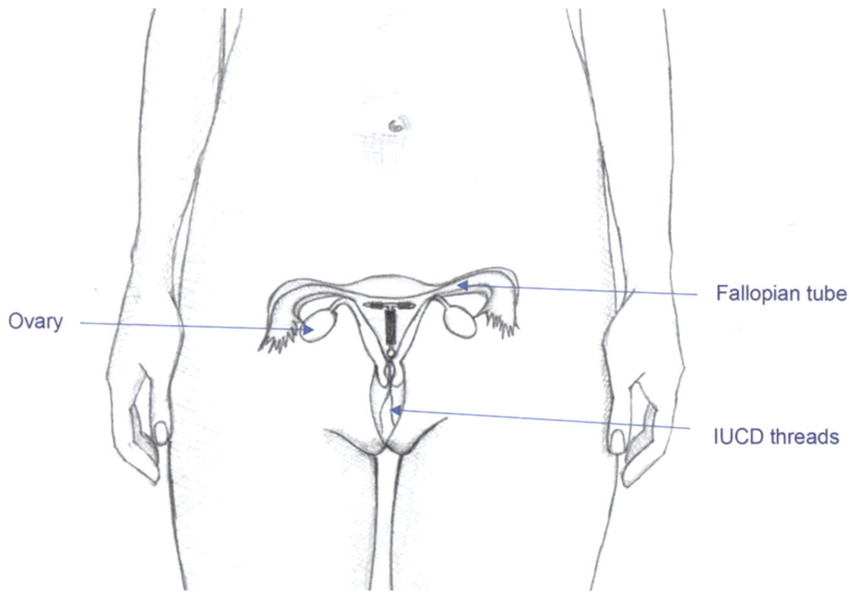

Fig. 7.3 Diagram of female sexual organs with IUCD in situ. (Courtesy of Jonathan Edache Otache)

want intrauterine devices or pills. I have discussed with my husband, and we are considering having BTL after this pregnancy although I have some fears concerning the procedure: I think BTL may affect my general well-being and my menses may stop after the surgery. I am afraid I may even die during such a major surgery.

7.3.2 Instruction to the Candidate

Mrs. GA is a 42-year-old G7P6 + 0 6 alive (3 boys and 3 girls). She booked for antenatal care 2 weeks ago at 20 weeks gestation, and the couple do not want further babies after the index pregnancy. She has aversion for IUCD and hormonal contraceptives.

She and her husband are willing to consider BTL but they are afraid that:

- She could become sick after the procedure
- She also feels her menses may stop after the procedure
- That she may die from such a major surgical procedure

Your task

1. Counsel Mrs. GA so that she can have enough information to favourably consider having a BTL
2. Address the other concerns raised above
3. Also educate her on when the BTL will be carried out and why at such a time

7.3.3 Instruction to the Examiners

The patient is a 42-year-old G7P6 + 0 6 alive who booked for antenatal care 2 weeks ago at 20 weeks gestation. She was counselled for contraception after this pregnancy, and she is considering having BTL after she delivers. However, she is concerned that the procedure may affect her subsequent well-being and stop her menses. She even thinks she could die from the procedure, which she thinks is a major surgery.

The candidate is supposed to counsel her to favourably consider accepting the BTL and address the fears she has raised. Use the checklist provided to score the candidate.

Checklist for counselling for BTL

Tasks	Well done	Fairly done	Poorly done	Not done
Greets patient and introduces self		2	1	0
Opening statement: Mrs. Aniobi, I understand you have a need for counseling on permanent method of family planning. I hope I can be of help to you		2	1	0
Counseling points - briefly explain what BTL involves; minor surgery, blocking the tubes, prevents sperm from reaching the egg - common procedure, used by millions of women all over the world, shown to be safe - general or local anaesthesia can be used - considered permanent, but in extreme cases reversal can be attempted - uses posters/charts to show anatomy of uterus and tubes	4 4 4 4 4	2 2 2 2 2	1 1 1 1 1	0 0 0 0 0
Ask couple to give you feedback of what they understand by what you said		2		0
Addressing their concerns: - BTL does not make women sick, puerperium is normal. - Menses will resume and continue normally. - The procedure is a minor surgery, women hardly die from it - The procedure to be carried out within 48 hours of delivery when the tubes are easily accessible. - Will be discharged home the following day like any normal delivery		2 2 2 2 2	1 1 1 1 1	0 0 0 0 0
Ask couple what they understand by your explanations		2		0
Closing: Thank the couple for letting you be of help and hope they can make informed decision		2		0
Communication skill: audible, eye contact, clarity, interactive, sensitive, confident.	4	2	1	0
Maximum score	42			
Candidate's score .../42				
Weighted score				

Examiner's signature Date

7.4 Station 7.4 Insertion of Intrauterine Contraceptive Device

Subject: Gynaecology.
Subspecialty: Family planning.
Domain of clinical competence: Therapeutic procedure.
Station: Demonstrating the insertion of CuT380A device for the purpose of contraception.
Station objective: To test the candidate's ability to correctly insert CuT380A intrauterine contraceptive device.
Requirements: A mannequin (or model) of the pelvis fitted with uterus and cervix (a model of the uterus will also suffice), samples of copper T IUCD, Cusco's speculum (if mannequin will be used), latex gloves, a table or dressed bed for the mannequin, a table and 2 chairs for the examiners, enough copies of the checklist, pencils and erasers, a chair for the candidate, and a chaperon to clear the table after each examination.

7.4.1 Instruction to the Candidate

Provided is a model of the uterus and a package of CuT380A intrauterine device. Demonstrate, step by step, while running commentary, how to insert CuT380A for use (Fig. 7.4).

7.4.2 Instruction to the Examiners

Provided is a uterine model and a package of CuT380A intrauterine contraceptive device. The candidate is supposed to demonstrate the insertion of the IUCD for use while running commentary. Use the checklist provided to score the candidate

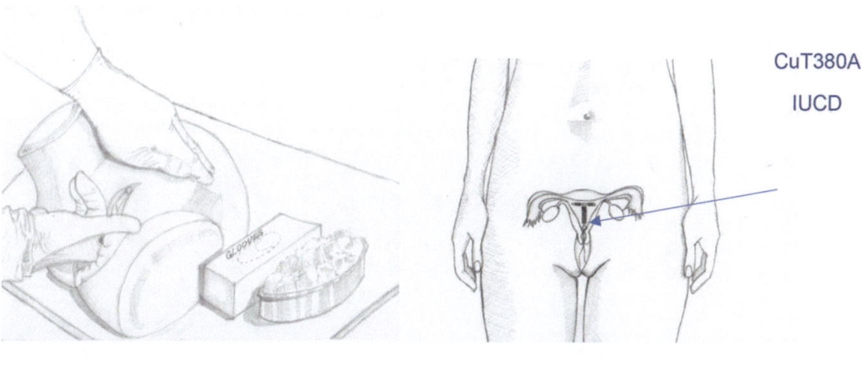

Fig. 7.4 Performing vaginal examination before insertion of IUCD. (Courtesy of Jonathan Edache Otache)

Checklist—IUCD insertion

Task	Well done	Fairly done	Poorly done	Not done
Correctly identifies CuT30A IUCD		2		0
Says patient will be in lithotomy position, cleaned and draped VE done to assess size, and position of uterus	4	2	1	0
Cervix will be exposed with bivalve speculum, anterior lip held with tenaculum and uterus sounded	4	2	1	0
Device opened on a sterile tray; fold arms and push into barrel, and adjust stopper to uterine depth on the uterine sound	4	2	1	0
Inserting device:				
- Steady uterus with vulsellum or tenaculum		2		0
- Insert loaded device transcervically without touching vaginal wall.		2		0
- Withdraw barrel while keeping plunger in position.		2		0
- Remove barrel and plunger leaving device in-utero.		2		0
- Tuck strings in posterior fornix, you may cut to 3cm length.		2		0
- Remove speculum and patient to lie on her side		2		0
Tell patient she may feel some cramps for a few hours		2		0
Tell her to feel the threads with the tip of her finger		2		0
Tell her menstrual flow may increase for the first 2-3 cycles		2		0
Prescribe antibiotics if she was menstruating during insertion		2		0
Reassure and give 6 weeks appointment		2		0
Penalty: non-sequential steps, clumsy, cannot load device	-4	-2	-1	0
Total score	34			
Candidates score .../34				

Examiner's name and signature Date

7.5 Station 7.5 Insertion of Jadelle Contraceptive Implants

Subject: Gynaecology.
Subspecialty: Family planning.
Domain of clinical competence: Therapeutic procedure.
Station: Insertion of Jadelle implants.
Station objective: To assess the candidate's ability to correctly insert Jadelle implants for the purpose of contraception.
Requirements: A plastic or wooden model of the arm wrapped with mackintosh or rubber, samples of Jadelle and insertion trocar, latex gloves, a vial of 1% Xylocaine (water for injection can be used), 5 mL syringe and needles, wet and dry swabs, galipot containing spirit, sterile gauze, dressing plaster, sponge holding forceps, a table and 2 chairs for examiners, enough copies of checklist, pencils and erasers, and a chair for the candidate.

7.5.1 Instruction to the Candidate

Mrs. GL is a 35-year-old P5 + 0 A5 who was counselled on family planning methods in the postnatal clinic. She chose to have Jadelle implant inserted. She is 6 weeks post-partum.

Demonstrate using the model provided with commentaries how to insert Jadelle implant (Fig. 7.5).

7.5.2 Instruction to Examiners

The candidate is to use the model of the arm provided to demonstrate, while running commentary, how to insert Jadelle implant using the samples provided. Use the checklist below to score the candidate.

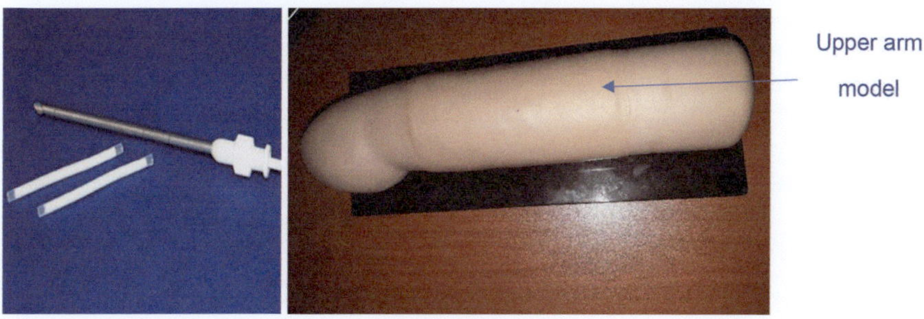

Fig. 7.5 Jadelle capsules and trocar, plastic model of upper arm

Jadelle implant insertion checklist

Task	Well done	Fairly done	Poorly done	Not done
Greets patient, introduces self		2		0
Inform patient he is to insert the implant as scheduled and obtains her permission	4	2	1	0
Reviews her case note; LMP within 7 days or client within 3 weeks of puerperium		2		0
Explains the procedure to client; site of insertion, analgesia etc.	4	2	1	0
Confirms assistant and consumable are ready; gloves, syringes and needles, gauze, 1% xylocaine, 2 packs of Jadelle etc.	4	2	1	0
Patient in supine position, non-dominant hand stretched over side tray, insertion site cleaned and draped	4	2	1	0
Chaperon to open the insertion pack, Jadelle pack, trocar pack, 5ml syringe and needle.	4	2	1	0
Procedure				
- Mark a point 8-10cm on medial aspect of upper arm and infiltrate with 2-4ml 1% xylocaine		2		0
- Stretch the skin and pierce at 30^0 with the beveled part of the trocar pointing upwards.		2		0
- As the trocar enters the skin, advance it horizontally till the proximal dark circular mark.		2		0
- Remove the plunger, load a rod of Jadelle, replace the plunger and push gently till you feel a resistance.		2		0
- Gently withdraw the plunger till you see the distal dark circular mark.		2		0
- Steady the first rod and change the direction of the trocar by 30^0 and advance subdermally.		2		0
- Insert the second rod as described for the first; clean the site and apply a small piece of gauze		2		0
Postoperative care				
- Ask patient to palpate the rods and to keep the site dry for 3 days.			1	0
- Prescribe analgesics and antibiotics.			1	0
- Fill appointment form			1	0
- Write your procedure			1	0
Total score	36			
Candidate's score .../36				

Examiner's signature Date

7.6 Station 7.6 Counselling for Emergency Contraception

Subject: Gynaecology.
Subspecialty: Family planning.
Domain of clinical competence: Communication and counselling.
Station: Counselling for emergency contraception.
Station objective: To test the candidate's ability to correctly counsel a client who is at risk of pregnancy for emergency contraception.
Requirements: Samples of Postinor 2, copper IUCD, COCP, a plastic model of the uterus may be useful, standardized patient (Role player), a comfortable chair or dressed bed for the Role player, a chair for the candidate, a table and 2 chairs for the examiners, enough copies of checklist, and pencils and erasers (Fig. 7.6).

7.6.1 Instruction to the Role Player

I am a 25-year-old, Corper, serving with the Bauchi state chapter. I was posted to Federal Government Girls College Bauchi to teach Biology (I am a graduate of zoology). Last night I went out with my boyfriend and had sexual intercourse without using any condom. My last menstrual period was about 10 days ago.

I am aware of modern methods of contraception but have never used any. I am sexually active and have used the male condom before, but this episode of sexual intercourse was not protected. I have never been pregnant before. I have come to the family planning clinic of Abubakar Tafawa Balewa University Teaching Hospital for assistance.

7.6.2 Instruction to the Candidate

The lady before you has come to the family planning clinic for contraception. Your task is to counsel her.

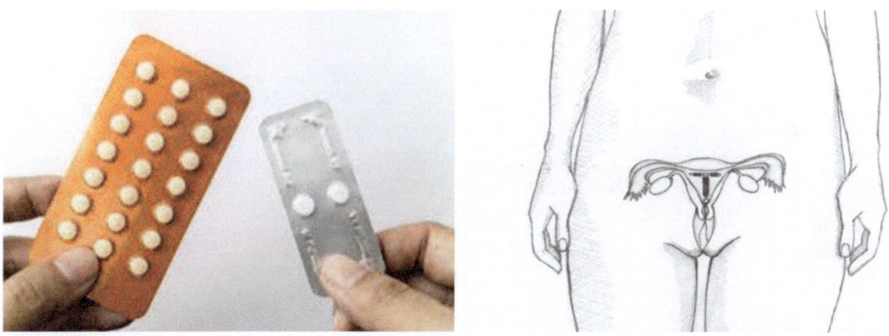

Fig. 7.6 Varieties of emergency contraceptives. (Drawing in the right—Courtesy of Jonathan Edache Otache)

7.6.3 Instruction to the Examiner

Ms. CP is a 25-year-old corper serving at FGGC Bauchi. She had an unprotected sexual intercourse last night and has come to the family planning clinic for an emergency contraception. The candidate is supposed to counsel her on emergency contraception. Use the checklist provided to score the candidate.

Checklist for emergency contraception

Task	Well done	Fairly done	Poorly done	Not done
Greets the patient and introduces self		2	1	0
Obtains Biodata: name, age, address, occupation, tribe, religion	4	2	1	0
Parity, LMP		2	1	0
Presenting complaint		2		0
History of presenting complaint - About how many hours ago did she have sexual intercourse? - What does she know about emergency contraception? - Has she used any contraceptive before?		 2 2 2		 0 0 0
Explains available methods				
Postinor 2 - 2 tablets of levonorgestrel 0.75mg - Can take the 2 tablets stat within 72 hours of unprotected sexual intercourse or one table about 12 hours apart - Delays ovulation and impairs sperm transport through the cervix - About 99% effective if taken correctly		 2 2 2 2		 0 0 0 0
Combined oral contraceptive pills - 2 pills containing oestradiol and norethisterone on 2 consecutive days - Like postinor 2 the earlier taken after sexual intercourse the more effective - Nausea and vomiting worse than with postinor 2 - Like postinor 2 it also delays ovulation and impair transport of sperm through the cervix - About 98% effective		 2 2 2 2 2		 0 0 0 0 0
Copper T IUCD - Inserted into the uterus within 7 days of unprotected sexual intercourse. - More effective than the other methods - Can prevent implantation even if fertilization has taken place. - Can be left in-situ for long term contraception		 2 2 2 2		 0 0 0 0
Allow patient to ask questions or seek for clarifications		2		0
Ask her which method she prefers and provide her with the method accordingly		2		0
Thank her for coming		2		0
Communication skill	4	2	1	0
Maximum score	52			
Candidate's score .../52				

Examiner's name and signature Date

Ethics and Medico-Legal Issues in Gynaecology OSCE Stations

8

8.1 Station 8.1 Rape-Related Pregnancy

Subject: Gynaecology.
Subspecialty: Ethics and medico-legal issues.
Domain of clinical competence: Counselling.
Station: Counselling an adolescent with rape-related pregnancy.
Station objective: To test the candidate's ability to counsel an adolescent with rape-related pregnancy with the aim of helping to decide how best to manage the pregnancy.
Requirements: An adolescent in the presence of a trusted guardian as standardized patient, dressed bed or comfortable chair for the SP. Instructions to the SP, candidate, and examiners. A table and chairs for examiners and candidate, sufficient checklists, pencils and erasers, and a chaperon.

8.1.1 Instructions to the Standardized Patient (SP)

I am a 16-year-old class 2 senior secondary school student who was raped by my uncle last month. My parents were advised to bring me to the hospital 5 days after the incident. I was examined and given postinor 2 for emergency contraception while blood samples and vaginal swabs were taken for analysis. The case is already with the police, and I am supposed to appear in court next week for hearing. However, it is 6 weeks now since I last saw my menses and I think I might be pregnant. I have come to see the gynaecologist who saw me after the rape incident to discuss what next to do concerning my situation.

C. Chama, *OSCE and VIVA VOCE in Obstetrics and Gynaecology*,
https://doi.org/10.1007/978-3-031-77262-7_8

8.1.2 Instruction to the Candidate

The adolescent who is here with her mother was seen 3 weeks ago after being raped by her uncle. She has come for follow-up, and her last menses was 6 weeks ago. How would you counsel her concerning a possible rape-related pregnancy?

8.1.3 Instructions to the Examiners

The patient is a 16-year-old SS-2 student who was seen as a case of rape 3 weeks ago in this hospital. Her case is being handled in conjunction with the police, and she is scheduled to appear in court for hearing next week. She has come for follow up, having missed her menses for 2 weeks. The candidate is supposed to counsel her for a possible rape-related pregnancy. Use the checklist provided to score the candidate as he counsels the patient and her mother who has accompanied her to the clinic.

Checklist for counselling on rape-related pregnancy

Tasks	Well done	Fairly done	Poorly done	Not done
Greets the patient and her mother, introduces self and obtains permission to talk to her	4	2	1	0
Assures her of confidentiality and asks if they could talk in the presence of her mother		2	1	0
Obtains her biodata: name, age, address, school, religion etc.		2	1	0
Asks her how she has been doing since the last visit 3 weeks ago		2	1	0
Patient discloses her LMP was 6 weeks ago and she is worried she might be pregnant despite taking the postinor 2.				
Asks her if she has pregnancy symptoms		2	1	0
Asks her sexual history before the rape, use of contraception		2	1	0
Requests for results of previous investigations including pregnancy test, reviews the results.	4	2	1	0
Asks patient what she would like to do if she is pregnant		2	1	0
Would like to request for the following tests to confirm pregnancy:				
- Pregnancy test		2		0
- Pelvic USS, preferably TVS		2		0
- Re-emphasize rescreening for HIV, HBV, HCV after another 3 weeks		2		0
Allows patient to ask any question or clarification.		2		0
If it turns out she is pregnant:				
- The court will give a ruling as to whether the pregnancy can be terminated or not.		2	1	0
- CVS and paternity test to be done to confirm that assailant fathered the pregnancy.		2	1	0
- She may have to drop from school		2	1	0
Allows her to digest the information and ask questions		2		0
If the pregnancy will continue, court will decide who will be responsible for her ANC and child care.	4	2	1	0
Thanks her for coming and gives her appointment, documents the discussion.	4	2	1	0
Communication skills: empathy, clarity, emphasis, listening	4	2	1	0
Penalty: judgmental, indecent language, etc	-4	-2	-1	0
Total scores	48			
Candidate's score .../48				

Examiner's signature Date

8.2 Station 8.2 Vaginal Examination in a Rape Victim (Fig. 8.1)

Subject: Gynaecology.

Subspecialty: Ethics and medico-legal issues.

Domain of clinical competence: Physical examination.

Station: Vaginal examination in a rape victim.

Station objective: To assess the candidate's ability to conduct vaginal examination in a prepubertal girl with the aim of assessing the degree of physical injuries and collect specimens for both medical and forensic examinations.

Requirements: Mannequin of a prepubertal girl, standardized patient as mother of the girl, swab sticks, culture medium for gonococcus, an examination couch for the mannequin and the SP, sufficient checklists, pencils and erasers, and a chaperon.

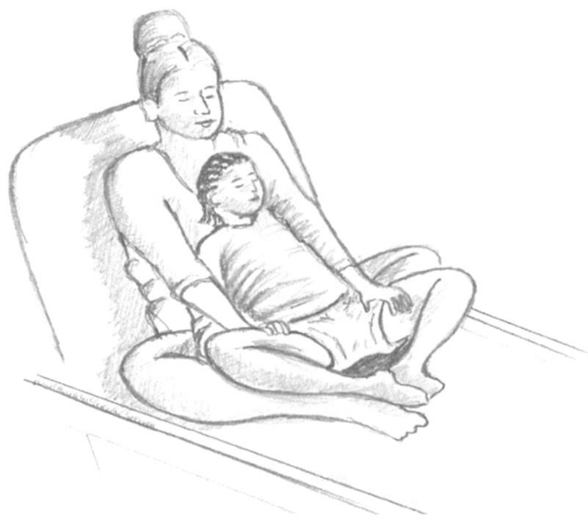

Fig. 8.1 Frog-leg position for examining a child. Courtesy of Jonathan Edache Otache

8.2.1 Instructions to the Standardized Patient (Mother of Child)

It is assumed that I am the mother of this 9-year-old girl child who has just been raped by her uncle who was supposed to take her home from school. I have brought her to the hospital, and the doctor has interviewed me concerning what has happened. With my consent, the police have been invited into the matter. The doctor is examining the child, and he has asked me to hold her in my lap so that her private part will be examined. He has demonstrated to me how he wants me to hold the child.

8.2.2 Instruction to the Candidate

The patient is a 9-year-old girl who has been raped by her uncle about 2 h ago. She has been brought to the hospital by her mother, and the police have been invited. Your task is to demonstrate step by step, how you would carry out a vaginal examination on this girl who has just been raped. Run your commentary to the hearing of the examiners as you perform the task.

8.2.3 Instructions to the Examiners

The patient is a 9-year-old schoolgirl who has been raped by her uncle. She has been brought to the hospital, and she is being assessed. The task of the candidate is to demonstrate using the mannequin how to perform vaginal examination on this girl. Study the checklist and use it to score the candidate as he performs the task to your hearing and observation.

Checklist for vaginal examination of a rape victim

Tasks	Well done	Fairly done	Poorly done	Not done
Greets the patient and her mother and introduces self		2	1	0
Explains the procedure and obtains permission to examine her		2	1	0
Requests the presence of female chaperon to assist		2		0
Helps the mother to position the child in frog-leg position		2	1	0
Inspects: - The external genitalia, perineum, anus, inner thighs for - Oedema, bruises, abrasions, lacerations, bleeding.	 4 4	 2 2	 1 1	 0 0
Gently holds the labia majora in both hands, moves them posteriorly and anteriorly to expose vaginal introitus and hymen.	4	2	1	0
- Inspect for tears to hymen and fourchette. - Use swab sticks to collect secretions, other forensic materials for MCS and DNA analysis. - NO DIGITAL or speculum vaginal examinations. - Insert lubricated small finger to assess anal sphincteric tone. - If colposcope available, may obtain still or video images for forensic purposes.		2 2 2 2 2	1 1 1 1 1	0 0 0 0 0
If there is significant haemorrhage or laceration, patient should be booked for repair under anaesthesia		2		0
If patient is also anxious or uncooperative, should have EUA		2		0
Thank the patient, reposition her, explain findings.	4	2	1	0
Document your findings, give appointment		2	1	0
Total marks	40			
Candidate's score .../40				

Examiner's signature Date

8.3 Station 8.3 Counselling on Assisted Reproductive Technology for a Lesbian

Subject: Gynaecology.
Specialty: Ethics and medico-legal issues.
Domain of clinical competence: Communication and counselling.
Station: Counselling for IVF-ET for a Lesbian.
Station objective: To assess the candidate's ability to counsel a lesbian for IVF with the aim of making her understand the ethical and legal issues involved in our country.
Requirements: Standardized patient as lesbian, a dressed bed or comfortable chair for the SP, instructions to the SP, candidate, and examiners, a table and chairs for the examiners and candidate, sufficient checklists, pencils and erasers, charts, and literature handouts for SP to read at home, and a chaperon.

8.3.1 Instructions to the Standardized Patient

I am a 32-year-old businesswoman who imports and sells textile materials. I have been seeing a consultant gynaecologist in this hospital for the purpose of achieving a pregnancy. I am a lesbian with a steady partner, but we cannot get married due to the legal constraints in this country. The doctor has explained the options of getting pregnant for me and I have come to receive further counselling on in vitro fertilization with donor sperm and embryo transfer.

I am the only female among four children of my parents. I have always been attracted to women but found it difficult to express my feelings until after I graduated from the university. I have had heterosexual sex a few times as an undergraduate but now in a faithful lesbian relationship. There is no history of diabetes, hypertension, or sickle cell disease in my family. I do not take alcoholic beverages or smoke cigarettes.

8.3.2 Instructions to the Candidate

The patient present is a lesbian who is planning to get pregnant. Your task is to counsel her for IVF-ET with donor sperm.

8.3.3 Instructions to the Examiners

The patient is a lesbian who is planning to get pregnant. She has come for counselling on IVF-ET with donor sperm. The candidate is supposed to counsel for this procedure. Use the checklist provided to score the candidate.

Checklist for counselling a lesbian for IVF-ET

Tasks	Well done	Fairly done	Poorly done	Not done
Greets the patient and introduces self		2	1	0
Assures her of confidentiality and obtains permission		2	1	0
Obtains biodata: name, age, address, occupation, marital status,	4	2	1	0
Parity, LMP		2	1	0
PC: wants to get pregnant		2		0
HPC:				
- Is your partner aware of your decision?		2		0
- Do you have a heterosexual relationship?		2		0
- Do you know the legal implication of lesbianism in this country?		2		0
- You know a donor sperm has to be sourced?		2		0
Explains how donor sperm is obtained:				
- Volunteers are invited.			1	0
- They are screened for STIs.			1	0
- Semen obtained by masturbation.			1	0
- Semen stored for use.			1	0
- Donors are paid.			1	0
- Donors sign legal papers to forfeit disclosure or claim of paternity.			1	0
Allows patient to ask questions		2		0
Explains how she will be prepared for the procedure:				
- To be screened for any infections or uterine abnormality that will affect pregnancy.		2		0
- She will be stimulated to produce many eggs which will be harvested.		2		0
- Her eggs will be fertilized using the donor sperm in the laboratory.		2		0
- 2 of the fertilized eggs will be transferred into her womb to achieve pregnancy.		2		0
- The chances of achieving pregnancy is about 25-30%.		2		0
Allows her to ask for clarifications		2		0
Further explains:				
- Drugs will be given to support the pregnancy.		2		0
- Pregnancy test will be done 2 weeks after IVF.		2		0
- Pregnancy can be seen on USS 4 weeks after IVF.		2		0
- If successful, she will book for antenatal care.		2		0
Asks her what she understands by the explanations so far.		2		0
Further explains:				
- Child outside wedlock are stigmatized in our society.		2		0
- The child may ask for the father as he/she grows.		2		0
- The identity of the father cannot be disclosed.		2		0
Makes any clarification on her comments		2		0
Thanks her for coming and gives her appointment.		2		0
Communication skills: audible, clear, empathic, listens.	4	2	1	0
Total marks	58			
Candidate's score .../58				

Examiner's signature Date

8.4 Station 8.4 Unruptured Ectopic Pregnancy

Subject: Gynaecology.
Subspecialty: Ethics and medico-legal issues.
Domain of clinical competence: Interpretation of abnormal test finding (IATF).
Station: Left unruptured ectopic pregnancy on transvaginal ultrasound scan.
Station objective: To test the candidate's ability to manage an unruptured tubal ectopic pregnancy in a patient who has suffered infertility for 10 years.
Requirements: A standardized patient, a dressed bed for the SP, investigation results, instructions to the SP, candidate, and examiners. A table and chairs for the examiners and candidate, sufficient checklists, pencils and erasers, and a chaperon.

8.4.1 Instructions to the Standardized Patient

I am a 40-year-old housewife who has never been pregnant in a 10-year-old marriage. I am a devout Christian who believes in the sanctity of life. My husband is a lecturer with a federal polytechnic in this town. We had two unsuccessful IVF cycles before but this time around I missed my menses for 2 months, and a pregnancy test done last week was positive. I have been having lower abdominal pains for the past 2 days. The school clinic doctor did a scan and referred me to see a specialist in this hospital. Some investigations were requested, and I have come with the results.

Investigation Results
Haematology

PCV = 34% (*n* 33–42%)
Hb = 12 g/dL (*n* 11–16 g/dL)
Blood group A Rh positive
HbAA
Serum B-hCG = 10,600 IU/mL (*n* < 5 IU/mL)

Transvaginal ultrasound scan

- Normal size empty uterus with secretory endometrium of 11 mm thickness.
- Both ovaries appear normal with a corpus luteum cyst of 26 mm diameter on the right.
- There is a left adnexal gestational sac containing an embryo of CRL 16 mm = 8 weeks.
- The foetus shows cardiac activity, and a yolk sac is seen.
- No free fluid in the pouch of Doughlas.

8.4.2 Instructions to the Candidate

The patient is a 40-year-old nullipara who missed her menses and a pregnancy test done in the Federal Polytechnic clinic was positive. She was referred to the gynaecology clinic in this hospital, and some tests were requested. She has been having lower abdominal pain for 2 days. Study her investigation results and discuss further management with her.

8.4.3 Instruction to the Examiners

The patient is a 40-year-old nullipara who had infertility for 10 years despite 2 cycles of IVF-ET. She missed her menses, and a pregnancy test was positive. However, a transvaginal ultrasound shows left unruptured tubal pregnancy. The candidate is supposed to discuss further management with the patient. Use the checklist provided to score the candidate.

Checklist for unruptured ectopic pregnancy

Tasks	Well done	Fairly done	Poorly done	Not done
Greets the patient introduces self		2	1	0
Introduces purpose of interaction and obtains permission		2	1	0
Obtains biodata: Name, age, address, marital status, occupation,	4	2	1	0
Parity, LMP		2	1	0
Studies the results of investigations and tells patient he has bad news for her.	4	2	1	0
Allows patient to absorb the shock and ask questions.		2		0
Explains further: - She is pregnant but located outside the womb. - If allowed to grow it will rupture, which is dangerous. - She must be operated to remove the pregnancy,		 2 2 2	 1 1 1	 0 0 0
Prompting: what will happen to my baby?				
Answer: if it ruptures the baby mostly dies and your life is in danger because of the internal bleeding.	4	2	1	0
Prompting: Isn't there a chance the baby will grow?				
Answer: the chances are infinitesimally small, almost no.		2	1	0
Prompting: But I don't want to kill my baby!				
Response: - Yes, saving your life will kill the baby. - And yes, the baby has the moral right to life. - But your life is more important than that of the baby. - And the baby will not survive if you die anyway		 2 2 2 2	 1 1 1 1	 0 0 0 0
Allows her to absorb the response.		2		0
Explains the options of treatment: - The pregnancy can be removed by laparoscopy. - She can also be treated medically but the live fetus and high B-hCG titer means the success rate is reduced. - Recovery is faster if she is treated laparoscopically. - She will require contraception for 3 months if treated medically.		 2 2 2 2	 1 1 1 1	 0 0 0 0
Allows her to choose mode of treatment, then admits her to the ward.	4	2	1	0
Communication skill: empathy, frank, clear, interactive	4	2	1	0
Total score	54			
Candidate's score .../54				

Examiner's signature Date

9 Preconception Care OSCE Stations

9.1 Station 9.1 Premarital Counselling and Testing for Human Immunodeficiency Virus (HIV) Infection

Subject: Obstetrics.
Theme: Preconception care.
Domain of clinical competence: Communication and counselling.
Station: Voluntary counselling and testing for HIV.
Station objective: To assess the candidate's ability to counsel an intending couple for HIV screening with the aim of knowing their HIV status before marriage.
Requirements: Standardized couple (or real intending couple), comfortable chairs or dressed bed for the couple (Fig. 9.1), a chair for the candidate, a table and two chairs for the examiners, enough copies of the checklist, pencils, and erasers, and a chaperon.

9.1.1 Instructions to the Intending Couple

You are intending to get married in a few weeks, and the officiating pastor has requested that both of you be screened for HIV infection. You have not had sexual intercourse since you started courting but both of you were sexually active before you started going out. You have never had a HIV screening test. No previous pregnancies before you started your friendship even though you were sexually active. Both of you will be asked some sensitive questions about your sexual lives and you may wish to be counselled separately first before coming together.

C. Chama, *OSCE and VIVA VOCE in Obstetrics and Gynaecology*,
https://doi.org/10.1007/978-3-031-77262-7_9

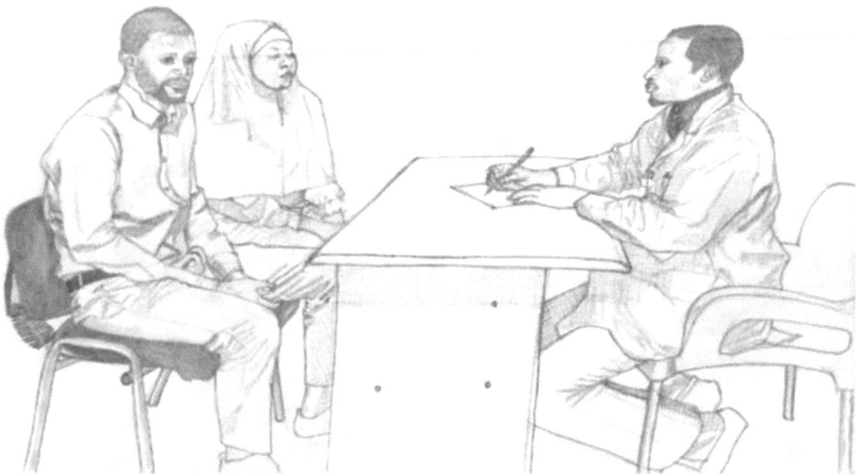

Fig. 9.1 Counselling a couple. Courtesy of Jonathan Edache Otache

9.1.2 Instruction to the Candidate

Mr. A and Miss F are courting and intend to get married in a month's time. They have come to the preconception care clinic and would like to have HIV testing. Your task is to counsel them to have a HIV screening test.

9.1.3 Instruction to Examiners

The candidate is supposed to conduct a premarital counselling for HIV testing for this intending couple. Use the score sheet provided to mark the candidate.

Checklist for HIV test counselling

Task	**Well done**	**Fairly done**	**Poorly done**	**Not done**
Greets couple and welcomes them, introduces self	4	2	1	0
Asks how he may be help		2		0
Informs the intending couple he may ask sensitive questions about their personal life, and they may wish to be interviewed separately first before the joint counselling	4	2	1	0
Asks about their sexual history including number of sexual partners	4	2	1	0
Probes their knowledge of HIV	4	2	1	0
Builds on couple's knowledge: - HIV are germs mainly transmitted through sexual intercourse. - Can also be transmitted through transfusion of infected blood, sharing needles and other sharp objects. - An infected mother can transmit the germ to her baby		2 2 2		0 0 0
Allows the couple to ask questions or seek clarifications		2		0
Further discusses: - The window period and the need for repeat test after 6 weeks - A newly infected person can remain healthy for 7-10 years before signs and symptoms of disease appear. - Available drugs can control the illness but no cure yet. - Healthy children can be born if couple are on treatment and care		2 2 2 2		0 0 0 0
Asks couple if they understood and may seek any clarification		2		0
HIV testing: - Rapid test for screening, can obtain result in 20-30 minutes. - Need confirmatory test if screening is positive		2 2		0 0
Asks intending couple if they are willing to take a screening test		2		0
Thanks couple for listening and for taking a decision to screen		2		0
Communication skills; sensitive, interactive, non-judgmental	4	2	1	0
Total score	48			
Candidate's score .../48				

Examiner Date

9.2 Station 9.2 Post-Test Counselling for Discordant Couple

Subject: Obstetrics.
Theme: Preconception care.
Domain of clinical competence: Communication and counselling.
Station: Post-test counselling of intending couple with discordant screening results.
Station objective: To assess the candidate's ability to disclose a bad news and help manage any crisis that may arise between the intending couple with discordant HIV screening results.
Requirements: Comfortable chairs for the intending couple, a chair for the candidate (counsellor), a table and two chairs for the examiners, enough copies of the checklist, and pencils and erasers.

9.2.1 Instruction to the Candidate

The intending couple you counselled on the last station agreed to have HIV screening test. They have come to receive the test result. The prospective bride tested negative while her fiancé tested positive for HIV 1. Your task is to disclose the screening results to the couple and counsel them on further steps to be taken.

9.2.2 Instruction to the Examiners

The candidate counselled a couple on the last station to have premarital HIV screening. They have come to receive the test results, and the intending bride is HIV negative while the intending bridegroom is positive. The candidate is supposed to disclose the results and counsel the intending couple on further steps to be taken. Use the checklist provided to score the candidate.

Checklist for HIV post-test counselling

Tasks	Well done	Fairly done	Poorly done	Not done
Greets couple, introduces self and welcomes them to the clinic		2	1	0
Softens the ground by asking how they have been since the screening test		2	1	0
Asks couple if they would prefer to receive the result together or separately		2	1	0
Discloses the result exactly; the man tested positive and the woman negative		2	1	0
Allows time for them to absorb the shock, then asks them what they understand by the result	4	2	1	0
Explains further the implications of the results:				
- The positive result needs to be confirmed by another test.		2	1	0
- If confirmed positive, he will be evaluated for treatment.		2	1	0
- Drugs are available that will make him live a normal life.		2	1	0
- The woman needs to be rescreened after 6 weeks since she is sexually active		2	1	0
Asks couple what they understand by what he has told them so far		2	1	0
Further discusses sex and reproduction if they get married:				
- They should use condoms during sexual intercourse till the husband's viral load is suppressed.		2	1	0
- They can achieve pregnancy using IUI or take a chance when the man's viral load is suppressed.		2	1	0
- When the viral load is undetectable, the chances of infecting your partner is almost zero		2	1	0
Allows the couple to ask questions		2		0
Further emphasizes the fact that HIV still has no cure, but one can live normal quality of life with treatment	4	2	1	0
Discusses linkage with support groups and spiritual leaders	4	2	1	0
Thanks them and gives appointment		2	1	0
Total marks	40			
Candidate's score .../40				

Examiner's signature Date

9.3 Station 9.3 History Taking for a Diabetic Woman

Subject: Obstetrics.
Theme: Preconception care.
Domain of clinical competence: History taking.
Station: Focused history taking of a diabetic planning to be pregnant.
Station objective: To test the candidate's ability to take a focused history of a diabetic lady who is planning to get pregnant soon with the aim of optimizing her health condition for a good pregnancy outcome.
Requirements: Standardized patient (Role player), a comfortable chair or dressed bed for the role player, a chair for the candidate, a table and two chairs for the examiners, pencils and erasers, plain papers for rough use by the candidate, and a chaperon.

9.3.1 Instruction to Standardized Patient (SP)

Biodata

Name: MB	Tribe: Kanuri
Age: 25 years	Religion: Islam
Address: Mairi village, Maiduguri	Education: Ordinary diploma in accounting
Occupation: Banker	Marital status: Single

Presenting Complaint
I am a diabetic and want to get married soon.

History of Presenting Complaint
I am 25 years old and was diagnosed diabetic when I was 15 years old and currently on mixed insulin 20 units before breakfast and 10 units before dinner. I am conversant with the use of glucometer and inject myself daily. My fasting glucose this morning was 7 mmol/L. I am planning to get married soon, and the endocrinologist referred me to see the gynaecologist. That's why I came. I have no other complaint.

PMH
I was treated for urinary tract infection three times this year with Augmentin injections and tablets. I have not been operated on before and I have no drug allergies.

Gynaecological History
I started seeing my menses when I was 13 years of age and I menstruate for 4 days in a month. I use 2–3 sanitary pads a day during menses and do not experience pains with menses. I occasionally have sexual intercourse with my fiancé and we use the male condom for preventing pregnancy. I have never been pregnant and my last menstrual period was 2 weeks ago. I did a Pap smear 6 months ago, and the result was negative.

Obstetric History
I have never conceived.

Family and Social History
I am the second of four children of my parents and all of us are alive and well. My mother is a diabetic and being managed by the same endocrinologist looking after me. There is no family history of hypertension or sickle cell disease. I occasionally take beer and smoke three sticks of cigarette a day. I am engaged to be married to a university lecturer in the next 6 weeks.

Systemic Review
I have no complaints.

9.3.2 Instruction to the Candidate

Miss MB is a 25-year-old nullipara who is a known type 1 diabetic. She is planning to get married, and her endocrinologist referred her to the preconception clinic.

Your task: Take her history.

9.3.3 Instruction to the Examiners

The patient is a 25-year known type 1 diabetic on insulin who is planning to get married. She has been referred by her endocrinologist to the preconception clinic. She is irregular with her follow-up, and her glucose level is poorly controlled. She smokes cigarettes and occasionally takes alcohol.

The candidate is supposed to take her history in the preconception clinic. Use the checklist below to mark the candidate.

Checklist for history of a diabetic

Task	Well done	Fairly done	Poorly done	Not done
Greets patient, introduces self and obtains permission	4	2	1	0
Take Biodata: name, age, address, occupation, marital status	4	2	1	0
Parity, LMP		2		0
Presenting complaints: referred for preconception care		2		**0**
History of presenting complaint:				
- Known type 1 diabetic for 10 years.		2		0
- On insulin; mixtard 20 IU morning, 10 IU evening		2		0
- Checks FBS weekly		2		0
- FBS today 7mmol/L		2		0
- Treated for UTI x 3 this year.		2		0
- Pap smear 6 months ago negative		2		0
PMH as above, no previous surgery, no drug allergy		2		0
Family and social history				
- Mother diabetic		2		0
- In courtship, engaged.		2		0
- Sexually active, uses male condoms.		2		0
- Smokes 3 sticks of cigarette a day		2		0
- Drinks alcohol occasionally		2		0
Summary of history	4	2	1	0
Communication skill	4	2	1	0
Total score	44			
Candidate's score .../44				

Examiner Date

9.4 Station 9.4 Preconception Counselling of a Diabetic Woman

Subject: Obstetrics.
Theme: Preconception counselling.
Domain of clinical competence: Communication and counselling.
Station: Preconception counselling of a diabetic woman preparing for pregnancy.
Station objective: To test the candidate's ability to counsel a diabetic woman with the aim of obtaining euglycaemia as well as eliminating the risk factors for poor pregnancy outcome in the mother.
Requirements: Standardized patient (role player), a comfortable chair or a dressed bed for the role player, a chair for the candidate (counsellor), a table and two chairs for the examiners, pencils and erasers, plain papers for use by the candidate, enough copies of the checklist for examiners, and a chaperon.

9.4.1 Instruction to the Candidate

Give a summary of the patient you clerked on the last station.

How would you counsel the patient you clerked?

9.4.2 Instruction to the Examiners

The candidate has clerked a 25-year-old known type 1 diabetic who is nulliparous and is planning to get married soon. She was referred to the preconception clinic by her endocrinologist. She has been infrequent in her visits to diabetic clinic, and her blood sugar is poorly controlled with a FBS 7 mmol/L today on 20:10 IU mixtard insulin. She smokes about three sticks of cigarettes a day and occasionally takes alcohol.

The candidate is supposed to counsel her on her condition before she gets pregnant. Use the checklist below to score the candidate.

Checklist for post encounter to diabetic

Task	Well done	Fairly done	Poorly done	Not done
Summary of the patient to include the following information:				
- 25-year-old known type 1 diabetic		2	1	0
- Nullipara, hoping to get pregnant soon.		2	1	0
- Referred to the preconception clinic by an endocrinologist.		2	1	0
- On insulin; mixtard 20 IU mornings and 10 IU evenings		2	1	0
- Poorly controlled blood sugar; FBS 7mmol/L today		2	1	0
- Smokes 3 sticks of cigarette daily		2	1	0
- Occasionally takes alcohol		2	1	0
Introduction: outlines issues to be addressed:				
- The need to control diabetes before pregnancy.		2	1	0
- Dangers of alcohol and smoking in pregnancy		2	1	0
- Need for multidisciplinary management.		2	1	0
- Necessary investigations; HbA1C, 4-point blood sugar etc.		2	1	0
To stop smoking because of:				
- Risk of miscarriage, IUGR, IUFD, SB		2	1	0
- Risk of ischaemic heart disease		2	1	0
- Risk of peripheral vascular disease		2	1	0
- Risk of respiratory disease including lung cancer		2	1	0
To stop alcohol consumption because:				
- Affects blood sugar control.		2	1	0
- Affects the fetus adversely.		2	1	0
- No safe level of alcohol in pregnancy		2	1	0
Need to start folic acid because:				
- Reduces risk of neural tube defects		2		0
- Improves haemoglobin level		2		0
To be screened for some infections; HIV, Rubella, Syphilis, HBV, HCV	4	2	1	0
Urine MCS, IVU may suggest need for prophylactic antibiotics in pregnancy	4	2	1	0
HbA1C, 4-point blood sugar to guide adjustment of insulin dosage and regimen	4	2	1	0
Routine prenatal investigations; FBC, Hb genotype, blood grouping,		2	1	0
Adherence counselling for optimal control	4	2	1	0
Communication skills	4	2	1	0
Total score	60			
Candidate's score .../60				

Examiner's signature Date

9.5 Station 9.5 History Taking of a Sickle Cell Disease Patient

Subject: Obstetrics.
Theme: Preconception care.
Domain of clinical competence: History taking.
Station: Focused history taking of a sickle cell disease patient planning pregnancy.
Station objective: To assess the candidate's ability to take a focused history of a patient with sickle cell disease with the aim of optimizing her health to carry pregnancy with good outcome.
Requirements: Standardized patient (SP), instructions to the SP, instructions to the candidate, instructions to the examiners, a dressed bed for the SP (Fig. 9.2). A table and chairs for the examiners, sufficient checklists, pencils and erasers, a plain sheet for candidate's use, and a chaperon.

9.5.1 Instructions to the Standardized Patient

Biodata

Name: SS	Tribe: Kilba
Age: 24 years	Religion: Christian
Address: Uba, Adamawa state	Educational status: Tertiary
Occupation: Secondary school teacher	Marital status: Married

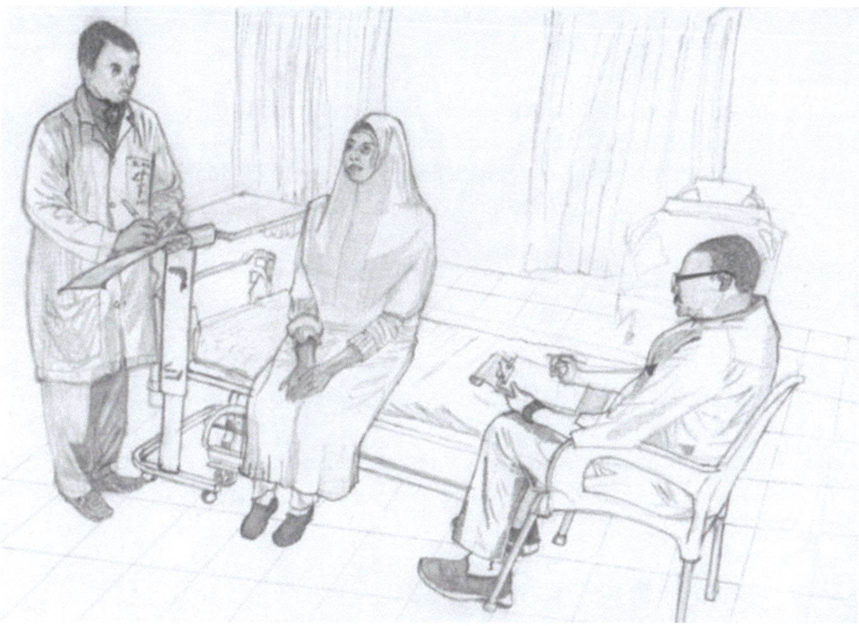

Fig. 9.2 History taking during OSCE examination. Courtesy of Jonathan Edache Otache

Presenting Complaints
I was referred by my doctor to see a gynaecologist when I got married.

History of Presenting Complaint
I am a 24-year-old sickle cell disease patient diagnosed since childhood. I have been attending sickle cell disease clinic at Mubi General Hospital since I was a child. I was placed on folic acid and paludrine tablets which I take daily. I used to have recurrent joint swelling and pain when I was a child which led to my diagnosis, as I grew up the frequency of crisis reduced and now, I occasionally experience bone-pain crisis, the last episode of crisis was more than a year ago. I do not have any bony deformity or sores on my body. On average, my Hb is 7–8 g/dL. When I got married my doctor asked me to see a gynaecologist before I get pregnant, and this is why I have come.

Gynaecological History
I attained menarche at the age of 15 years and menstruate for 2–3 days in a cycle length of 30–32 days. The menstrual flow is moderate and associated with mild lower abdominal pains. I am aware of modern methods of family planning but have never used any. I got married 3 months ago, and my husband is my only life-time sexual partner.

Obstetric History
I have never had sexual intercourse before marriage, and I desire to get pregnant soon.

Past Medical and Surgical History
Have been admitted severally at General Hospital Mubi for bone-pain crisis; the last episode was more than 1 year ago. No previous surgery.

Family and Social History
I am the second of four children of my parents: two males and two females. My younger brother is also a sickle cell disease patient. None of my parents is a sickler. I am the only wife of my husband who is a lecturer with Federal Polytechnic Mubi. I teach geography at the Government Secondary School, Mubi. I do not smoke cigarette or drink alcohol.

Systemic Review
I have no complaints today.

9.5.2 Instructions to the Candidate

This couple have been married for only 3 months. They have come to the preconception clinic. Your task is to take the history of the woman to the hearing of the examiners.

9.5.3 Instruction to the Examiners

The candidate has been instructed to take the history of this woman who is a known sicker, married 3 months ago, and is planning to get pregnant, use the checklist provided to score the candidate.

Checklist for history of a sickler

Tasks	**Well done**	**Fairly done**	**Poorly done**	**Not done**
Greets the patient and introduces self		2	1	0
Explains purpose of interaction and obtains permission		2	1	0
Obtains biodata: name, age, address, occupation, tribe, etc.	4	2	1	0
Parity, LMP		2	1	0
Presenting complaint – referred to see a gynaecologist		2		0
History of presenting complaint				
- When did she get married?		2		0
- Why were you advised to see a gynaecologist?		2		0
- When were you diagnosed Sickler?		2		0
- What medications are you taking?		2		0
- How often do you have crisis?		2		0
- When was the last crisis?		2		0
- Any bony deformity?		2		0
- Any chronic ulcer?		2		0
- What is your average Hb or PCV?		2		0
Gynae history: menarche, periods, cycles, flow, contraception, etc.	4	2	1	0
Obstetric history - nulligravida		2		0
PMH: as above, no previous surgery		2		0
Systemic review: no fever, no body pains, no urinary symptom		2	1	0
Summarizes history of the patient to examiners	4	2	1	0
Penalties: not sequential, poor rapport, inaudible,	-4	-2	-1	0
Total marks	44			
Candidate's score .../44				

Examiner's signature Date

9.6 Station 9.6 Preconception Counselling of a Patient with Renal Transplant

Subject: Obstetrics.
Theme: Preconception care.
Domain of clinical competence: Communication and counselling.
Station: Preconception counselling of a patient with renal transplant.
Station objective: To test the candidate's ability to counsel a woman who had renal transplant, in order to optimize her for a successful pregnancy outcome.
Requirements: A standardized patient, a comfortable chair or dressed bed for the patient, a chair for the candidate, plain paper for use by the candidate, a table and two chairs for the examiners, pencils and erasers, enough copies of the checklist, and a chaperon.

9.6.1 Instructions to the Role Player

I am a 24-year-old married woman who had chronic renal disease in childhood. At the age of 18, I started receiving regular dialysis until the age of 21 when I had renal transplant in a hospital in the United Kingdom. The kidney was donated by one of my brothers.

The transplant was successful, and I was placed on prednisolone and azathioprine tablets to prevent rejection. I am also taking atenolol for hypertension. I have been doing well since the transplant. I started menses at the age of 16 and menstruates for 3 days in a regular cycle of 28–30 days. I stopped seeing my menses for about 6 months after the surgery, otherwise my cycles have been regular. I have not had a Pap smear even though I am aware of the need.

I am the last and fourth child of my parents. My father is a general in the Nigerian Army, and I was married to a Captain in the Nigerian Army last year. My husband has been supportive to me. I do not take alcoholic beverages or smoke cigarettes.

The doctor who has been looking after me (Nephrologist) has referred me to the gynaecologist because I am planning to get pregnant.

9.6.2 Instruction to the Candidate

Mrs. EG is a 24-year-old married woman who had renal transplant in the United Kingdom 3 years ago. She got married to an army Captain last year and she wants to try getting pregnant. Her nephrologist has referred her to the preconception clinic.

Your task is to counsel her for optimization for pregnancy.

9.6.3 Instruction to the Examiners

The patient is a 24-year-old P0+0 who had renal transplant 3 years ago. She was referred to the gynaecologist because she is planning to get pregnant. The candidate is supposed to counsel her for optimization before getting pregnant. Use the checklist provided to score the candidate.

Checklist for preconception counselling following renal transplant

Task	Well done	Fairly done	Poorly done	Not done
Greets patient, introduces self and obtains permission to discuss her health issue	4	2	1	0
Introduces the subject matter; I understand you had renal transplant, and you are planning to get pregnant ………	4	2	1	0
Parity, LMP		2	1	0
Past medical history:				
- Type and duration of renal disease		2	1	0
- Where transplant was done, post-surgery drugs.		2	1	0
- Who is the Nephrologist looking after.		2	1	0
- Current medications		2	1	0
- Last investigations (RFTs) whether they are normal or not		2	1	0
Ask patient what implications of pregnancy she knows		2		0
Pre-pregnancy advice:				
- Should not be pregnant within 2 years of surgery to avoid risk of rejection.		2		0
- Pregnancy advisable only when HT is controlled and RFT are normal.		2		0
- Switch atenolol to labetalol or aldomet to avoid IUGR.		2		0
- To start folic acid to reduce risk of congenital anomalies		2		0
Ask patient if she needs further clarification		2		0
Explain the risk of pregnancy in renal transplant:				
- Risk of rejection 2-5%		2		0
- Risk of developing PIH 30%		2		0
- Risk of IUGR 1/3 of cases		2		0
- Risk of preterm delivery 50%		2		0
Investigations to guide further action:				
- E/U/Cr		2		0
- MSU for urinalysis and MCS		2		0
- 24-hour urinary protein and creatinine		2		0
- Pap smear due to immunosuppression		2		0
Ask patient for clarifications if any		2		0
Thank patient for coming and give appointment to see with results of investigation	4	2	1	0
Communication skills	4	2	1	0
Total score	58			
Candidate's score …/58				

Examiner's signature Date

Antenatal Care OSCE Stations 10

10.1 Station 10.1 Managing Pre-Eclampsia with Renal Transplant

Subject: Obstetrics.
Theme: Antenatal care.
Domain of clinical competence: Interpretation of abnormal test finding.
Station: Managing pre-eclampsia in a patient with renal transplant.
Station objective: To assess the candidate's ability to manage pregnancy complication in a patient with renal transplant for the purpose of obtaining a healthy mother and baby.
Requirements: Standardized patient, dressed bed for standardized patient, a chaperon to attend to the patient, a chair for the candidate, plain papers for use by the candidate, a table and two chairs for.

10.1.1 Instruction to the Candidate

The patient with renal transplant (station 1.6) eventually got pregnant and booked for antenatal care. At 30 weeks gestation, she was admitted into the antenatal ward with pre-eclampsia. You are the registrar on call and have been called by the midwife to come and review her with some investigation results which were earlier requested that day. When you saw her, her BP170/110 mmHg, PCV 21%, platelets 40, ALT 460, AST 360, proteinuria 3+, and creatinine 260umol/L: Answer the questions which follow to the examiners.

1. What is your diagnosis?
2. Outline your emergency intervention
3. How would you subsequently manage her?

C. Chama, *OSCE and VIVA VOCE in Obstetrics and Gynaecology*,
https://doi.org/10.1007/978-3-031-77262-7_10

10.1.2 Instructions to the Examiners

The patient is a 24-year-old primigravida at 30 weeks of gestation who was admitted earlier today with the working diagnosis of pre-eclampsia. She had renal transplant 3 years ago in the United Kingdom. Some investigation results have just been retrieved, and the candidate is supposed to review her with the results. The results show severe hypertension with proteinuria, low PCV and platelets, and elevated liver enzymes. He is specifically to make a diagnosis, outline emergency intervention and how he would subsequently manage the patient. Use the score sheet provided to mark the candidate's performance.

Answer Outline

1. The diagnosis **(2 marks each)**
   (a) HELLP syndrome
   (b) Complicating severe pre-eclampsia
2. Immediate interventions include **(2 marks each)**
   (a) Set an IVL access
   (b) Give loading dose of MgSO4 according to protocol
   (c) Give IV hydralazine or labetalol according to protocol
   (d) Send blood specimen for grouping and cross matching of 4 units of fresh whole blood
   (e) Transfer to labour ward
3. Subsequent management **(2 marks each)**
   (a) Contact your consultant, haematologist, neonatologist, nephrologist, and anaesthesiologist
   (b) Book theatre for EMCS
   (c) Counsel patient for the procedure; informing her the foetus is unlikely to survive at this gestational age
   (d) Spinal anaesthesia not suitable due to risk of bleeding
   (e) Will require hydrocortisone cover during CS
   (f) Close monitoring of renal functions post-op

Checklist for HELLP syndrome

Task	Well done	Fairly done	Poorly done	Not done
Diagnosis: - HELLP syndrome - Complicating PE in renal transplant		 2 2		 0 0
Immediate intervention - Set IVL - Give loading dose of MgSO4 according to protocol. - Give IV hydralazine or labetalol according to protocol. - Urgent PCV, grouping and cross matching of 4 pints fresh whole blood - Transfer to labour ward		 2 2 2 2 2 2		 0 0 0 0 0 0
Subsequent management - Request for FBC, LFT, EUC - IM dexamethasone 12mg - Contact your consultant, haematologist, neonatologist, nephrologist, anaesthesiologist. - Book theatre for EMCS - Counsel patient for the procedure; poor prognosis for the baby - Spinal anaesthesia not suitable due to bleeding - Will require hydrocortisone during CS. - Monitor RF postoperatively		 2 2 2 2 2 2 2 2	 1 1 1 1 1 1 1 1	 0 0 0 0 0 0 0 0
Routine postoperative management - IVF nutrition - Analgesia - Antibiotics - Input and output chart		 2 2 2 2		 0 0 0 0
Before discharge - Counsel on prognosis of subsequent pregnancy (poorer) - The need for nephrology and haematology follow-up - Give appointment for PNC		 2 2 2		 0 0 0
Total score	46			
Candidate's score .../46				

Examiner's signature   Date

10.2 Station 10.2 Counselling a Mother with Twin Gestation

Subject: Obstetrics.
Theme: Antenatal care.
Domain of clinical competence: Communication and counselling.
Station: Counselling a pregnant woman with twin gestation.
Station objective: To test the candidate's ability to counsel a twin-carrying mother to understand the risks of twin gestation and how to cope with the pregnancy and delivery.
Requirements: Standardized patient (or real mother carrying twin pregnancy), a comfortable chair or dressed bed for the patient, a chair for the candidate, plain papers for use by the candidate, a table and two chairs for the examiners, enough copies of the checklist, pencils and erasers, some charts of twin gestation may be useful if available.

10.2.1 Instructions to the Role Player

I am carrying my third pregnancy, having had two previous normal deliveries, both of them boys and alive and well. The last childbirth was 2 years ago, and both previous pregnancies were supervised in the General Hospital, Damaturu. I have been referred to the Teaching Hospital for antenatal care in this pregnancy because I am carrying twins this time around.

I am the only wife of my husband who is a lecturer with the Federal Polytechnic Damaturu. I am also a graduate in English language and teaches in the staff school of the same institution. I neither smoke cigarettes nor drink alcoholic beverages.

Although I have carried two pregnancies before, I am concerned about this one as to:

- What additional things do I need to do?
- What are the risks of twin gestation?
- Would I be able to deliver the twins normally like the previous pregnancies?

10.2.2 Instructions to the Candidate

Mrs. RA is a 32-year booked G3P2+0 A2 who was earlier referred to this hospital for antenatal care due to twin gestation. She has had two previous normal vaginal deliveries. An early ultrasound in this pregnancy showed dichorionic, diamniotic (DCDA) twins at 16 weeks gestation. She is now 20 weeks pregnant and has come for follow-up. She has some concerns about twin pregnancy she would like to discuss with you.

Your task is to counsel her concerning her fears.

10.2.3 Instruction to the Examiners

The patient is a 32-year-old G3P2+0 A2 who is currently carrying twin pregnancy. She has come for antenatal follow-up and would like to share some concerns about twin pregnancy with the doctor. She is particularly concerned about what additional things she needs to do in this pregnancy, the risks of twin pregnancy and whether she would be able to deliver normally like her two previous pregnancies. The candidate is supposed to counsel her concerning her fears. Use the check list provided to score the candidate.

Checklist for counselling on twin gestation

Task	Well done	Fairly done	Poorly done	Not done
Greets patient, introduces self and obtains permission to talk about her pregnancy	4	2	1	0
Obtains her Biodata: name, age, address, occupation, education etc.	4	2	1	0
Obtains her Parity, LMP, EDD, GAD		2	1	0
Introduces the discussion and asks the patient about her concerns		2	1	0
Allows patient to express her concerns		2		0
Addresses additional things she needs to do:				
- Be more faithful with taking antenatal drugs		2		0
- Need for more rest, may require additional support		2		0
Explains maternal risks of twin pregnancy:				
- Exaggerated pregnancy symptoms		2		0
- APH possible due to placenta praevia		2		0
- Medical conditions; pre-eclampsia, anaemia, DM, etc.		2		0
Allows patient to ask questions or seek clarification		2		0
Explains fetal risks of twin pregnancy:				
- Risk of miscarriages higher		2		0
- Perinatal morbidity due to preterm delivery, IUGR, etc.		2		0
- Perinatal death due to prematurity, congenital anomalies		2		0
Explains intrapartum risks; increased operative delivery, trauma to baby	4	2	1	0
Postpartum risks; PPH, breastfeeding problems, maternal depression	4	2	1	0
PROMPT (patient asks): am I going to deliver normally?				
- Depends on absence of complications and presentation of first twin.		2		0
- Experts are available to attend to you.		2		0
- Most twins are delivered vaginally but CS rate is higher		2		0
Thanks patient for coming to discuss with him, gives her appointment		2		0
Communication skills	4	2	1	0
Total score	52			
Candidate's score .../52				

Examiner's signature Date

10.3 Station 10.3 Managing a Patient with Intrauterine Foetal Death (IUFD) of One Twin

Subject: Obstetrics.
Theme: Antenatal care.
Domain of clinical competence: Communication and counselling—breaking bad news.
Station: Management of IUFD of one twin.
Station objective: To test the candidate's ability to manage a mother carrying twin gestation with intrauterine death of one twin before term with the aim of achieving delivery of a viable co-twin.
Requirements: Standardized patient, a comfortable chair or dressed bed for the patient, a chair for the candidate, plain papers for use by the candidate, a table and 2 chairs for the examiners, pencils and erasers, and a chaperon to attend to the patient.

10.3.1 Instruction to the Candidate

The patient you counselled on the last station presents at 34 weeks gestation for follow-up and was found to have IUFD of the first twin on ultrasound scan. Outline your management of the patient.

10.3.2 Instruction to the Examiners

The patient is a booked G3P2+0 A2 carrying DCDA twins confirmed by ultrasound scan at 16 weeks. She has come for follow-up at 34 weeks gestation and found to have IUFD of the first twin. The candidate is supposed to outline his line of management of the patient. Use the checklist provided to score the candidate.

Answer Outline

1. Tactfully breaks the bad news to the patient **(4 marks)**
2. Reassures her everything will be done to save the co-twin **(4 marks)**
3. Request for investigations **(2 marks each)**
   (a) Antenatal CTG
   (b) Obstetric USS to confirm diagnosis
   (c) PCV, cross matching of 2 units of whole blood
   (d) Plasma fibrinogen and fibrin degradation products
4. Since pregnancy is DCDA, the co-twin is unlikely to be lost but is at risk of preterm delivery and neurological deficit occurs in <1% of cases **(4 marks)**
5. If the CTG is reactive, manage conservatively and deliver co-twin at term **(4 marks)**
6. Coagulopathy is rare and if occurs will resolve spontaneously **(4 marks)**
7. Immediate delivery only necessary if the CTG is abnormal **(4 marks)**

Total marks …/32

Checklist for management of IUFD of one twin

Task	Well done	Fairly done	Poorly done	Not done
Greets the mother and introduces self		2	1	0
Tactfully break the bad news to the mother or couple	4	2	1	0
Allows the mother a moment to absorb the shock		2		0
Reassures the mother everything will be done to save the co-twin		2		0
Request for investigations: - Obstetric USS to confirm diagnosis. - Antenatal CTG - PCV, group and cross match 2 units of whole blood - Plasma fibrinogen and fibrin degradation products		 2 2 2 2		 0 0 0 0
Explains that since pregnancy is DCDA, the cotwin is not likely to be affected but is at risk of preterm delivery	4	2	1	0
If CGT is reactive, manage conservatively and deliver at term		2		0
Coagulopathy is rare and if it occurs resolves spontaneously		2		0
Immediate delivery is only necessary if the CTG is abnormal	4	2	1	0
Allows the mother to ask any questions		2	1	0
Admits mother to antenatal ward for close observation	4	2	1	0
Total score	36			
Candidate's score .../36				

Examiner's signature Date

10.4 Station 10.4 Obstetric Examination to Detect Intrauterine Growth Restriction (IUGR) (Fig. 10.1)

Subject: Obstetrics.
Theme: Antenatal care.
Domain of clinical competence: Physical examination.
Station: Abdominal examination to detect intrauterine growth restriction.
Station objective: To test the candidate's ability to detect intrauterine growth restriction based on correlating the findings on obstetric examination and the dates of the patient.
Requirements: Standardized patient, dressed bed for the patient, a chair for the candidate, tape measure in centimetres, Pinnard's stethoscope, plain papers for use by the candidate, a table and two chairs for the examiners, enough copies of the checklist, pencils and erasers, and a chaperon to attend to the patient.

10.4.1 Instruction to the Role Player

I am carrying my first pregnancy, which I booked for antenatal care (ANC) at 14 weeks gestation. I had ultrasound scan at 16 weeks gestation, which confirmed the gestational age and the fact that I am carrying a single foetus. Even though the size of my pregnancy is 28 weeks and is compatible with my dates, for the purpose of this examination, I assume that I saw my menses 1 month earlier than my true LMP; I am therefore to assume I am 32 weeks pregnant. There has been no problem with the pregnancy since I booked for ANC, and I have been regular with my appointments.

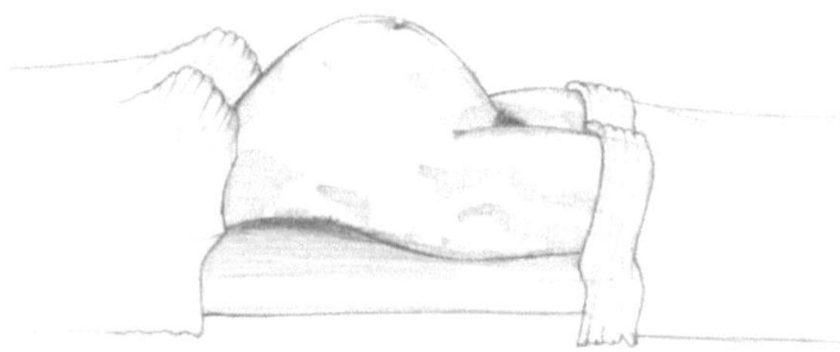

Fig. 10.1 Appropriate exposure for obstetric examination. Courtesy of Jonathan Edache Otache

10.4.2 Instruction to the Candidate

Mrs. HB is a booked primigravida who presents to the ANC for follow-up at a gestational age of 32 weeks. An ultrasound dating done at 16 weeks was compatible with her dates. Your task is to examine her abdomen.

10.4.3 Instruction to the Examiner

The patient provided is 32 weeks pregnant, but her SFH is 28 cm. The candidate is supposed to examine her abdomen in order to detect intrauterine growth restriction. Use the checklist provided to score the candidate.

Checklist for abdominal examination for IUGR

Task	Well done	Fairly done	Poorly done	Not done
Greets patient		2		0
Introduces self		2		0
Takes permission to examine patient		2		0
Asks patient to lie down and expose her abdomen as he assists her	4	2	1	0
On inspection - Abdominal enlargement - Moves with respiration. - Linear nigra - Striae gravidarum		 2 2 2 2		 0 0 0 0
On palpation - Asks for area of tenderness. - Light palpation sequentially - Deep palpation-liver, spleen, kidneys		 2 2 2		 0 0 0
Obstetric palpation - Correct measurement of SFH in cm, correlates with GAD. - Lie of the fetus - Presentation of the fetus - Position of the fetus - Attitude of the fetus - Descent of PP in fifths above pelvic brim		 2 2 2 2 2 2		 0 0 0 0 0 0
Auscultation - Chooses the correct quadrant. - FHR synchronized with maternal pulse		 2 2		 0 0
Asks the patient to lie on her side		2		0
Thanks the patient and covers her appropriately		2		0
Gives a summary of his findings	4	2	1	0
Communication skill – audible, gentle, eye contact, interactive	4	2	1	0
Maximum score	52			
Candidate's score .../52				
Weighted score				

Examiner's name and signature Date

10.5 Station 10.5 Management of IUGR

Subject: Obstetrics.
Theme: Antenatal care.
Domain of clinical competence: Diagnostic and therapeutic skill.
Station: Management of a patient with intrauterine growth restriction.
Station objective: To test the candidate's ability to manage a patient with intrauterine growth restriction before term with the aim of delivering the baby when the risk of intrauterine life outweighs the risk of extrauterine survival.
Requirements: Clearly written questions addressing the findings on the last station, may be laminated to prevent staining and squeezing, plain papers as answer sheets to be used by the candidates, a chair for the candidate, a table and two chairs for the examiners, marking scheme for the examiners, and pencils and erasers.

10.5.1 Instruction to the Candidate

1. Give a summary of your findings on the last station
2. What is your diagnosis?
3. What are the possible causes of the condition?
4. Give 5 relevant investigations you would request
5. When would you deliver the patient?

10.5.2 Instruction to the Examiners

The candidate examined a patient with IUGR on the last station. He is supposed to give a summary of his findings on the last station and answer the questions that follow. Use the marking scheme provided to score the candidate.

Answers

1. Good summary (**4 marks**) poor summary (**2 marks**)
2. Diagnosis IUGR (**4 marks**)
3. Possible causes of the IUGR
   (a) Maternal (**maximum of 3 = 6 marks**)
   - Constitutional
   - Malnutrition
   - Medical disorders—HT, RF, collagen disorders, HD, anaemia
   - Toxins—alcohol, smoking, cocaine

   (b) Foetal (**maximum of 3 = 6 marks**)
   - Structural anomalies like CV or renal
   - Chromosomal anomalies like trisomies
   - Infections—TORCH
   - Multiple pregnancy

   (c) Placental (**maximum of 3 = 6 marks**)
      - Praevia
      - Abruption
      - Circumvallate
      - Infarction
      - Mosaicism
   (d) Idiopathic in 40% of cases (**4 marks**)
4. Relevant investigations (**maximum of 5 = 10 marks**)
   (a) FBC
   (b) EUC
   (c) USS growth assessment
   (d) CTG
   (e) Biophysical profile
   (f) Doppler USS
   (g) Foetal kick count
5. Time of delivery
   (a) At 34 weeks for severe IUGR if maternal and foetal conditions are stable (**4 marks**)
   (b) At 37 weeks for mild IUGR (**4 marks**)
   (c) Immediately if (**maximum of 3 = 6 marks**)
      - Foetal demise is imminent
      - Foetus not growing
      - Congenital anomaly
      - Maternal organ failure

Checklist for management of IUGR

Task	Well done	Fairly done	Poorly done	Not done
Summary of the history (Max 10 marks):				
- Mrs. Hajara Bitrus is 22 years old.		2		0
- Primigravida		2		0
- Ultrasound at 16 weeks gestation compatible with dates		2		0
- At 32 weeks of gestation today and		2		0
- SFH is 28cm which is small for gestational age.		2		0
- The pregnancy has been uneventful		2		0
The diagnosis is intrauterine growth restriction, IUGR	4			0
Possible causes of IUGR				
- Maternal; constitutional, medical disorders, toxins, malnutrition	4	2	1	0
- Fetal; chromosomal, structural anomalies, infections (TORCH), multiple gestation	4	2	1	0
- Placental; infarction, circumvallate, praevia, mosaicism.	4	2	1	0
- Idiopathic (40% of cases)	4	2	1	0
Relevant investigations				
- FBC to rule out maternal anaemia or sepsis.		2	1	0
- EUC to rule out maternal renal disease.		2	1	0
- Screen for TORCH to rule out maternal infection.		2	1	0
- USS for growth assessment; to know degree of growth retardation.		2	1	0
- Biophysical profile/fetal doppler for fetal well being		2	1	0
Timing of delivery				
- At 34 weeks if severe IUGR		2	1	0
- At 37 weeks if mild IUGR		2	1	0
- Immediately if fetal demise imminent, fetus not growing, congenital anomaly, maternal organ failure		2	1	0
Total marks	46			
Candidate's score .../46				

Examiner's signature Date

10.6 Station 10.6 History Taking for One Previous Caesarean Section

Subject: Obstetrics.
Theme: Antenatal care.
Domain of clinical competence: History taking.
Station: History taking of a patient with one previous caesarean section.
Station objective: To assess the candidate's ability to take a focused history of an antenatal client with one previous caesarean section, who has come to book for antenatal care.
Requirements: Standardized patient or real patient, a comfortable chair or dressed bed for the patient, a table and two chairs for examiners, pencils and erasers, enough copies of the checklist, a chair for the candidate, and A4 plain papers for the candidate's jottings.

10.6.1 Instruction to the Standardized Patient

Biodata

Name: SH	Tribe: Kilba
Age: 24 years	Religion: Christianity
Address: Low-cost estate, Hong	Educational level: Tertiary
Occupation: Teacher	Marital status: Married

Presenting Complaint
I have been referred to register for antenatal care in this hospital.

Reason for booking (if the candidate asks) is one previous caesarean section.

History of Presenting Complaint
I am a 26-year-old mother carrying my second pregnancy which I have come to register for antenatal care. My last menses started on ……………; about 3 months ago. Apart from occasional nausea and vomiting which I consider normal in pregnancy, I do not have any problem with this pregnancy. My first pregnancy was 3 years ago, and I booked for antenatal care at 3 months of pregnancy at General Hospital Mubi. The pregnancy was carried to 9 months without problem, but I was delivered by a planned caesarean section because the baby was coming by the buttocks (breech presentation). I was delivered of a live male baby weighing 3.7 kg who cried immediately after delivery. The recovery period was uneventful, and I was discharged home after 3 days. I did not receive blood transfusion during or after the surgery. My baby is alive and doing well.

Obstetric History
As above.

Gynaecological History
I started to menstruate when I was 13 years old. I bleed for 3–4 days every 26–28 days. I use about three sanitary pads per day during menses and experience some lower abdominal discomfort the first day of the menses. I am aware of modern methods of family planning but have not seen the need to use any yet. I did a Pap smear in this hospital 2 years ago after a health talk in my church and it turned out to be negative.

Past Medical and Surgical History
Apart from the CS earlier discussed, I do not have any medical condition and do not have any drug allergy.

Family and Social History
I do not smoke or drink alcohol. I have never been diagnosed to have hypertension, diabetes, or sickle cell disease, and none of my close relatives have such conditions. I am the only wife of my husband who is a civil engineer with a private firm. I hold a master's degree in English language and currently teach in a Federal Government College.

Systemic Review
I have no other complaint today.

10.6.2 Instruction to the Candidate

Mrs. SH has come to book for antenatal care in this hospital. Your task is to take her history.

10.6.3 Instructions to the Examiners

The patient is a 26-year-old G2P1+0A1 who has come to book for antenatal care. She had elective caesarean section at terms due to breech presentation in her last pregnancy. The candidate is expected to take a focused history in a case of previous caesarean section coming to book for antenatal care. Use the checklist provided to score the candidate.

Checklist for history taking of a previous CS

Task	Well done	Fairly done	Poorly done	Not done
Greets patient, introduces self and gets consent	4	2	1	0
Biodata – name, age, address, education, occupation	4	2	1	0
Parity, LMP, EDD, GAD		2	1	0
Presenting complaint				
- I have been referred to come and book for ANC.		2		0
- Indication is one previous CS		2		0
History of presenting complaints – occasional nausea, no vomiting, no dizziness.		2		0
Obstetric history				
- Last pregnancy was 3 years ago.		2	1	0
- Received antenatal care at General Hospital Mubi		2	1	0
- Pregnancy carried to term, uneventful.		2	1	0
- Delivered by ELCS		2	1	0
- Indication for ELCS was breech presentation.		2	1	0
- Birthweight 3.7Kg, cried immediately after delivery.		2	1	0
- Recovery from surgery uneventful		2	1	0
- Child alive and well		2	1	0
Gynaecological history – menarche, period, cycle, contraception, history of pap smear	4	2	1	0
PMH/PSH – apart from above CS, nil of note		2		0
Drug history – no known drug allergy		2		0
FSH – Husband civil engineer with private firm. No family history of HT, DM, SCD. Does not smoke or take alcoholic beverages	4	2	1	0
Systemic review – nil of note		2		0
Summary of history	4	2	1	0
History not taken in sequence attracts a penalty of 4 marks	-4			
Total score	52			
Candidate's score .../52				

Examiner's signature Date

10.7 Station 10.7 Uterovaginal Prolapse in Pregnancy

Subject: Obstetrics.
Theme: Antenatal care.
Domain of clinical competence: Virtual sign identification (picture test).
Station: Picture test on uterovaginal prolapse in pregnancy.
Station objective: To test the candidate's ability to recognize uterovaginal prolapse in pregnancy and manage it with the aim of achieving safe delivery.
Requirements: A laminated picture of uterovaginal prolapse in advanced pregnancy, clearly written set of questions on uterovaginal prolapse in pregnancy, three chairs and a table for the examiners and the candidate, pencils and erasers for the examiners, enough copies of the check list or marking scheme, plain A4 papers for the candidate to answer the questions on, a chaperons to ensure the picture is not mutilated before the next candidate comes and to replenish supplies to candidate and examiners.

10.7.1 Instructions to the Candidate

A 32-year-old G8P7+0 7 alive presented to antenatal clinic at 28 weeks gestation with vaginal protrusion of 10 days duration. She did not notice vaginal protrusion prior to pregnancy or during her previous pregnancies. Vaginal examination revealed the Fig. 10.2.

1. What is the diagnosis?
2. Enumerate the possible causes of this condition

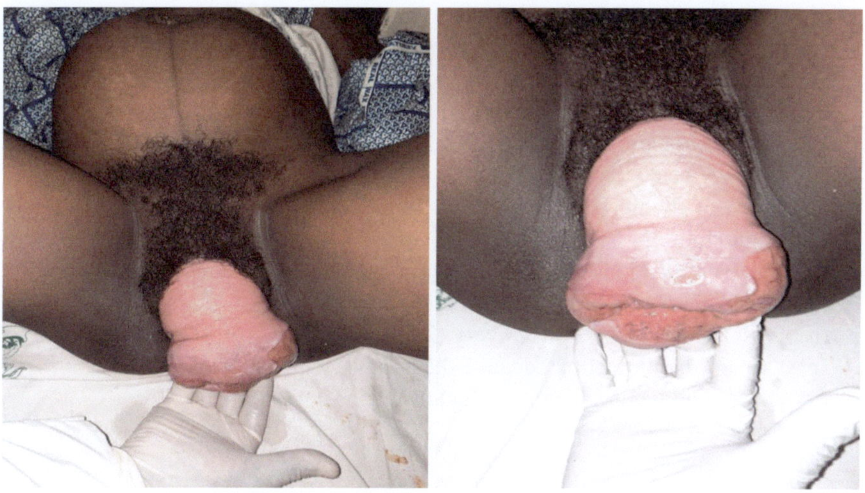

Fig. 10.2 Uterovaginal prolapse in pregnancy, Chama et al. (2020)

3. How would you manage this patient?
4. What are the possible complications you will watch out for?

10.7.2 Instructions to the Examiners

The candidate is provided with a picture showing uterovaginal prolapse in pregnancy at 28 weeks gestation. Printed below the pictures are four questions which the candidate is supposed to answer. Please study the questions and use the marking scheme provided to score the candidate.

Answer Outline

1. The diagnosis is uterovaginal prolapse in pregnancy (**4 marks**)
2. The possible causes are as follows:
   (a) Previous difficult vaginal deliveries (**max = 4 marks**)
   - A grand multipara, first delivery might have been at early age (**2 marks**)
   - Might have had instrumental vaginal delivery (**2 marks**)
   - Might have had prolonged labour (**2 marks**)

   (b) Intra-abdominal pressure (**max = 4 marks**)
   - Ovarian tumour in pregnancy (**2 marks**)
   - Uterine fibroid co-existing with pregnancy (**5 marks**)
   - Chronic cough (**2 marks**)

   (c) Congenital weakness of pelvic floor (**max = 2 marks**)
   - Connective tissue disorder as in Marfan's syndrome (**2 marks**) or Ehlers-Danlos syndrome (**2 marks**)
3. Her management could include:
   (a) Conservative (**max = 4 marks**)
   - Genital hygiene (**2 marks**)
   - Bed rest in slight Trendelenburg position (**2 marks**)
   - Use of vaginal silicone pessaries to hold the cervix in place (**2 marks**)

   (b) Surgical (**max = 4 marks**)
   - Caesarean section and uterine suspension at term (**2 marks**)
   - Laparoscopic suspension in early pregnancy but this patient is unsuitable at 28 weeks (**2 marks**)

   (c) Delivery should be ELCS because she is likely to have cervical dystocia (**2 marks**)
4. Possible complications to watch out for in this patient include: (**max = 6 marks**)
   (a) Sepsis because there is cervical ulceration (**2 marks**)
   (b) PPROM and premature delivery (**2 marks**)
   (c) Urinary tract infection because she has cystocele (**2 marks**)
   (d) Obstructed labour due to cervical dystocia (**2 marks**)

Total marks = 80

Checklist for uterovaginal prolapse in pregnancy

Task	Well done	Fairly done	Poorly done	Not done
Diagnosis: Uterovaginal prolapse (2) in pregnancy (2)	4	2		0
Possible causes				
- previous difficult vaginal delivery (2) as in obstructed labour, instrumental deliveries, grandmultipara (2)		2	1	0
- intra-abdominal pressure (2) as in fibroids in pregnancy, ovarian tumor in pregnancy, chronic cough (2)		2	1	0
- congenital weakness of pelvic floor (2) as in Marfan's syndrome, Ehlers-Danlos syndrome (2)		2	1	0
The management of this patient could include:				
- conservative; genital hygiene, bed rest, vaginal pessaries		2	1	0
- surgical; ELCS at term, definitive surgery after puerperium		2	1	0
- vaginal delivery followed by definitive surgery after puerperium (cervical dystocia a risk)		2	1	0
Possible complications to watch out for include:				
- sepsis because there is cervical ulceration.		2	1	0
- PPROM and premature delivery		2	1	0
- UTI due to cystocele and kinking of ureters		2	1	0
- Obstructed labour due to cervical dystocia		2	1	0
Total score	24			
Candidate's score .../24				

Examiner's signature Date

Foetal Diagnosis and Therapy OSCE Stations

11

11.1 Station 11.1 Transvaginal Ultrasound Scan for Dating Pregnancy

Subject: Obstetrics.
Theme: Foetal diagnosis and therapy.
Domain of clinical competence: Diagnostic procedure.
Station: TVS for foetal dating.
Station objective: To test the candidate's ability to correctly perform a transvaginal ultrasound scan for the purpose of dating a first trimester pregnancy.
Requirements: Ultrasound machine with transvaginal probe, scan gel, latex gloves, half-body female mannequin, male condoms, a table or dressed bed for the mannequin, an office chair for the candidate, a table and two chairs for examiners, plain papers for reporting by candidates, sufficient checklists, pencils and erasers, and a chaperon (Fig. 11.1).

11.1.1 Instructions to the Candidate

Provided is a transvaginal ultrasound probe. Using the mannequin provided, demonstrate step by step how you would perform a transvaginal ultrasound to date a pregnant woman who present at about 10 weeks of gestation. Comment on the procedure to the hearing of the examiners, as you proceed.

11.1.2 Instructions to the Examiners

The candidate has been provided with a female mannequin and a transvaginal ultrasound probe. He is supposed to demonstrate how to perform a transvaginal ultrasound scan for dating a first trimester pregnancy. Study the checklist provided and use it to score the candidate.

C. Chama, *OSCE and VIVA VOCE in Obstetrics and Gynaecology*,
https://doi.org/10.1007/978-3-031-77262-7_11

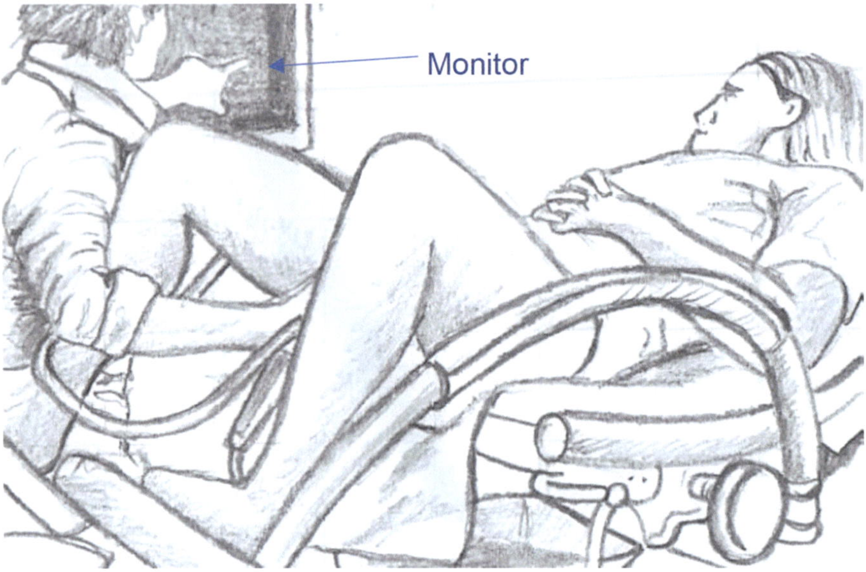

Fig. 11.1 Transvaginal ultrasound scan procedure. Courtesy of Jonathan Edache Otache

Checklist for TVS for dating pregnancy

Tasks	**Well done**	**Fairly done**	**Poorly done**	**Not done**
Greets the patient and introduces self		2	1	0
Explains the procedure and obtains permission		2	1	0
Request the chaperon to screen patient		2	1	0
Positions patient supine, knees flexed, hips flexed and abducted, foot of the bed broken (lowered at 90°)	4	2	1	0
Wears gloves, squeezes gel into condom tip, rolls it over the probe with the rolled side out.	4	2	1	0
Sets the orientation of the monitor, anterior objects on the right of screen	4	2	1	0
Applies gel to tip of probe, parts labia and introduces the probe into the vagina	4	2	1	0
Using pushing and pulling, rotational, rocking and panning movements, the following is done:	4	2	1	0
- Obtain clear view of the GS with longitudinal axis of the fetus. - Freeze the image by tapping freeze button. - Go to menu, select obstetrics, select CRL and press set. - Drag the caliper to the tip of the crown, press set, drag the second caliper to the rump and press set. - Save the measurement displayed.		2 2 2 2 2	1 1 1 1 1	0 0 0 0 0
Check the yolk sac, myometrium and adnexa for any pathology	4	2	1	0
Get longitudinal view of the cervix and measure cervical length and internal os diameter	4	2	1	0
Tell patient you are removing the probe		2		0
Press the report button to display findings		2		0
Thank patient, offer her tissue paper to clean herself		2		0
Document your report and explain to the patient, give appointment	4	2	1	0
Total marks	54			
Candidate's score .../54				

Examiner's signature Date

11.2 Station 11.2 The Quadrivalent Test

Subject: Obstetrics.
Theme: Foetal diagnosis and therapy.
Domain of clinical competence: Interpretation of abnormal test finding (IATF).
Station: Interpreting the quadrivalent test.
Station objective: To test the candidate's ability to correctly interpret the results of the quadrivalent test for the purpose of managing a pregnancy at risk of carrying a foetus with Down's syndrome.

11.2.1 Instruction to the Candidate

Mrs. JJ is a 41-year-old lawyer who is G5P1+3 who had 3 consecutive first trimester miscarriages after her first childbirth. She was seen in the booking clinic last week, and the quadrivalent test was requested. She has brought the results which is shown below:

1. What does MoM mean?
2. What does the quad test result indicate and why?
3. At what gestational age is this test done?
4. Name the most appropriate diagnostic test Mrs. JJ should be counselled to do.
5. List four complications of this test (four above)
6. What alternative test could she have done and at what gestational age to obtain a numerical risk?

Test	Result	Normal range	MoM
MSAFP	4.90	10-150 ng/mL	0.49
UE3	2.40	>4 nmol/L	0.83
Free B-hCG	56,000 IU/mL	1400–53,000 IU/mL	2.56
Inhibin A	195 pg/mL	41.0–69.0 pg/mL	1.24

11.2.2 Instruction to the Examiners

The candidate has been given the results of the quadrivalent test requested for a patient who had three consecutive first trimester miscarriages probably due to aneuploidy. The candidate is supposed to study the results and answer the questions which follow. Use the checklist provided to score the candidate as he answers the questions to your hearing.

Checklist

Tasks	**Well done**	**Fairly done**	**Poorly done**	**Not done**
What does MoM in this result mean? - Multiples of median		2		
What does the test result indicate and why? - Test result screen positive for aneuploidy (2),particularly trisomy 21 or Down's syndrome. - Because MSAFP and unconjugated estriol are low and free B-hCG and Inhibin A are high	 4 4	 2 2	 1	 0 0
The quad test is done between 14 -21 weeks of gestation		2		0
The most appropriate diagnostic test is amniocentesis		2		0
The reasons for choosing amniocentesis are: - Her age is 41 - She had 3 previous first trimester miscarriages - The quadrivalent test is positive - She is in the second trimester			 1 1 1 1	 0 0 0 0
List 4 complications of the test above - Miscarriage or pregnancy loss - Leakage of amniotic fluid or PROM - Chorioamnionitis/infection - Fetal trauma - Vaginal bleeding			 1 1 1 1 1	 0 0 0 0 0
What alternative test could she have had and at what gestational age? - Nuchal translucency measurement (2) in combination with free B-hCG and pregnancy associated plasma protein-A - Done 11-14 weeks GA or CRL45-84mm	4	2 2		0 0
Total score	28			
Candidate's score …/28				

Examiner's signature Date

11.3 Station 11.3 Chorionic Villus Sampling for Karyotyping

Subject: Obstetrics.
Theme: Foetal diagnosis and therapy.
Domain of clinical competence: Diagnostic procedure.
Station: Chorionic villus sampling for karyotyping.
Station objective: To test the candidate's ability to perform chorionic villus sampling for karyotyping, for the purpose of foetal diagnosis of sickle cell disease and further management.
Requirements: Ultrasound scanning machine with both transabdominal and transvaginal probes, a half-body female mannequin with uterus (Fig. 11.2), a table for the mannequin. A laboratory scientist, Grave's or Cusco's speculum, 20 mL syringe, 18 or 20G spinal needle, culture medium, sterile gloves, wet swabs, sponge holding forceps, checklists, pencils and erasers, and a chaperon.

11.3.1 Instructions to the Candidate

Mrs. GP is a 26-year-old primigravida and a known sickle cell disease (HbSS) patient who booked for antenatal care last week. Her husband's haemoglobin genotype is AS (HbAS). They have been counselled about the possibility of having a HbSS child and they opted for chorionic villus sampling for early diagnosis of the baby's status.

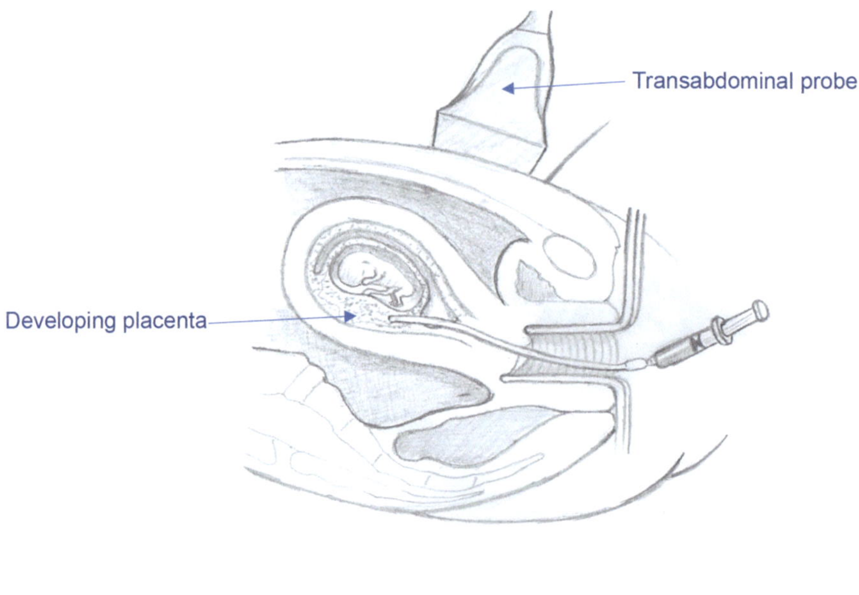

Fig. 11.2 Chorionic villus sampling procedure. Courtesy of Jonathan Edache Otache

Using the ultrasound machine provided and the female mannequin demonstrate step by step, how you would perform CVS under ultrasound guidance.

11.3.2 Instruction to the Examiners

The candidate is provided with a scenario of a 10-weeks pregnant woman who is a HbSS whose husband is HbAS carrier. The couple was counsel about the possibility of bearing a baby with sickle cell disease. The opted to have CVS to know the status of the baby and decide on further line of management.

The candidate is supposed to use the mannequin and the ultrasound machine to demonstrate how to perform CVS. Study the checklist provided and score the candidate accordingly.

Checklist for chorionic villus sampling

Tasks	Well done	Fairly done	Poorly done	Not done
Pre-procedure preparation: - Confirm HbAS in both couple. - TVS for dating and location of chorion frondosum - HVS for MCS; treat any infection		 2 2 2	 1 1 1	 0 0 0
Greets patient or couple and introduces self		2	1	0
Explains the procedure and obtains permission		2	1	0
Checks investigation results to rule out any problem		2	1	0
Scrubs, gowns and gloved		2	1	0
Patient in lithotomy position, exposes cervix with Grave's speculum	4	2	1	0
TAS to locate chorion frondosum (Future placenta) by assistant		2		0
Inserts needle through cervix to placenta under USS guidance	4	2	1	0
Removes stellate and aspirate about 1ml tissue into syringe containing culture medium	4	2	1	0
Removes needle under USS guidance, examines for cervical bleeding	4	2	1	0
Cleans and thanks patient. Reassures her and give appointment		2	1	0
Document findings, label specimen and send to the laboratory	4	2	1	0
If mother is Rh-Negative, give 50ug of ant-D globulin		2	1	0
Total marks	40			
Candidate's score .../40				

Examiner's signature Date

11.4 Station 11.4 Intrauterine Transfusion

Subject: Obstetrics.
Theme: Foetal diagnosis and therapy.
Domain of clinical competence: Therapeutic procedure.
Station: Intrauterine transfusion in alloimmunized anaemic foetus.
Station objective: To test the candidate's ability to perform intrauterine blood transfusion in a foetus showing features of moderate to severe anaemia.
Requirements: Ultrasound machine with Doppler facility, mannequin of a pregnant woman, dressed bed for the mannequin, an assistant conversant with obstetric ultrasound, a haematologist, a nurse counsellor, 23G spinal needle, washed, irradiated and packed maternal blood, 20 mL syringes, sterile gloves, sterile drapes, chlorhexidine solution, sterile gauze pack, methylated spirit, Gali pot and kidney dish, checklist, pencils and erasers, and a chaperon (Fig. 11.3).

11.4.1 Instruction to the Candidate

Mrs. AS is a booked G2P1+0 A1 who is D-negative but did not receive anti-D immunoglobin after her last delivery. She booked at 16 weeks with a positive indirect Coob's test result. Her husband is D-positive. She has been having serial MCA Doppler ultrasound scan and at 32 weeks, the peak systolic velocity was 70 cm/s which was >1.5 multiples of median for the gestational age. She is scheduled for foetal blood sampling and possible intrauterine transfusion. Using the mannequin provided, demonstrate step by step, how you would perform intrauterine transfusion on the foetus.

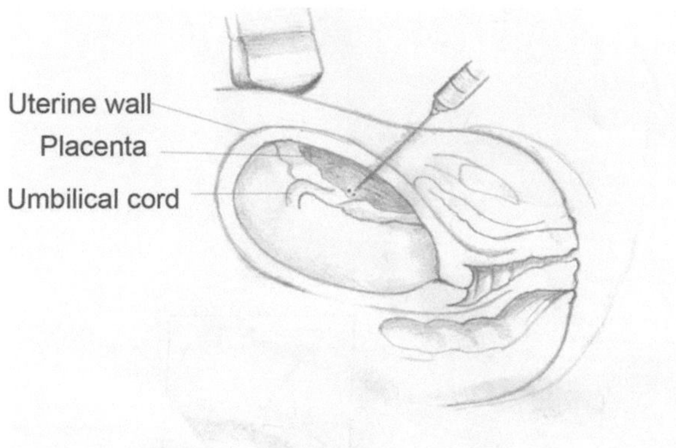

Fig. 11.3 Cordocentesis procedure. Courtesy of Jonathan Edache Otache

11.4.2 Instruction to the Examiners

The candidate has been given a scenario of a sensitized D-negative mother whose husband is D-positive. She has been followed up by serial MCA Doppler examinations and the foetus is assessed to be severely anaemic at 32 weeks gestation for which reason she has been scheduled for foetal blood sample and possible intrauterine transfusion. Using the mannequin provided, the candidate is supposed to demonstrate step by step how to conduct intrauterine blood transfusion. Observe and listen to the candidate and use the checklist provided to score his performance.

Checklist for intrauterine transfusion (Fig. 11.3)

Tasks	Well done	Fairly done	Poorly done	Not done
Greets the patient and introduces self		2	1	0
Reassures patient, explains procedure, and obtain permission		2	1	0
Switches on USS machine to boot, checks completeness of other requirements on the tray.		2	1	0
Asks chaperon to screen patient and position her supine		2	1	0
Performs USS to estimate fetal weight, locate placenta and confirm diagnosis	4	2	1	0
Explains findings to patient and further reassures her		2	1	0
Scrubs and gowns, cleans patient's abdomen, and apply sterile drape leaving window for the procedure	4	2	1	0
Infiltrates puncture site with 1% xylocaine and introduces spinal needle transplacental, to near insertion of the cord.	4	2	1	0
Bring the needle close to the umbilical vein, then advance sharply to enter the vein.	4	2	1	0
Assistant removes stylet and attaches 5ml syringe, withdraws 3ml of fetal blood for PCV, direct Coob's test, chemistry	4	2	1	0
Injects 0.1mg/Kg fentanyl to immobilize fetus		2	1	0
Calculates volume of blood needed based on EFW and fetal PCV to raise the PCV to 40-50%		2	1	0
Draw the prepared maternal blood in the 20ml syringe and slowly transfuse through the spinal needle under USS guidance	4	2	1	0
Withdraw the needle and perform USS to rule out bleeding at site of transfusion and fetal wellbeing.	4	2	1	0
Clean the mother and reposition in left lateral position		2	1	0
Write the procedure note		2	1	0
Thank the patient and give her appointment		2	1	0
Penalty: clumsy, rough, inadequate communication with patient	-4	-2		
Total marks	48			
Candidate's score .../48				

Examiner's signature Date

11.5 Station 11.5 Multifoetal Pregnancy Reduction

Subject: Obstetrics.
Theme: Foetal diagnosis and therapy.
Domain of clinical competence: Therapeutic procedure.
Station: Foetal reduction in a patient carrying quadruplet pregnancy following in vitro fertilization and embryo transfer.
Station objective: To assess the candidate's ability to perform foetal reduction in quadruplet pregnancy for the purpose of improving the pregnancy outcome.
Requirements: Full body female mannequin, dressed bed for the mannequin, ultrasound machine with Doppler facility, 22G spinal needle, 5 mL syringe and needle, a vial of 2 mE/mL KCL, sterile gloves, sterile drapes, Gali pot containing savlon solution, sterile gauze pack, sufficient checklists, pencils and erasers, a table and chairs foe examiners, and a chaperon.

11.5.1 Instructions to the Candidate

The patient is a 30-year-old primigravida carrying quadruplets following IVF-ET after a primary infertility of 6 years duration. She has been counselled and scheduled for foetal reduction to twins to improve the pregnancy outcome. Using the mannequin provided, demonstrate step by step, how you would conduct foetal reduction from quadruplets to twins. Explain the procedure to the hearing of the examiners as you proceed.

11.5.2 Instructions to the Examiners

The candidate has been given a scenario of a primigravida carrying quadruplet pregnancy following IVF-ET, who has been counselled for foetal reduction. The candidate is supposed to use the mannequin provided to demonstrate how to conduct foetal reduction. Study the checklist provided and use it score the candidate.

Checklist for multifoetal reduction

Tasks	Well done	Fairly done	Poorly done	Not done
Greets the patient and introduces self		2	1	0
Reassures patient, explains the procedure and obtains consent	4	2	1	0
Checks instrument tray to ensures all materials are available		2		0
Asks chaperon to screen patient		2		0
Performs TVS to confirm number of fetuses, chorionicity, viability, location of sacs and gross morphology	4	2	1	0
Scrubs, cleans and drapes patient with suprapubic window		2		0
Assistant opens 22G spinal needle, draws 3ml of 2mEq/ml KCL into 5ml syringe		2		0
Under USS guidance, insert spinal needle into the thorax of one of the upper fetuses, remove stellate, inject 2-3mEq of KCL and observe for asystole for several minutes	4	2	1	0
Withdraw needle and repeat procedure with a fresh needle to the other upper fetus	4	2	1	0
Confirm viability of the remaining 2 fetuses		2		0
Clean patient, reassure her, give appointment		2		0
Document procedure		2		0
Total marks	32			
Candidate's score .../32				

Examiner's signature Date

11.6 Station 11.6 Interpretation of Cardiotocograph

Subject: Obstetrics.
Theme: Foetal diagnosis and therapy.
Domain of clinical competence: Interpretation of abnormal test finding.
Station: Interpretation of abnormal CTG finding.
Station objective: To test the candidate's ability to interpret an abnormal CTG for the purpose of planning her management.
Requirements: A print out of abnormal CTG tracing, clearly written questions for the candidate, answer guide for the examiners, plain papers for use by the candidate, a table and chairs for the examiners, pencils and erasers, and a chaperon.

11.6.1 Instructions to the Candidate

A 20-year-old primigravida was referred from a Primary Health Centre (PHC) to this hospital 24 h after admission into the PHC. She was 38 weeks of gestation and had drained liquor for 2 days before going to the PHC where she had antenatal care. Vaginal examination revealed a 6 cm cervical dilatation, marked caput, and a foul-smelling liquor. No cord prolapse. Her CTG tracing is shown in Fig. 11.4.

Study the CTG tracing and answer the following questions:

1. What is your diagnosis?
2. How would you classify the abnormality on the CTG?

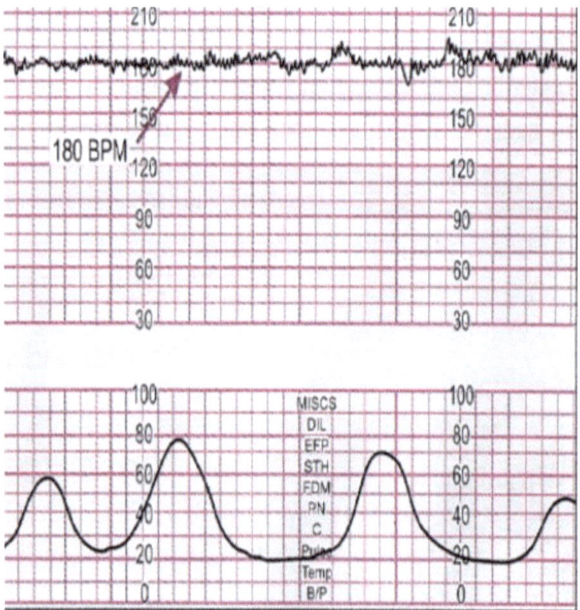

Fig. 11.4 A section of cardiotocograph (CTG)

3. List six causes of this type of abnormality.
4. Briefly outline the management of this patient.

11.6.2 Instructions to the Examiners

The candidate has been given a scenario of a primigravida referred with prolonged obstructed labour and chorioamnionitis. A print out of the patient's CTG is given, and he is supposed to interpret it and outline the management of the patient. Use the answer guide (checklist) provided to mark the candidate.

Answer Guide

1. The diagnosis is foetal tachycardia. This is defined as foetal heart rate >160 bpm, lasting 10 min or more.
2. Foetal tachycardia is divided into:
   (a) Mild foetal tachycardia → FHR 160–180 bpm.
   (b) Severe foetal tachycardia → FHR 180–200 bpm.
   (c) Ominous foetal tachycardia → FHR >200 bpm.
3. The causes of foetal tachycardia include:
   (a) Maternal medications—terbutaline, ritodrine, atropine.
   (b) Maternal/foetal infection (chorioamnionitis).
   (c) Maternal/foetal anaemia.
   (d) Maternal anxiety.
   (e) Prematurity.
   (f) Foetal movement or stimulation.
   (g) Early response to foetal hypoxia.
4. Outline of management of this patient:
   (a) Admit patient into labour ward.
   (b) Set IVL and run a litre of normal saline.
   (c) Lie patient in left lateral position.
   (d) Administer oxygen by face mask.
   (e) Give IV broad spectrum antibiotics.
   (f) Take blood sample for PCV, grouping, and cross matching.
   (g) Book for emergency caesarean section.

Checklist for interpretation of CTG

Tasks	**Well done**	**Fairly done**	**Poorly done**	**Not done**
Diagnosis: Fetal tachycardia because FHR around 180bpm.	4	2	1	0
Degree of fetal tachycardia:				
- Mild FHR 160-180bpm.		2	1	0
- Severe FHR 180-200bpm.		2	1	0
- Ominous FHR >200bpm.		2	1	0
Causes of fetal tachycardia (Max. 5):				
- Maternal medications; terbutaline, atropine.		2		0
- Maternal/fetal infection (Chorioamnionitis).		2		0
- Maternal/fetal anaemia.		2		0
- Maternal anxiety.		2		0
- Prematurity.		2		0
- Fetal hypoxia.		2		0
Outline of management:				
- Admit patient into labour ward.		2		0
- Set IVL, give 1L normal saline fast.		2		0
- Left lateral position.		2		0
- Oxygen by face mask.		2		0
- Broad spectrum antibiotics parenterally.		2		0
- PCV, grouping and cross matching.		2		0
- Book for EMCS.		2		0
Total marks	34			
Candidate's score …/34				

Examiner's signature Date

11.7 Station 11.7 Ultrasound for Growth Assessment and Foetal Well-being

Subject: Obstetrics.
Theme: Foetal diagnosis and therapy.
Domain of clinical competence: Interpretation of abnormal test finding.
Station: Interpretation of result of obstetric ultrasound for growth assessment and foetal well-being.
Station objective: To test the candidate's ability to interpret the findings of obstetric ultrasound in a patient with severe IUGR and pre-eclampsia.
Requirements: Report of the obstetric ultrasound including pictures captured, clearly written instructions to the candidate and examiners, a table and chairs for the examiners and candidates, plain papers for use by the candidates, sufficient checklists if candidates are answer verbally, a chaperon.

11.7.1 Instructions to the Candidate

Mrs. AA is a 25-year-old G2P1+0 A1 who's last childbirth was 2 years ago. She booked this pregnancy at 16 weeks gestation with a BP140/90 mmHg. She is currently 34 weeks gestation on 100 mg atenolol twice a day and BP140/90 mmHg. An obstetric ultrasound done today showed a live singleton weighing 1.1 kg and AFI 6.5 cm. The estimated foetal weight 2 weeks ago was 1.1 kg. the Doppler velocimetry of the umbilical artery is shown in Fig. 11.5.

Answer the following questions:

1. What is your diagnosis of this pregnancy?
2. What are the two most important abnormal findings on ultrasound scan today?
3. What other investigation would you request for the management of this patient?
4. When would you prefer to deliver the patient?
5. What are the options of delivery and why?

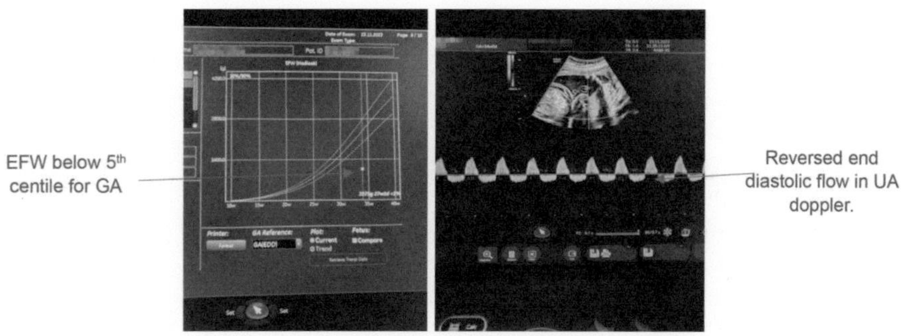

Fig. 11.5 Doppler study of umbilical artery, Chama et al. (2023)

11.7.2 Instructions to the Examiners

The candidate been given a patient who is diagnosed to have IUGR and pre-eclampsia. He has been given the result of an obstetric ultrasound done today and is supposed to study the scan report and answer the questions which follow. Use the checklist provided to score the candidate.

Answer Outline

1. The diagnosis is severe IUGR with reversed end-diastolic flow in the umbilical artery.
2. The abnormalities seen on the ultrasound report are as follows:
   (a) Severe IUGR, below one-percentile.
   (b) Reversed end-diastolic flow in umbilical artery on Doppler scan.
3. Another important investigation is CTG since the foetus is 34 weeks gestation.
4. I would like to deliver the baby immediately because it has not gained weight over the past 2 weeks and the presence of end-diastolic flow suggest increased perinatal mortality (30–40%) and cerebral palsy of about 8% among survivors compared with 1% in the normal population.
5. The options of delivery are as follows:
   (a) Induction of labour and vaginal delivery if the CTG is reactive.
   (b) Elective caesarean section if the CTG is non-reassuring.

Checklist for obstetric USS

Tasks	Well done	Fairly done	Poorly done	Not done
Diagnosis: severe IUGR (2) with reversed end-diastolic flow (2)	4	2	1	0
Important abnormalities on USS: - IUGR below one-percentile. - Reversed end-diastolic flow in umbilical artery doppler.		 2 2		 0 0
CTG is important in deciding whether the baby can withstand labour	4	2	1	0
Immediate delivery, the fetus is not growing and stands the risk of intrauterine death anytime	4	2	1	0
Options of delivery: - Induction of labour if CTG is reactive. - ELCS if CTG non-reassuring.		 2 2		 0 0
Total marks	22			
Candidate's score .../22				

Examiner's signature Date

Medical Disorders in Pregnancy OSCE Stations 12

12.1 Station 12.1 History Taking of Cardiac Disease in Pregnancy

Subject: Obstetrics.
Theme: Medical disorders in pregnancy.
Domain of Clinical Competence: History taking.
Station: Focused history of a patient with cardiac disease in pregnancy.
Station Objective: To test the candidate's ability to take a focused history of patient with cardiac disease who has come to book for antenatal care.
Requirements: Standardized patient, a comfortable chair or dressed bed for the patient, a table and two chairs for the examiners, pencils and erasers, enough copies of the checklist, a chair for the candidate, plain papers for the candidate.

12.1.1 Instructions to the Standardized Patient (Role Player)

Biodata

Name: FN	Tribe: Ibo
Age: 25 years	Religion: Christianity
Address: New GRA, Enugu	Educational level: Tertiary
Occupation: Teacher	Marital status: Married

Presenting Complain
I have come to book for antenatal care.

C. Chama, *OSCE and VIVA VOCE in Obstetrics and Gynaecology*,
https://doi.org/10.1007/978-3-031-77262-7_12

History of Presenting Complaint
I am a 25-year-old secondary school teacher with tertiary level of education who lives in New GRA, Enugu, Enugu state. I am carrying my first pregnancy and my LMP (GA = 8 weeks). I have come to register for antenatal care today. I have had no problem with the pregnancy so far; I have no dizziness, no tiredness, shortness of breath, and do not hear my heart beating. I can do my normal daily activities.

When I was 14 years old, I had a surgery to replace my heart valves. I had noticed some difficulty with breathing especially when lying flat, tiredness, leg swelling, and hearing my heartbeat. I also had cough (NYHA Class 2). I was then taken to the hospital and so many tests were done. I do not know the names of some of them but was told I had rheumatic heart disease, which had affected some of my heart valves. So, I was operated on, and the heart valves were replaced with artificial ones. Since the operation, I have been on drugs to prevent my blood from clotting. I was also placed on some antibiotics, but I have stopped them after 2 years. I was given a wristband that I wear to alert people that I am on the anti-blood clot drug. Since the surgery, I have not had bleeding from the nose or any other site. I have been seeing my doctor (cardiologist) regularly and I have been okay.

I got married 2 years ago, and initially I used condoms to prevent pregnancy. When I was ready to try for a baby, I mentioned it to the cardiologist, and he stopped the particular anti-blood clot drug (warfarin) I was taking and changed to injections (low-molecular-weight heparin). He also advised me to register early for antenatal care whenever I got pregnant hence my coming today.

Gynaecological History
I started to menstruate when I was 13 years old. My periods are regular, they last 4 days and I see it every 28 days. No menstrual abnormalities. I used condom for contraception. I have not done a Pap smear although I am aware it.

Past Medical and Surgical History
As above.

Family and Social History
I am the second of four children of my parents. There is no family history of DM, HT, SCD, or twinning. I am married to a 35-year-old business man who deals in automotive spare parts. I do not drink alcohol nor smoke cigarettes.

Systemic Review
I feel well and have no other complaints. (If asked, no shortness of breath, no feeling of heart beat, no tiredness, no bleeding from any part of the body).

12.1.2 Instruction to the Candidate

Obtain a focused obstetric history from this patient who came to book for antenatal care today.

12.1.3 Instruction to the Examiners

The patient is a primigravida who had valvular heart surgery at the age of 14 years due to rheumatic heart disease. The cardiologist has switched her regular drug from warfarin to low-molecular-weight heparin because of the pregnancy. She has come to book for antenatal care today. The candidate is supposed to take a focused obstetric history from the patient. Use the checklist provided to score the candidate.

Checklist for history of valvular heart disease

Task	Well done	Fairly done	Poorly done	Not done
Greets patient, introduces self and obtains consent to talk to her	4	2	1	0
Obtains Biodata; name, age, address, occupation, tribe, etc.	4	2	1	0
Parity, LMP, EDD, GAD		2	1	0
Presenting complaint came to book for antenatal care		2		0
History of presenting complaint: no nausea, no vomiting, no dizziness, can do my normal activities, no shortness of breath		2	1	0
Obstetric history: first pregnancy				
Gynaecological history: menarche, periods, cycles, flow, dysmenorrhea, contraception, pap smear	4	2	1	0
Past medical and surgical history: - Diagnosed to have heart disease at the age of 14 years. - Several tests were done, and my heart valves said to be damaged. - Had artificial heart valves inserted the same year. - Placed on daily warfarin for which I received wrist band. - Placed on antibiotics for 2 years. - Cardiologist changed warfarin to heparin when I got pregnant and referred me for ANC		 2 2 2 2 2 2		 0 0 0 0 0 0
Family and social history: second of children of parents, no family history of HT, DM, SCD, twining. My husband is a businessman. I don't smoke or drink alcoholic beverages	4	2	1	0
Systemic review: no shortness of breath, no feeling of heartbeat, no bleeding from any part of the body, no tiredness.		2	1	0
Summary of history	4	2	1	0
Total marks	40			
Candidate's score .../40				

Examiners name/signature Date

12.2 Station 12.2 Management of Valvular Heart Disease in Pregnancy

Subject: Obstetrics.
Theme: Medical disorders in pregnancy.
Domain of Clinical Competence: Diagnostic and therapeutic procedures.
Station: Management of complication of valvular heart disease in pregnancy.
Station Objective: To test the candidate's ability to manage a patient with valvular heart disease in pregnancy.
Requirements: Clearly written questions for the candidate, preferably laminated to prevent staining and squeezing, plain papers as answer sheets for the candidate, marking scheme for examiners, a table and two chairs for the examiners, pencils and erasers, a chair for the candidate.

12.2.1 Instructions to the Candidate

1. Provide a summary of the history taken on the last station.
2. What are the routine and specific investigations to be done for this patient?
3. List the prerequisites for a safe vaginal delivery.

Answers to the Questions

1. Summary of history
   (a) _________, a 25-year-old primigravida (**2 marks**) who had prosthetic valve replacement for valvular heart disease in childhood. (**2 marks**)
   (b) Referred to the antenatal clinic for booking by her cardiologist at 8 weeks gestation. (**2 marks**)
   (c) She was on prolonged warfarin therapy that was changed to LMWH just before conception (**2 marks**). She is Stage 1 NYHA classification. (**2 marks**)
   (d) She has no complaints today. (**2 Marks**)
2. Investigations to be done
   (a) Routine investigations—HB/PCV, blood group and haemoglobin genotype (**2 marks**), routine Infection screening (HIV, HBSAg, HCV, VDRL), urine MCS, pelvic ultrasound scan (**2 Marks**)
   (b) Specific—ECG, echo cardiogram, clotting profile, anomaly scan at 20 weeks (**4 marks**), serial growth scans from 24 weeks (**4 Marks**)
3. Prerequisites for safe delivery
   (a) Multi-disciplinary team–Consultant obstetrician, cardiologist, anaesthesiologist, trained cardiology midwives should be involved (**2 marks**).
   (b) Perform general and specific systemic examinations including thorough check for cardiac murmurs and classify patient using NYHA criteria (**4 marks**).
   (c) Nurse patient in semi-recumbent position with a lateral tilt (**2 marks**).

(d) Establish IV access, maintain adequate fluid but avoid fluid overload (**2 marks**). Do FBC, urinalysis, and cross match blood (**2 marks**).
(e) IV antibiotics according to unit protocol (**2 marks**) and give oxygen via intranasal route (**2 marks**).
(f) Monitor patient carefully with CTG for continuous electronic foetal monitoring (**2 marks**), BP, pulse, temperature, oxygen saturation (**2 marks**), CVP if available. Also, thromboembolic deterrent (TED) stockings should be worn if indicated (**2 marks).**
(g) Do ARM and monitor labour closely on partograph. Minimal vaginal examinations and maintain strict asepsis while examining (**2 marks**).
(h) Ensure adequate obstetric analgesia (**4 marks**).
(i) Deliver patient preferably in left decubitus position avoiding lithotomy position (**2 marks**).
(j) Shorten second stage with use of forceps (**2 marks**).
(k) Manage third stage actively using Oxytocin, early cord clamping/cutting, additional Oxytocic if need be (**2 marks**). Repair any episiotomy promptly (**2 marks**).

Total marks = 60

Checklist for management of valvular heart disease in pregnancy

Task	Well done	Fairly done	Poorly done	Not done
Summary of history:				
- 25-year-old primigravida		2	1	0
- With prosthetic valves due to valvular heart disease		2	1	0
- Referred for ANC by cardiologist at 8 weeks gestation.		2	1	0
- Had warfarin changed to LMWT heparin just before pregnancy.		2	1	0
- She has no complaints today		2	1	0
Routine ANC investigations:				
- PCV, grouping, genotype or FBC.		2		0
- Serology for HIV, HBV, HCV, syphilis		2		0
- Urine MCS, stool parasitology		2		0
- Early USS for dating, viability		2		0
Specific investigations for valvular heart disease in pregnancy				
- Cardiology; ECG and echocardiogram		2		0
- Hematology; clotting profile		2		0
- Obstetric; anomaly and growth USS at 20 weeks and beyond		2		0
The prerequisites for safe delivery entails team management:				
Obstetrician:				
- IVL and give prophylactic antibiotics.		2		0
- Continue LMWT heparin.		2		0
- Continuous CTG		2		0
- ARM and open partograph for close monitoring		2		0
- Assist second stage with forceps or vacuum.		2		0
- Active management of third stage		2		0
Anaesthesiologist:				
- Insert epidural analgesia.		2		0
- Monitor maternal vitals including oxygen saturation.		2		0
- May set central venous line (CVP)		2		0
Cardiologist:				
- Thorough CVS examination and classify patient based on NYHA.		2		0
- Maintain adequate fluid intake and avoid fluid overload		2		0
Hematologist:				
- Do clotting profile, cross match blood		2		0
Trained midwife:				
- Monitor vitals closely, alert obstetrician as needed.		2		0
- Nurse in left lateral position.		2		0
- Intranasal oxygen		2		0
Neonatologist to resuscitate baby if need be		2		0
Postpartum care: routine immunization, can switch anti-coagulant to oral warfarin, avoid fluid overload, establish breastfeeding	4	2	1	0
Refer back to cardiologist after puerperium, to see in preconception clinic	4	2	1	0
Total score	64			
Candidate's score .../64				

Examiners name/signature Date

12.3 Station 12.3 History Taking in Pre-Eclampsia

Subject: Obstetrics.
Theme: Medical disorders in pregnancy.
Domain of Clinical Competence: History taking.
Station: Focused history taking of a patient with pre-eclampsia.
Station Objective: To assess the candidate's ability to take a focused history of a patient with pre-eclampsia with the aim of planning her management.
Requirements: Standardized or real patient, a comfortable chair or dressed bed for the patient, a table and two chairs for the examiners, pencils and erasers, enough copies of the checklist, a chair for the candidate, plain papers for use by the candidate.

12.3.1 Instructions to the Role Player

Biodata

Name: CS	Tribe: Kilba
Age: 20 years	Religion: Christianity
Address: Kubwa ward, Abuja	Educational level: Secondary
Occupation: Tailor	Marital status: Married

Presenting Complaint
Headache
Duration of 1 day (if asked).

History of Presenting Complaint
I am a 20-year-old housewife carrying my first pregnancy. I have started attending antenatal clinic at about 4 months of pregnancy and all the investigations carried out are normal. I have been regular with my follow-up visits and prescribed drugs. I am about 36 weeks pregnant now and yesterday I had headache which was severe, throbbing, affecting mainly the frontal part of my head. It did not affect my vision. I took paracetamol tablets which gave me some relief. This morning I went to Kubwa General Hospital where I attend antenatal clinic and I was referred to this hospital because my blood pressure is very high. I have no abdominal pain, vaginal bleeding, or any problem passing urine.

Past Medical and Surgical History
I have never been hospitalized for any illness. I have been treated for malaria fever several times with tablets and I have no known drug allergy.

Gynaecological History
I started to menstruate when I was 14 years of age and I bleed for 4 days every 28 to 30 days. I experience some lower abdominal discomfort during menses and the flow is heavier the first 2 days. I am aware of modern methods of contraception but have not used any. I am not aware of Pap smear and have not done any.

Family and Social History
My mother had eclampsia (convulsions) in her first pregnancy. There is no person in my family with diabetes mellitus, sickle cell disease, or twinning. I am the only wife of my husband who is a National Certificate of Education (NCE) holder and teaches in a public primary school. I am a tailor. I do not smoke cigarettes or take alcoholic beverages.

Systemic Review
I have no other complaint.

12.3.2 Instruction to the Candidate

The patient was referred from a General Hospital to this hospital this morning. Your task is to take a focused obstetric history.

12.3.3 Instruction to the Examiners

The patient is a primigravida at 36 weeks gestation who was referred to this hospital this morning on account of high blood pressure. The candidate is to take a focused obstetric history from her. Use the checklist provided to score the candidate.

Checklist for obstetric history for pre-eclampsia

Task	Well done	Fairly done	Poorly done	Not done
Greets patient and introduces self, seeks consent of patient to talk with her about her health problem	4	2	1	0
Obtains Biodata; name, age, address, occupation, tribe, religion etc.	4	2	1	0
Parity, LMP, EDD, GAD		2	1	0
Presenting complaint with duration	4	2	1	0
History of presenting complaint				
- Frontal headache		2		0
- Throbbing in nature		2		0
- No visual symptoms		2		0
- No epigastric pain		2		0
- No nausea or vomiting.		2		0
- No convulsion		2		0
Past medical and surgical history; nil of note		2		0
Gynaecological history; menarche, periods, cycle, contraception, pap smear	4	2	1	0
Family and social history; married, husband's occupation, family history of HT, DM, CSD, twining	4	2	1	0
Systemic review		2	1	0
Summary of history		2	1	0
Penalty: History not sequential	-4	-2	-1	0
Total marks	38			
Candidate's score .../38				

Examiner's signature   Date

12.4 Station 12.4 Management of Severe Pre-Eclampsia

Subject: Obstetrics.
Theme: Medical disorders in pregnancy.
Domain of Clinical Competence: Diagnostic and therapeutic procedures.
Station: Post encounter to history of pre-eclampsia.
Station Objective: To assess the candidate's ability to synthesize the history of a patient for the management of the case.
Requirements: Clearly written instructions to the candidate, preferably laminated to prevent staining and squeezing, plain papers as answer sheets for the candidate, a table and two chairs for the examiners, marking scheme for examiners, pencils and erasers, a chair for the candidate.

12.4.1 Instruction to the Candidate

The patient you clerked on the last station was found to have BP160/110 mmHg and proteinuria 2+. Abdominal examination revealed SFH 36 cm and a live singleton foetus lying longitudinally and presenting cephalic. The pelvis was clinically adequate and the Bishop score was 4.

1. What relevant investigations would you want to request?
2. Prescribe the two most important drugs you want give immediately.
3. When and how would you deliver her?
4. List five possible complications in this patient if delivery is delayed.

12.4.2 Instructions to the Examiners

The patient is a primigravida at 36 weeks gestation, who was referred to this hospital this morning from a primary health centre due to high blood pressure. On examination, her BP160/110 mmHg. The FH is 36 cm, a singleton foetus is lying longitudinally and presenting cephalic. The decent of the presenting part is 4/5 and the FHR is 136 beats/min. Vaginal examination revealed a Bishop score of 4. The candidate is supposed to answer the questions provided concerning the management of this patient. Use the marking scheme provided to mark the candidate's answers.

Answers

1. Relevant investigations
   (a) full blood count including absolute platelet count (**2 marks**)
   (b) renal function tests; electrolytes, urea, creatinine and uric acid (**2 marks**)
   (c) liver function tests; alanine and aminotransferases (**2 marks**)
   (d) obstetric ultrasound (**2 marks**)
   (e) cardiotocograph (**2 marks**)
   (f) grouping and cross matching of 2 units of whole blood (**2 marks**)
2. Two most important drugs to be given are:
   (a) MgSO4 (**2 marks),** dosage according to regimen (**2 marks**)
   (b) Labetalol or hydralazine (**2 marks**), dosage depending on drug chosen (**2 marks**)
3. When and how to deliver this patient:
   (a) Once patient is stabilized, she should be delivered (**2 marks**)
   (b) If maternal condition is satisfactory and CTG is reactive, ripen the cervix and induce labour (**4 marks**). If CTG is non-reassuring and/or maternal chemistry deranged, deliver by emergency caesarean section (**4 marks**).
4. Possible complications (**2 marks** each):
   (a) Convulsion (Eclampsia)
   (b) Cerebral haemorrhage (stroke)
   (c) Acute kidney injury
   (d) Hypertensive heart failure
   (e) Placental abruption

Total marks = 40

Checklist for management of severe pre-eclampsia

Task	Well done	Fairly done	Poorly done	Not done
Relevant investigations				
- FBC including absolute platelet count to assess level of possible complications.		2	1	0
- RFT also assess level of possible renal complications,		2	1	0
- LFT to rule out possible HELLP syndrome,		2	1	0
- Obstetric USS for fetal wellbeing		2	1	0
- CTG also for fetal wellbeing		2	1	0
- Group and cross matching of blood for possible emergency use		2	1	0
Two most important drugs for this patient:				
- MgSO4 to prevent convulsion in this patient; dosage given.	4	2	1	0
- Hydralazine or Labetalol to prevent hypertensive complications; dosage given.	4	2	1	0
When and how to deliver this patient				
- Once this patient is stabilized, delivery should be by the fastest and safest route.		2	1	0
- If maternal condition is stable and CTG is reactive, ripen cervix and induce labour.		2	1	0
- If the CTG is non-reactive, deliver by elective CS.		2	1	0
Possible complications if delivery is delayed are (Max 5):				
- Convulsion (Eclampsia)		2		0
- Cerebral haemorrhage (stroke)		2		0
- Acute renal injury		2		0
- Placental abruption		2		0
- Hypertensive heart failure		2		0
- HELLP syndrome		2		0
Total score	36			
Candidate's score .../36				

Examiner's signature Date

12.5 Station 12.5 History Taking of Sickle Cell Disease (SCD) Patient

Subject: Obstetrics.
Theme: Medical disorders in pregnancy.
Domain of Clinical Competence: History taking.
Station: Focused history taking of a pregnant woman with sickle cell disease.
Station Objective: To assess the candidate's ability to take a focused history of pregnant a woman with sickle cell disease with the aim of achieving a healthy a baby and mother.
Requirements: Standardized patient, a comfortable chair or dressed bed for the patient, a table and two chairs for the examiners, enough copies of the checklist, pencils and erasers, a chair for the candidate, a chaperon, plain papers for use by the candidates.

12.5.1 Instructions to the Role Player

Biodata

Name: GP	Tribe: Birom
Age: 26 years	Religion: Christianity
Address: Riyom, plateau state	Educational level: Secondary
Occupation: Housewife	Marital status: Married

Presenting Complaint
No complaints; referred for antenatal care.

History of Presenting Complaint
I am 26 years old and diagnosed to have sickle cell disease since childhood. My genotype is SS and I have been looked after by the medical officers at the General Hospital Riyom, my hometown. The frequency of crisis has decreased with age and the last episode was about 3 years ago. I have had several blood transfusions in childhood also, but this has reduced with age; the last transfusion was about 5 years ago. I am on daily paludrine and folic acid tablets.

I got married last year and my last menses was about 2 months ago. My doctor has confirmed that I am 9 weeks pregnant by ultrasound scan and referred me to this hospital for expert care. I do not have any complaints today apart from nausea and occasional vomiting for about 1 month now.

Gynaecological History
I started to see my menses at the age of 16 years and menstruate for 3 days every 25 to 30 days. I use 2–3 sanitary pads per day and experience only mild lower abdominal discomfort during menses. I am aware of modern methods of family planning but have not used any before. I am aware of Pap smear but have not done any yet.

Obstetric History
This is my first pregnancy.

Past Medical and Surgical History
As above. No previous surgery and I am not aware of any drug allergy.

Family and Social History
I am the first of four children of my parents: all of us alive. The second child who is a boy is also a Sickler. There is no family history of HT, DM, or twinning. My husband is a secondary school teacher, and his genotype is AA. I don't smoke or drink alcoholic beverages.

Systemic Review
I have no other complaints.

12.5.2 Instructions to the Candidate

Mrs. GP is a 26-year-old primigravida who has come to book for antenatal care. Your task is to take her history.

12.5.3 Instructions to the Examiners

Mrs. GP is a 26-year-old primigravida who has come to book for antenatal care at 9 weeks gestation. She is a known sickle cell disease patient diagnosed since childhood. She has been managed by the Medical Officer in the General Hospital in her hometown who referred her to this hospital for antenatal care. The candidate is to take a focused history of the patient. Use the checklist provided to score the candidate.

Checklist for obstetric history of SCD in pregnancy

Task	Well done	Fairly done	Poorly done	Not done
Greets patient, introduces self and obtains permission to discuss her case	4	2	1	0
Obtains Biodata: name, age, address, occupation, tribe, religion, etc.	4	2	1	0
Obtains parity, LMP, EDD, GAD		2	1	0
Presenting complaint: referred for antenatal care		2		0
History of presenting complaint				
- Was pregnancy planned and wanted.		2		0
- Has pregnancy been confirmed.		2		0
- Any pregnancy symptoms		2		0
- Any illness since pregnant		2		0
Past medical history				
- Diagnosed sickle cell disease since childhood.		2		0
- Under medical supervision		2		0
- Frequency of crisis, last episode		2		0
- Previous blood transfusion, last episode		2		0
- Regular drugs; paludrine, folic acid		2		0
- Any bone infection (osteomyelitis)		2		0
Gynaecological history: menarche, periods, cycles, dysmenorrhea, contraception, pap smear	4	2	1	0
Systemic review; nausea, vomiting, fever, jaundice, easy fatigability		2	1	0
Family and social history: SCD among parents and siblings, husband's genotype, alcohol consumption, smoking	4	2	1	0
Summary of history	4	2	1	0
Total score	46			
Candidate's score .../46				

Examiner's name and signature Date

12.6 Station 12.6 Management of Sickle Cell Disease in Labour

Subject: Obstetrics.
Theme: Medical disorders in pregnancy.
Domain of Clinical Competence: Therapeutic procedure.
Station: Management of sickle cell disease in labour.
Station Objective: To assess the candidate's ability to manage a known patient of sickle cell disease presenting in labour, with the aim of preventing sickle cell crisis in labour and delivering a healthy baby.
Requirements: Clearly written instructions to the candidate, preferably laminated to prevent staining and squeezing, plain papers as answer sheets for the candidate, a table and two chairs for the examiners, marking scheme for the examiners, pencils and erasers, a chair for the candidate.

12.6.1 Instruction to the Candidate

The patient you clerked on the last station later presents in established labour at 37 weeks gestation. You are the Registrar in labour ward. Outline how you would manage her in labour.

12.6.2 Instructions to the Examiners

This is a post encounter station to a sickle cell disease mother presenting in established labour at 37 weeks gestation. The candidate is supposed to outline how he will manage the patient in labour. Use the checklist provided to score the candidate.

Checklist for management of sickle cell disease patient in established labour

Task	Well done	Fairly done	Poorly done	Not done
Will admits patient in labour ward		2		0
General examination: pallor, jaundice, PR, BP		2	1	0
Obstetric examination: lie, presentation, position, attitude, descent, FHR	4	2	1	0
Vaginal exam: effacement, dilatation, presenting part, station, caput, molding, adequacy of pelvis	4	2	1	0
Open partograph for close monitoring of labour, CTG monitoring		2		0
IVL access; maintain hydration with Ringer's lactate or normal saline		2		0
PCV, grouping and cross matching of 2 units of HbAA blood		2		0
Analgesia: epidural preferred, pethidine good option	4	2		0
Inform consultant Obstetrician, Haematologist, Anaesthesiologist, and neonatologist.	4	2	1	0
4-6 hourly PCV, liver USS to detect early sequestration crisis.		2		0
Second stage; assist second stage with vacuum delivery, if possible, avoid episiotomy		2		0
Immediately postpartum: continue serial PCV, Liver USS and hydration, analgesia and antibiotic cover.	4	2	1	0
Maximum score	34			
Candidate's score .../34				

Examiner's name and signature Date

13 Labour, Delivery, and Puerperium

13.1 Station 13.1 Mechanism of Normal Labour

Subject: Obstetrics
Theme: Labour and delivery
Domain of Clinical Competence: Therapeutic procedure (Understanding mechanism of normal labour)
Station: Demonstrating mechanism of normal labour
Station Object: To test the candidate's ability to demonstrate the mechanism of normal labour using a pelvic model and baby mannequin
Requirements: A model of the female pelvic bone and a baby doll, a table or dressed bed on which to place the pelvic model and the baby doll, a table and two chairs for the examiners, enough copies of the checklist, pencils and erasers, latex hand gloves, chaperon

13.1.1 Instruction to the Candidate

You are provided with a model of the female pelvis and a baby doll. Demonstrate using the mannequin, and running commentary, the mechanism of normal labour.

13.1.2 Instruction to the Examiners

The candidate is to demonstrate, while running commentaries, the mechanism of normal labour, using the model of the female pelvis and the baby doll. Use the checklist provided to score the candidate (Fig. 13.1).

C. Chama, *OSCE and VIVA VOCE in Obstetrics and Gynaecology*,
https://doi.org/10.1007/978-3-031-77262-7_13

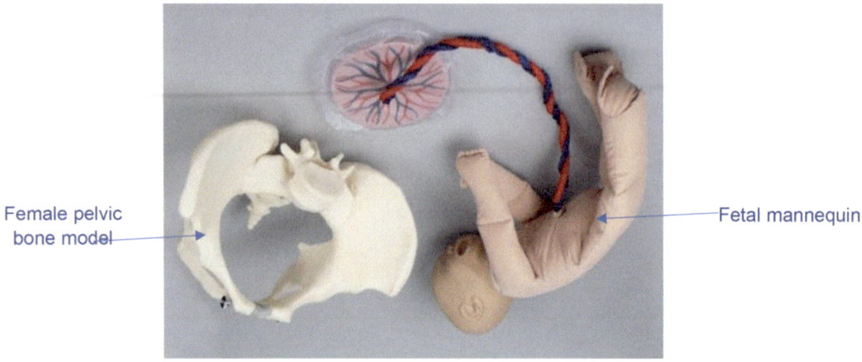

Fig. 13.1 Pelvic model and a baby doll

Checklist for mechanism of labour

Candidate's number

Task	Well done	Fairly done	Poorly done	Not done
Def; mechanism of labour is the series of changes in position (2) and attitude (2) that the fetus undergoes during its passage through the birth canal	4	2	1	0
Step 1: descent and engagement: - Fetal head enters pelvis in transverse diameter. - Engagement occurs when fetal head reaches ischial spines		2 2		0 0
Step 2: flexion: - Passive flexion as fetal head enters pelvic mid-cavity. - This minimizes presenter diameter		2 2		0 0
Step 3: internal rotation: - The occiput leads in well flexed attitude. - With further descent, levator ani rotates head to OAP. - If fetus engages in OPP, internal rotation occurs through 180°		2 2 2		0 0 0
Step 4: extension: - Fetal head extends to escape under pubic symphysis. - With further extension, face sweeps over perineum - Each step of extension presents smallest diameter to prevent tissue damage		2 2 2		0 0 0
Perineal trauma could be prevented at this stage by exerting downward pressure on the emerging occiput until crowning	4	2	1	0
Step 5: Restitution: - Fetal occiput rotates through 45°. - This aligns with the shoulders entering the pelvis obliquely		2 2		0 0
Step 6: External rotation: - As fetal shoulders descent, they rotate to AP position. - Accordingly, the delivered head further rotates 45°		2 2		0 0
Step 7: Delivery of the shoulders and the rest of fetal body: - Anterior shoulder slips under pubic symphysis by lateral flexion - Though passive, this movement can be assisted by pulling fetal head. - The rest of the body fall out easily		2 2 2		0 0 0
Penalty: non-sequential, clumsy	-4	-2		
Total score	42			
Candidate's score .../42				

Examiner's name and signature Date

13.2 Station 13.2 Vaginal Examination in Labour

Subject: Obstetrics
Theme: Labour and delivery
Domain of Clinical Competence: Physical examination
Station: Vaginal examination in established labour
Station Objective: To assess the candidate's ability to perform vaginal examination in labour with the aim of diagnosing labour and assessing the adequacy of the maternal pelvis for vaginal delivery
Requirements: Mannequins with inflatable uterus to simulate pregnancy (Fig. 13.2) and models of the uterine cervix at various diameters to simulate cervical dilatation in labour. A table or dressed bed on which to place the mannequin, latex hand gloves, gallipot with wet swabs, a table and two chairs for the examiners, enough copies of the checklist, pencils and erasers, a chaperon

13.2.1 Instruction to the Candidate

A 25-year-old G3P2+0, 2 alive, presents to the labour ward at term with a history of labour pain of 6 h duration. She had seen show but it's no drainage of liquor. Abdominal examination revealed a gravid uterus with an SFH 37 cm, a singleton foetus lies longitudinally and presenting cephalic in left occiput anterior position. The descent is three-fifth and the foetal heart rate 140 bpm. Your task is to perform a vaginal examination and comment on your findings as you go on.

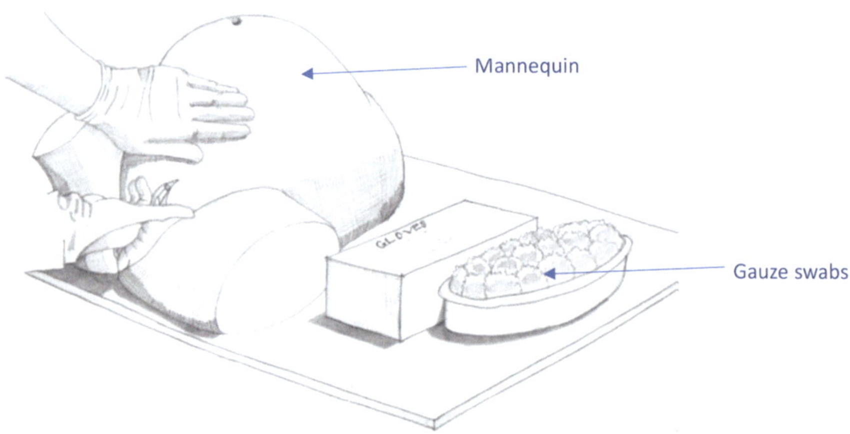

Fig. 13.2 Demonstrating vaginal examination in labour. Courtesy of Jonathan Edache Otache

13.2.2 Instruction to the Examiners

The candidate is provided with pregnant mannequin simulating a pregnant woman in established labour. The candidate is to perform vaginal examination and run commentary of his findings as he performs the examination. Use the checklist provided to score the candidate.

Checklist for vaginal examination in labour

Task	Well done	Fairly done	Poorly done	Not done
Will ensure a midwife is present for the examination		2		0
Will greet patient and introduces self		2		0
Will explain the procedure to the patient		2		0
Washes hand and wear sterile gloves		2		0
Patient positioned dorsally with the help of the midwife		2		0
Swabs vulvar and perineum with antiseptic swab from anterior to posterior	4	2	1	0
Parts the labia with non-dominant hand and inspects for liquor or bleeding.	4	2	1	0
Informs patient he is going to put his fingers into the vagina and correctly inserts index and middle fingers of dominant hand.	4	2	1	0
Assesses the cervix for: - Position - Consistency - Effacement - Dilatation		 2 2 2 2		 0 0 0 0
Assesses the fetus for: - State of the membranes - Presenting part - Position - Molding		 2 2 2 2		 0 0 0 0
Performs clinical pelvimetry correctly	4	2	1	0
Examines gloved fingers for meconium, blood, and color of liquor	4	2	1	0
Penalty: non-sequential, clumsy	-4	-2		
Total score	46			
Candidate's score .../46				

Examiners signature Date

13.3 Station 13.3 Understanding Obstetric Forceps

Subject: Obstetrics
Theme: Labour and delivery
Domain of Clinical Competence: Therapeutic procedure
Station: Describing parts of obstetric forceps and the conditions for their application to achieve assisted vaginal delivery
Requirements: Simpson's and Wrigley's obstetric forceps (Fig. 13.3), a tray or table to place the forceps, a table and two chairs for examiners, enough copies of the checklist, pencils and erasers, a chair for the candidate, a chaperon

13.3.1 Instruction to Candidates

Identify objects A and B.

Pick any of them and describe its parts.

A woman has been pushing in second stage of labour for 2 h and is exhausted; there is no head palpable per abdomen and the station is +2. Which of the instruments would you use to assist her delivery?

Give five prerequisites for its use.

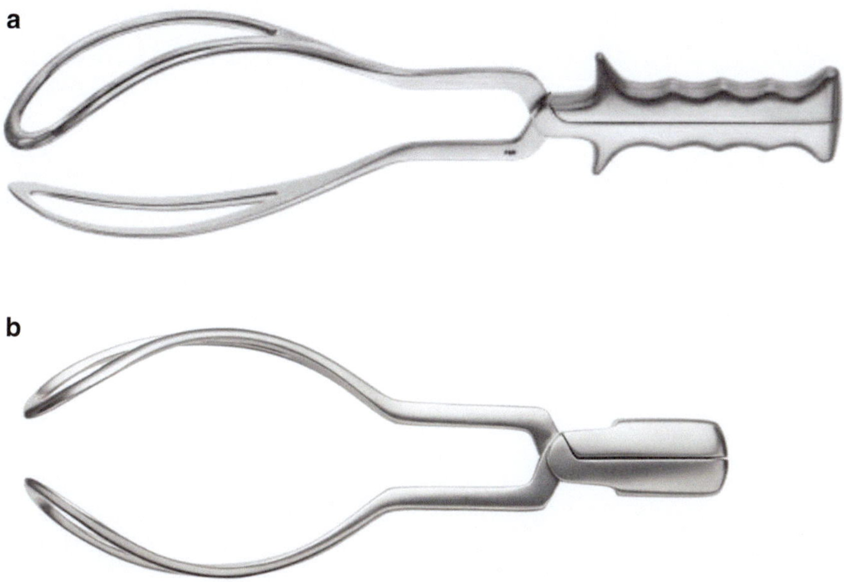

Fig. 13.3 Obstetric forceps. (**a**) Simpson's forceps, (**b**) Wrigley's forceps

13.3.2 Instruction to Examiners

Provided are a pair of Simpson's Obstetric forceps (object A) and a pair of Wrigley's Obstetric forceps (object B). The candidate is expected to identify the two forceps by name and describe the parts of any of them. A scenario of a woman in second stage of labour with station +2 is given and the candidate is supposed to choose the most appropriate forceps to assist the delivery of the patient.

Use the checklist provided to score the candidate.

Checklist for obstetric forceps

Task	Well done	Fairly done	Poorly done	Not done
Identity of objects				
- Object A: Simpson's (1) obstetric (1) forceps		2	1	0
- Object B: Wrigley's (1) obstetric (1) forceps		2	1	0
Parts of obstetric forceps				
- Toe		2		0
- Cephalic curve		2		0
- Pelvic curve		2		0
- Heel		2		0
- Fenestration		2		0
- Shank		2		0
- Lock		2		0
- Finger guide		2		0
- Handle		2		0
Simpson's forceps (2), being mid-cavity forceps (2) is more suitable	4	2		0
Prerequisites for application of obstetric forceps:				
- cephalic presentation		2		0
- presenting part engaged		2		0
- adequate pelvis		2		0
- membranes ruptured.		2		0
- bladder emptied.		2		0
- skilled operator		2		0
Sequential description of parts	4	2	1	0
Communication skill; confident, articulate	4	2	1	0
Total score	44			
Candidate's score .../44				

Examiner's signature Date

13.4 Station 13.4 Uterovaginal Prolapse in Labour

Subject: Obstetrics
Theme: Labour and delivery
Domain of Clinical Competence: Virtual sign identification (Picture test)
Station: Picture test of uterovaginal prolapse in labour
Station Objective: To test the candidate's ability to identify the picture of uterovaginal prolapse in established labour and suggest ways of managing the patient
Requirements: A picture of uterine prolapse in established labour, preferably laminated to prevent squeezing or staining, clearly written instructions to the candidate, plain papers, a chair for the candidate, a table and two chairs for the examiners, a marking scheme for the examiners, pencils and erasers

13.4.1 Instruction to Candidate

A G5P4+0 A4 presented with labour pains of 7 h duration and vaginal protrusion since early pregnancy. Inspection of the vulva revealed the features shown in the Fig. 13.4.

Study the Fig. 13.4 and answer the following questions:

1. What is the diagnosis?
2. The incidence of this condition in pregnancy is about:
   (a) 1/100 deliveries
   (b) 1/1000 deliveries
   (c) 1/10,000 deliveries
   (d) 1/100,000 deliveries
3. List four complications of this condition in pregnancy.
4. What are the options for delivery of this patient?

Answer Outline

1. Uterovaginal prolapse in labour (**4 marks**)
2. The incidence of uterine prolapse in pregnancy is about 1/10,000 deliveries (**2 marks**)
3. The complications of uterine prolapse in pregnancy include: (**2 marks each; max 8**)

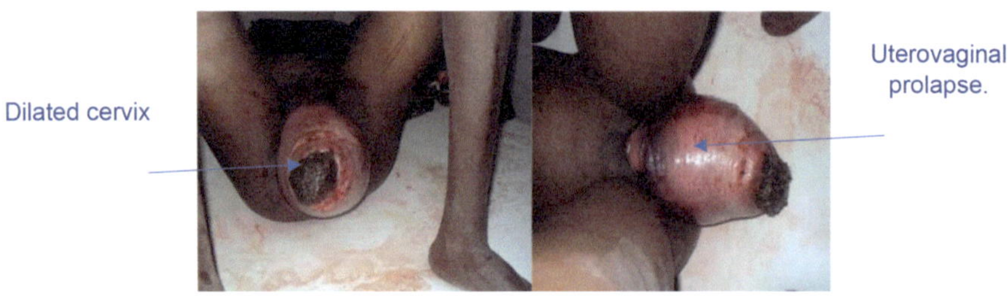

Fig. 13.4 Uterovaginal prolapse in labour, courtesy El-Nafaty and Chama (2014)

   (a) abortion
   (b) preterm delivery
   (c) urinary retention
   (d) cervical oedema
   (e) obstructed labour due to cervical dystocia
4. The options of delivery for this patient are: (**2 marks each**)
   (a) classical caesarean section (the lower segment is outside the introitus)
   (b) vaginal delivery following Duhrssen incision (longitudinal cervical incision)

Total marks = 18

Checklist for uterine prolapse in labour

Task	Well done	Fairly done	Poorly done	Not done
The diagnosis is Uterovaginal prolapse (2) in labour (2)	4	2		0
The incidence of this condition in pregnancy is 1/10,0000		2		0
Possible complications of UV prolapse in pregnancy are (Max 4): - miscarriage - preterm delivery - urinary retention - obstructed labour due to cervical dystocia - cervical oedema		 2 2 2 2 2		 0 0 0 0 0
The options of delivery for this patient are: - spontaneous vaginal delivery with risk of cervical dystocia - longitudinal cervical incision (Duhrssen incision) and VD - emergency classical caesarean section		 2 2 2		 0 0 0
Total marks	20			
Candidate's score .../20				

Examiner's signature Date

13.5 Station 13.5 Picture Test on Obstructed Labour

Subject: Obstetrics
Theme: Labour and delivery
Domain of Clinical Competence: Virtual sign identification
Station: Picture test on prolonged obstructed labour
Station Objective: To assess the candidate's ability to recognize the "three-tumour sign" as a feature of prolonged obstructed labour
Requirements: A clearly written instruction to the candidate with a laminated picture of a uterus with three-tumour sign (Fig. 13.5), a chair for the candidate, plain papers as answer sheets for the candidate, a table and two chairs for the examiners, a marking scheme for the examiners, pencils and erasers, a chaperon

13.5.1 Instructions to the Candidate

A grand multipara presents with prolonged obstructed labour at term. She was resuscitated and had emergency caesarean section. The picture below shows the finding at laparotomy. Answer the questions that follow:

1. Give the names of the structures labelled A, B, and C
2. What term is used to describe this feature of obstructed labour?
3. What uterine incision would you use to deliver the baby and why?
4. What were the possible pathological conditions in the mother at presentation?
5. What complications are anticipated in the baby if delivered alive?

Answer Outline
1. Names of the structures labelled (**2 marks each**)
   (a) uterine fundus
   (b) lower uterine segment
   (c) urinary bladder

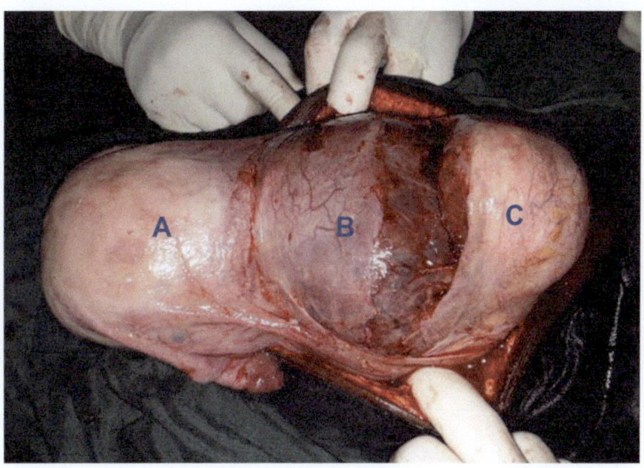

Fig. 13.5 Three-tumour sign in prolonged obstructed labour, Chama et al. (2018)

2. This feature is described as "three-tumour sign" (**4 marks**)
3. De-Lee incision (**2 marks**) so that it can be extended into the retraction ring when necessary (**2 marks**)
4. The possible pathological conditions in the mother are: (**2 marks each, max. 6 marks**)
   (a) Exhaustion
   (b) Dehydration
   (c) Metabolic acidosis
   (d) Chorioamnionitis
5. Possible complications in the baby if delivered alive are: (**2 marks each; max. 8 marks**)
   (a) Birth asphyxia
   (b) Acidosis
   (c) Intracranial haemorrhage
   (d) Sepsis
   (e) Perinatal death

Checklist for prolonged obstructed labour

Task	Well done	Fairly done	Poorly done	Not done
Names of the structures labelled A, B, and C				
- A = Uterine fundus		2		0
- B = Lower uterine segment		2		0
- C = Urinary bladder		2		0
The feature depicted in the picture is called "three-tumor sign'	4			0
The preferred uterine incision is De-Lee incision (2) so that it can be extended into the retraction ring if necessary (2)	4	2		0
The possible pathological conditions in the mother are (max. 4)				
- Exhaustion		2		0
- Dehydration		2		0
- Metabolic acidosis		2		0
- Chorioamnionitis		2		0
- Septicaemia		2		0
Possible complications in the baby if delivered alive (max.4)				
- Birth asphyxia		2		0
- Acidosis		2		0
- Intracranial haemorrhage		2		0
- Sepsis		2		0
- Perinatal death		2		0
Differentiating constriction ring from retraction ring abdominally (4):				
- Uterus feels normal and non-tender in constriction ring but tense and tender with retraction ring	4	2		0
- Constriction ring cannot be felt on abdominal examination while retraction ring is felt as a groove abdominally	4	2		0
- Fetal parts are easily felt with constriction ring but not easily felt with retraction ring	4	2		0
- Round ligaments cannot be felt with constriction ring but are taut and tender with retraction ring	4	2		0
- FHS is usually present with constriction ring but usually absent with retraction ring	4	2		0
Total score	50			
Candidate's score .../50				

Examiner's signature Date

13.6 Station 13.6 Postpartum Breast Examination

Subject: Obstetrics
Theme: Puerperium
Domain of Clinical Competence: Physical examination
Station: Breast examination in the puerperium
Station Objective: To test the candidate's ability to examine the breasts in the puerperium with the aim of establishing normal lactation and normal breastfeeding
Requirements: A lactating mother (a mannequin of a female chest with fully developed breasts can also be used) (Fig. 13.6), a table and two chairs for the examiners, a dressed bed for the mother or a table for the mannequin, enough checklists for the examiners, pencils and erasers, a chaperon

13.6.1 Instruction to the Standardized Patient

We are conducting medical examination as part of training obstetricians and gynaecologists. The candidates will be expected to examine your breasts as the examiners who are consultant obstetricians watch for correctness of the examination by the candidates. If a candidate is causing you any discomfort, do not hesitate to tell the candidate, chaperon, or the consultants. A maximum of five candidates will examine you and then another mother will be asked to replace you. Thank you for being part of this process of training future obstetricians for our country.

13.6.2 Instruction to the Candidate

The patient in front of you is a breastfeeding mother. Your task is to examine her breasts.

13.6.3 Instruction to the Examiners

Provided is a breastfeeding mother. The candidate is expected to examine her breasts for lactation and any lumps. Use the checklist provided to score the candidate.

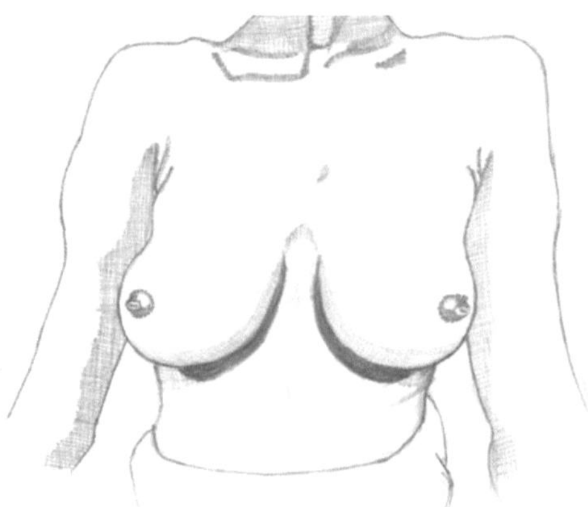

Fig. 13.6 Lactating breasts. (courtesy of Jonathan Edache Otache)

Checklist for breast examination

Task	Well done	Fairly done	Poorly done	Not done
Greets patient, introduces self		2		0
Explains breast examination and obtains permission to examine her breasts	4	2	1	0
Politely asks patient to undress down to middle abdomen		2	1	0
Asks patient to sit straight with hands akimbo		2		0
Inspection:				
- symmetry (sizes of both breasts)		2		0
- comments on fullness		2		0
- comments on areola		2		0
- comments on nipples		2		0
Palpation:				
- stabilizes breast with one hand.		2	1	0
- palpates the breast with the other hand.		2	1	0
- palpates the middle (areola) last.		2	1	0
- expresses the areola with 2 fingers for milk expression		2	1	0
Repeats the same palpation on the other breast	4	2	1	0
Asks patient for any discomfort		2		0
Thanks patient and helps her to dress up	4	2	1	0
Penalty: clumsy, causes discomfort to patient	-4	-2		
Total score	36			
Candidate's score .../36				

Examiner's signature Date

13.7 Station 13.7 Application of NASG

Subject: Obstetrics
Subspecialty: Labour, delivery, and puerperium
Domain of Clinical Competence: Therapeutic procedure
Station: Application of non-pneumatic anti-shock garment (NASG) in shock due to PPH
Station Objective: To test the candidate's ability to correctly apply the NASG on a patient in shock due to PPH for the purpose of transfer to tertiary health centre
Requirements: A full-size mannequin of a female, a pack of NASG (Fig. 13.7), dressed bed for the mannequin, latex gloves, Foley's catheter, urine bag, 5 mL syringes and needles, a table and chairs for the examiners, sufficient checklist, pencils and erasers, a chaperon

13.7.1 Instructions to the Candidate

Mrs. HH a 36-year-old P8+0 A8 who delivered in a primary health centre about 3 h ago and sustained primary postpartum haemorrhage. She is unconscious, BP90/50 mmHg, PR 120 bpm, and a respiratory rate of 24 cpm. She is being planned for transfer to the nearby teaching hospital. Provided is a non-pneumatic anti-shock garment. Using the mannequin provided, demonstrate step by step how you would apply the NASG before transferring the patient. Explain what you are doing to the hearing of the examiner as you perform the procedure.

13.7.2 Instructions to the Examiners

Provided is a mannequin depicting a grand multipara who is in shock following a primary postpartum haemorrhage. The candidate is supposed to demonstrate step by step how to apply the non-pneumatic anti-shock garment on the patient before transfer to a tertiary hospital. Use the checklist provided to score the candidate.

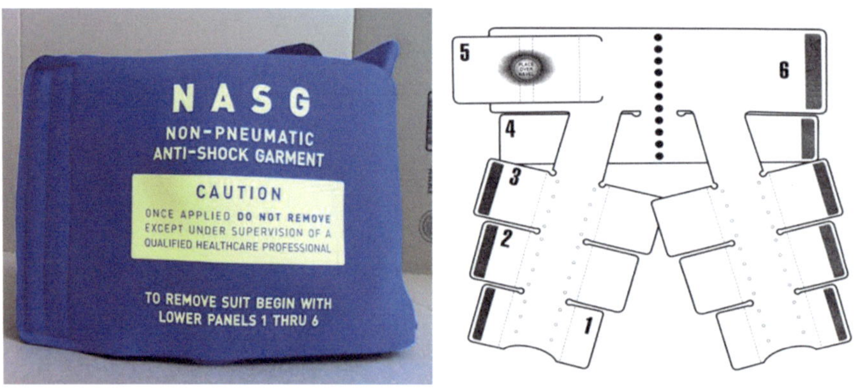

Fig. 13.7 Non-pneumatic anti-shock garment (NASG). Drawing in the right—Courtesy of Jonathan Edache Otache

Checklist for application of NASG

Tasks	Well done	Fairly done	Poorly done	Not done
Calls for help: nurses to bring IVF, 16G cannula, specimen bottles, oxygen concentrator or cylinder etc.	4	2	1	0
Opens the NASG, starting with S1 through S6		2	1	0
With the help of assistant, rolls the patient to her side to place NASG under her	4	2	1	0
With patient supine, closes the segments:				
- S1 to legs		2		0
- S2 to calf		2		0
- S3 to thighs		2		0
- S4 to pelvis		2		0
- S5&6 to abdomen; below lowest rib.		2		0
After closing each segment, insinuates finger, lift and release with a SNAP	4	2	1	0
Leaves a gap between S2 and S3 so knee can bend		2		0
Sets IVL, catharize patient to monitor urine output	4	2	1	0
One on one nursing care, monitor vitals continuously or ¼ hourly	4	2	1	0
Move patient on a trolley to the ambulance for transfer	4	2	1	0
Penalty: non-sequential application	-4	-2	-1	0
Total marks	38			
Candidate's score .../38				

Examiner's signature Date

Reference

1. Aliyu U El-Nafaty, Calvin M Chama, Habiba I Ismail, Saidu A Kadas. Uterine prolapse as an unusual cause of obstructed labour. J Cases Obstet Gynecol 2014;1(4):51–53.

Ethics and Medico-Legal Issues in Obstetrics

14

14.1 Station 14.1 Booking a Prostitute for Antenatal Care

Subject: Obstetrics
Theme: Ethics and medico-legal issues
Domain of Clinical Competence: History taking
Station: Booking a commercial sex worker for antenatal care
Station Objective: To test the ability of the candidate to take a focused history of the client and request appropriate investigations necessary for her care in this pregnancy
Requirements: Standardized patient, a comfortable chair or dressed bed for the SP, a table and chairs for the examiners and candidate, sufficient checklist, pencils and erasers, a chaperon

14.1.1 Instructions to the Standardized Patient

Biodata

Name: Miss XX	Religion: Christianity
Age: 25 years	Educational level: Secondary school
Address: Bayan gari, Bauchi	Marital status: Single
Occupation: Commercial sex worker	

Presenting Complaint
I want to register for antenatal care.

History of Presenting Complaint
I am about 3 months pregnant and have no problems. I suspected I was pregnant when I missed my period and last month, I had ultrasound scan to confirm the pregnancy. I was advised by my friends to come for antenatal care in this hospital.

C. Chama, *OSCE and VIVA VOCE in Obstetrics and Gynaecology*,
https://doi.org/10.1007/978-3-031-77262-7_14

Obstetric History
This is my third pregnancy. I terminated the first two pregnancies because I was not prepared to look after the kids. Now I do not want to keep terminating my pregnancies and one day I may not be able to get one.

Gynaecological History
I saw my first menses when I was 14 years of age and I bleed for 4 days every 26 to 28 days. I experience mild lower abdominal pains with menses and the flow is normal. I am aware of modern family planning methods and have occasionally used postinor (emergency contraception). My last menstrual period started on _______ (about 12 weeks ago).

Past Medical and Surgical History
I had appendicectomy in a General Hospital in my hometown 5 years ago. I am not allergic to any drug. I have been treated for malaria on a few occasions. I occasionally take Ampiclox capsules (ampicillin and cloxacillin combination) when a customer's condom breaks inside me.

Family and Social History
I am the first of six children of my parents who are farmers. There is no history of diabetes, hypertension sickle cell disease, or twinning in my family. I completed the secondary school in my hometown but could not progress due to financial constraints. I decided to come to this town to stay with my aunty who introduced me to prostitution which I have been doing for the past 5 years. I planned this pregnancy after I have set up a hair dressing saloon in this town. I know the father of my pregnancy because I allowed him to sleep with me without using condom. He is a soldier who has just been posted to Maiduguri. He has been my friend and customer for the past 1 year. I have not disclosed the pregnancy to him yet. I occasionally take stout beer when my boyfriend visits me. I don't smoke cigarettes.

Systemic Review
I do not have any problem today.

14.1.2 Instruction to the Candidate

The lady sitting on the bed has come to book for antenatal care. Your task is to take her history to the hearing of the examiners.

14.1.3 Instruction to the Examiners

The patient present is a commercial sex worker who is about 12 weeks pregnant. She has come to book for antenatal care. The candidate is supposed to take her history. Listen to the conversation and use the checklist to score the candidate.

Checklist for history taking of a commercial sex worker

Tasks	Well done	Fairly done	Poorly done	Not done
Greets the patient and introduces self		2	1	0
Explains purpose of interaction, obtains permission		2	1	0
Biodata: name, age, address, occupation, religion, etc.	4	2	1	0
Parity, LMP, calculates EDD and tells patient her GAD	4	2	1	0
Presenting complaint		2	1	0
History of presenting complaint		2	1	0
Obstetric history: 2 previous TOPs, unwanted pregnancies	4	2	1	0
Gynaecological history: menarche, periods, cycle, contraception,	4	2	1	0
Past medical and surgical history:				
- Occasional malaria			1	0
- No drug allergy			1	0
- Appendicectomy 5 years ago.		2		0
- Ampiclox for post-exposure prophylaxis.		2		0
Family and social history:				
- First of 6 children of her parents who are farmers.		2	1	0
- No family history of DM, HT, SCD, or twinning.		2	1	0
- Currently lives with her aunty but works in a brothel.		2	1	0
- Attends to 5-10 customers per day.		2	1	0
- Uses male condoms except her boyfriend.		2	1	0
- Boyfriend is a soldier.		2	1	0
- Thinks boyfriend is father to the pregnancy.		2	1	0
- Has not disclosed pregnancy to boyfriend.		2	1	0
- Pregnancy confirmed by USS.		2	1	0
Systemic review			1	0
Summary of history to the examiners	4	2	1	0
Penalty: use of inappropriate language, judgmental, etc.	-4	-2	-1	0
Total marks	50			
Candidate's score .../50				

Examiner's signature Date

14.2 Station 14.2 Abnormal Test Finding: Follow-up for Pregnant Prostitute

Subject: Obstetrics
Theme: Ethics and medico-legal issues
Domain of Clinical Competence: Interpretation of abnormal test findings
Station: Antenatal follow-up of a commercial sex worker with test results
Station Objective: To assess the ability of the candidate to manage a pregnant, single, commercial sex worker who is HIV positive and has genital gonococcal infection as well
Requirements: Standardized patient, a comfortable chair or dressed bed for the SP, trained HIV counsellor, a table and chairs for examiners and candidate, instructions to the SP, candidate, and examiners, sufficient checklist, pencils and erasers, a chaperon

14.2.1 Instructions to the Standardized Patient

You were earlier seen in the booking clinic of this hospital with 3 months pregnancy whose presumed father is yet to be aware. Some investigations were requested, and you have come for follow-up today with the results of the investigations. The doctor will study the results and have a discussion with you concerning the subsequent management of your pregnancy.

14.2.2 Investigation Results

Haematology
- PCV = 28% (normal range 33–42%)
- Hb = 9.3 g/dL (normal range 11–14 g/dL)
- Blood group A Rhesus positive
- Hb genotype AA

Immunology
- Retroviral screening = HIV 1 positive
- HBV screening = negative
- HCV screening = negative
- VDRL test = non-reactive
- Chlamydia antibodies = negative

Microbiology
- Urine MCS = no growth
- HVS/ECS = *Neisseria gonorrhoeae* isolated
- Rectal swab = no growth
- Pharyngeal swab = no growth

Pelvic Ultrasound

Live singleton foetus 12W+3D. Placenta posterior fundal, no gross abnormality seen.

14.2.3 Instruction to the Candidate

Miss XX is a commercial sex worker who was booked for antenatal care last week. She has come for follow-up with the investigation results. Your task is to study the investigation results and answer the questions which follow.

1. What is your diagnosis?
2. What further investigations would you request?
3. What additional prescriptions would you give at this second visit?
4. What issues would you like to address in counselling her at this visit?

Answer Outline

1. The diagnosis is HIV in pregnancy (**2 marks**) with anaemia and gonococcal infection (**2 marks**).
2. Further investigations to be requested include: (**2 marks each**)
   (a) FBC including blood film to elucidate the type of anaemia
   (b) Serum ferritin and stool parasitology, looking for the possible cause of anaemia
   (c) Baseline viral load and CD4 count for subsequent monitoring of the treatment of HIV
   (d) Baseline EUCr as the ARVs may affect the kidneys
   (e) OGTT or 75 g oral glucose test as some ARV can trigger diabetes
   (f) LFT as some ARVs are hepatotoxic
   (g) Serum lipids as these may be affected by some ARVs
3. What prescriptions would you give at this visit? (**4 marks** each)
   (a) Dolutegravir (DTG) + Tenofovir (TDF) + Lamivudine (3TC) for the treatment of HIV
   (b) Multivitamins containing essential amino acids, zinc, and selenium as these may be depleted in HIV infection
   (c) Ceftriaxone or Amoxicillin-clavulanic acid for gonorrhoea in pregnancy
4. Issues to be counselled on this visit include (**2 marks** each):
   (a) Adherence counselling on ARV and haematinics
   (b) Birth preparedness
   (c) Contact tracing for screening and treatment for STDs including HIV
   (d) Possible conflict with paternity acceptance including partner violence
   (e) Denial of investigation results

Checklist for antenatal follow-up of HIV-positive prostitute

Tasks	Well done	Fairly done	Poorly done	Not done
Diagnosis: HIV in pregnancy (2) with anaemia and gonorrhea	4	2		0
Further investigations to be requested:				
- FBC with blood film.		2		0
- Serum ferritin and stool parasitology.		2		0
- Viral load and CD4 count.		2		0
- Electrolytes, urea, and creatinine.		2		0
- OGTT or 75g oral glucose test.		2		0
- LFT: liver enzymes, serum proteins, bilirubin.		2		0
- Serum lipids.		2		0
Prescriptions:				
- DTG + 3TC + TDF	4	2		0
- Multivitamins containing essential amino acids, zinc and selenium	4	2		0
Issues to be addressed in counselling:				
- Adherence counselling for ARV and haematinics.		2		0
- Birth preparedness.		2		0
- Contact tracing for screening for STDs including HIV.		2		0
- Conflict with paternity and partner violence.		2		0
- Denial of investigation results		2		0
Total marks	36			
Candidate's score .../36				

Examiner's signature Date

14.3 Station 14.3 Elective Caesarean Section on Maternal Request

Subject: Obstetrics
Theme: Ethics and medico-legal issues
Domain of Clinical Competence: Counselling
Station: Counselling a mother requesting for elective caesarean section for social reasons
Station Objective: To assess the ability of the candidate to counsel a mother requesting for elective caesarean section on social grounds with the aim of balancing between respect for her autonomy and her best interest based on clinical experience
Requirements: A standardized patient (pregnant woman), a dressed bed for the SP (Fig. 14.1), a table and chairs for the examiners and candidate, instructions to the SP, candidate, and examiners, sufficient checklists, pencils and erasers for examiners, a chaperon

14.3.1 Instructions to the Standardized Patient (SP)

I am 35 years old and carrying my third pregnancy, having had two normal deliveries before, the last delivery about 3 years ago. I booked for antenatal care at 12 weeks of gestation and am 36 weeks pregnant today. My PhD dissertation defence has been scheduled to hold 3 weeks from today. I am afraid I may go into labour around

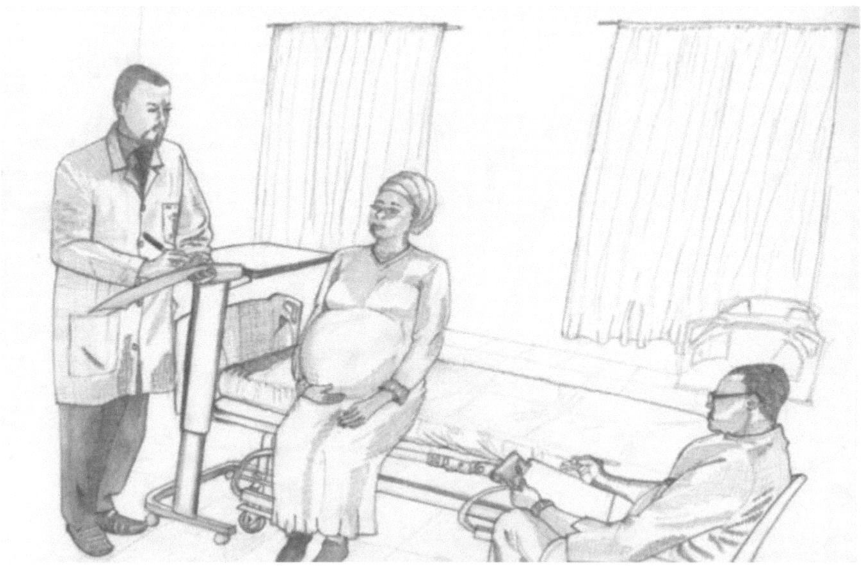

Fig. 14.1 Counselling for caesarean section. Courtesy of Jonathan Edache Otache

the time for my dissertation defence and would like to be delivered by elective caesarean section now so that I can recover before the defence. The advantages of induction of labour and the risks of caesarean section have been explained to me but I prefer to be delivered by caesarean section now.

14.3.2 Instructions to the Candidate

The patient is a booked 35-year-old G3P2+0, 2 alive at 36 weeks gestation. She is requesting for elective caesarean section so that she can prepare for her dissertation defence in 3 weeks' time. Your task is to counsel her concerning the request.

14.3.3 Instructions to the Examiners

The candidate is supposed to counsel this booked patient who is 36 weeks pregnant and requesting for elective caesarean section to enable her prepare for her dissertation defence in 3 weeks' time. Use the checklist provided to score the candidate.

Checklist for counselling for ELCS

Tasks	**Well done**	**Fairly done**	**Poorly done**	**Not done**
Greets patient and introduces self		2	1	0
Introduces the subject and obtains permission	4	2	1	0
Obtains biodata: name, age, address, occupation, religion etc.	4	2	1	0
Parity, LMP		2	1	0
Asks why she is requesting for ELCS		2	1	0
Explains implications of ELCS now on the baby: - Small chance baby may suffer complications of prematurity. - Even term babies may suffer birth asphyxia.		2 2	1 1	0 0
Explains implication to mother: - She must spend a few days on admission post-surgery. - Any surgery may suffer complication, she may still miss the defense. - ELCS has not been shown to be safer than labour.		2 2 2	1 1 1	0 0 0
Asks what she understands by the information given so far.		2		0
Prompting: I still prefer to have ELCS				
Explains the option of induction of labour: - The cervix can be ripened, and labour induced. - Can go home after few hours of successful IOL. - There is a small chance IOL may fail leading to EMCS.		2 2 2	1 1 1	0 0 0
Allows patient to ask questions and whether she has changed her mind.		2	1	0
Reminds her of the alternative of deferring the defense: - She can be given medical report to defer her defense. - She may go into labour and deliver before the defense date.		2 2	1 1	0 0
Prompting: Doctor, I still prefer to have ELCS.				
Thanks patient, requests investigations and asks her to come for admission tomorrow.	4	2	1	0
Total score	42			
Candidate's score …/42				

Examiner's signature Date

14.4 Station 14.4 Breaking Bad News: Non-identical Twins with Dual Paternity

Subject: Obstetrics
Theme: Ethics and medico-legal issues
Domain of Clinical Competence: Communication and counselling
Station: Breaking a social problem; possible dual paternity
Station Objective: To test the candidate's ability to handle a highly sensitive matter; informing a married mother of the possibility of dual paternity of her twin babies
Requirements: Standardized patient (mother of twins) who just delivered and is due for discharge home, dressed bed for the SP (Fig. 14.2), a table and chairs for the examiners and candidate, instructions to the SP, candidate, and examiners. Sufficient checklists, pencils and erasers, nurse counsellor, and a chaperon

14.4.1 Instructions to the Standardized Patient

I am a 25-year-old mother who delivered a set of twins 3 days ago and waiting for discharge home today. It was my first pregnancy and I have been married for the past 2 years. I hold a high national diploma in hotel and catering and I'm currently working with a 5-star hotel in this town. My husband is a 35-year-old Civil Engineer with a private firm. I did go out with a white tourist at about the time I got pregnant and when the doctor confirmed I was carrying twins, little did I know the white man was also involved. I had vaginal birth of the twins 3 days ago and the second twin looked like a white baby. The paediatrician who attended the delivery thinks the

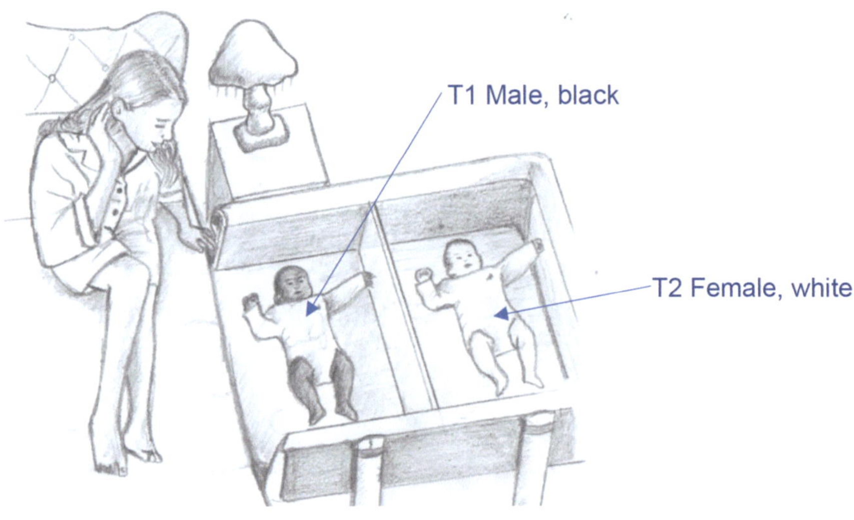

Fig. 14.2 Twins with different fathers. Courtesy of Jonathan Edache Otache

baby is normal and not an albino as was thought by some health workers in attendance. What do I do now?

14.4.2 Instruction to the Candidate

The patient delivered a set of twins 3 days ago but the second twin has straight blond hair like the white race. Your task is to counsel the mother concerning the possibility of dual paternity in this set of twins.

14.4.3 Instruction to the Examiners

This mother delivered a set of twins 3 days ago and is about to be discharged home. One of the twins appears to be fathered by a white man. The candidate is supposed to counsel the mother about the possibility of dual paternity. The mother admits having had a sexual relation with a white man about the time she conceived, use the checklist provided to score the candidate.

Checklist for dual paternity twins

Tasks	Well done	Fairly done	Poorly done	Not done
Greets patient and introduces self		2	1	0
Introduces the issue of non-identical twins and obtains permission to talk with her.		2	1	0
Obtains biodata: Name, age, address, occupation, marital status	4	2	1	0
Confirms parity and LCB		2	1	0
Asks of possible of extramarital affair with empathy.	4	2	1	0
Mother admits having sex with a white man.		2		0
Explains possibility of double fertilization in one cycle	4	2	1	0
Asks what she thinks her husband will do		2		0
Explains to her the options of what to do:				
- She may disclose the possibility of dual paternity to her husband.		2	1	0
- Disclosure may reduce conflict and relieve her psychological burden.		2	1	0
- She should also contact the white man and disclose the matter to him.		2	1	0
- Paternity test may be required to confirm the diagnosis.		2	1	0
Allows her ask for further clarifications.		2		0
Informs her that:				
- The child may also want to know who his father is when he grows up.		2	1	0
- He may suffer stigmatization in school.		2	1	0
- The twins may need to attend different schools in the future.		2	1	0
Tells mother he is willing to talk to her and her husband if she wants		2	1	0
Thanks her for talking with him and gives her appointment to PNC	4	2	1	0
Total score	44			
Candidate's score .../44				

Examiner's signature Date

Introduction to Viva Voce 15

15.1 Viva Voce

Viva voce which means "by word of mouth" in Latin was the earliest form of formal assessment in medical training dating back to the Middle Ages. Although the invention of the printing press and consequent increase in popularity of mass-produced textbooks have since reduced the dependence on the spoken word, oral examination method (viva voce) remains an important method of assessment in many fields of medical training to date. While oral examinations are almost a continuous and an on-going exercise during lectures and ward rounds, they usually take the form of supplementary tests during the final or exit examinations. The oral examination is usually the last paper, supplementing the written and clinical aspects of the examination. These probing questions, and some situations cross-questioning, dig out the degree of real assimilation of learning where a student cannot easily dodge.

In medical examination, grammatical accuracy, pronunciation, vocabulary, and usage are downplayed because medicine tends to have its own language. Candidates are assessed mainly on ideational content and its organization, delivery, and effect. The main tools of evaluation are checklists and rating scales. The aim of the oral examination is to assess the candidate's cognitive knowledge, psychomotor skills, and best attitude for good outcome (affective domain) in the chosen specialty. Because of the few stations and the limited time allocated, SBAs and OSCE are superior to viva voce in assessing these domains of clinical competence. However, oral examinations can test many things which written examinations cannot.

Currently, the Faculty of Obstetrics and Gynaecology of the West African College of Surgeons (WACS) uses the structured viva voce examination (SVVE). There are four questions (two Obstetrics and two Gynaecology), each constituting an independent station with independent group of examiners. All candidates rotate through all the four stations and spend the same amount of time; 5 min for membership and 7.5 min for fellowship examination (a total of 20–30 min). Each question (station) has a structured answer outline in the form of checklist with rating scales ranging from well done, fairly done, poorly done, and not done.

C. Chama, *OSCE and VIVA VOCE in Obstetrics and Gynaecology*,
https://doi.org/10.1007/978-3-031-77262-7_15

Compared with the traditional viva voce examination (TVVE), the SVVE has been shown to be more objective, with higher reliability and validity [1]. Student-teacher and student-topic bias are removed. Chance and luck factors get minimized and there is more uniformity, transparency, and fairness of examination results.

The viva voce examination requires fewer staff and resources when compared to the OSCE. Both examiner and candidate fatigue are less, and it gives a measure of the candidate's depth of knowledge and practical concepts on the topic discussed. Preparation for examination requires little effort by the examiners as they simply study the checklist provided.

The disadvantage of the viva voce is that it has a narrow scope (only four questions in 20–30 min). This narrow scope may be compensated by the in-depth probing of the topic in question, but the validity of the examination remains low. Another setback of the viva voce examination is the "difficult first question". This can throw-off even a good candidate and affect the entire examination. In the faculty of obstetrics and gynaecology examinations, the candidate is allowed to start with either obstetrics or gynaecology, depending on his choice but, this only relieves the candidate temporarily, as all questions must be answered.

15.2 Characteristics of Structured Viva Voce

The disadvantages of the traditional viva voce include:

- Poor content validity
- Low inter-rater and inter-case reliability
- Inconsistency in marking
- Lack of standardization

Structured viva voce (SVV) was probably used in medical education before 1989, but properly described as a separate assessment tool by Oakley and Hencken in 2005 [2, 3]. Because of the disadvantages of the traditional viva voce (TVV), the SVV was designed to be more reliable, valid, and acceptable. According to the standards in medical education, validity, reliability, and acceptability are considered parts of the criteria used for determining the usefulness of a particular method for assessment. Together with the feasibility and educational impact, these five elements constitute the characteristics of a good assessment tool [4].

Validity

Validity is the ability of an assessment tool to measure what it is supposed to measure. Mathematically, it is estimated by the correlation coefficient, which is the linear relation to a criterion variable. A recent meta-analysis showed a highly significant correlation coefficient between the results of SVV and MCQs [5]. This means a positive linear relationship between SVV and MCQs. The MCQ is considered a standard assessment tool in validity and reliability in medical education. A similar positive correlation was found between SVV and OSCE [6]. These findings of positive correlation with standard assessment tools give SVV a good validity.

Reliability

This is the ability of an assessment tool to produce the same results if repeated for a similar group of candidates. It is measured by the ratio of the true score variance to the observed score variance. Mathematically, either the Cronbach alpha ($a = 0.8$ is very reliable) or the reliability coefficient is used to measure the reliability of an assessment tool. A meta-analysis of the validity and reliability of SVV in medical examinations showed a Cronbach alpha of 0.8 (range 0.75–0.80), the Cronbach for MCQs were >0.8 [7]. The reliability of SVV was good for each pair of examiners and for each question.

Acceptability

In modern medical training, especially postgraduate training, the "adult learning theory" has to be applied. According to the adult learning theory, the learners are self-motivated, problem-based, aware, and have the right to be involved in the curriculum delivery and assessment tools [8]. It is vital for the educational procedure that the learners should be involved and highly accept learning methods and assessment tools. Learners' acceptability to the new assessment tool, for example, structured viva compared to the traditional or conventional viva vary from a high acceptance rate to a low acceptance rate throughout the published studies [7]. Compared to the TVV, the SVV has a significantly higher acceptance rate of about 80% in the meta-analysis quoted above. Thus, in addition to the traditional value of testing higher cognitive levels, problem-solving, and communication skills, the SVV has high acceptability, good validity, and reliability.

15.3 Preparing for the Viva

Viva voce can be unpredictable as there are no routines that can be practised and very little familiar territory for the average candidate to fall back on. As well as assessing clinical knowledge, viva voce also assesses the candidate's ability to think on the spot and react under pressure, both of which are vital skills for the clinician to possess. Even seasoned exam veterans have frozen up and gone blank in vivas. For this reason, the viva is probably the most dreaded of all the different types of examinations that medical students are faced with. Fortunately, viva usually carries a small proportion of the total marks for the examination. In some faculties, like the faculty of obstetrics and gynaecology, WACS, the viva voce is a stand-alone paper that must be passed, and has recently been a source of casualty for many candidates.

Like any other medical examination, preparation for viva should start early. Try to get a feel for the sort of questions that are likely to come up by talking to colleagues and consulting any available textbook on the subject matter. Although mock viva voce should be conducted by trainers before the real examination, candidates should also practise group work by creating exam conditions for themselves so that they can get used to the stress and anxiety that the viva can induce. Burning the candle is good but reading and understanding does not guarantee true comprehension, the ability to recall, and give back a set of facts in a form that is clearly understood by its recipients. Although viva voce presents undue advantage to gifted speakers, brain block or tongue-tie is more common and remains the most dreaded problem for candidates. There are reports of some candidates going on drugs like B-blockers to calm them down on the morning of the examination.

It is very common to be asked to give definitions or give lists, and these should be a source of easy marks for the candidate. These are often used as opening questions and should be second nature to the candidate by the time the viva is sited. When reciting lists, you should try to start with the commonest causes first. It will be helpful if the candidate can make a list of common definitions and practise them before the real examination.

Candidates should dress the same way they would for a job interview in smart but comfortable clothing. Men should wear a conventional dark coloured suit (black or navy blue), conservative shirt, and a dark coloured tie. Women should wear a conventional skirt or trouser suit but avoid low cut tops, short skirts, and excessive make-ups.

As you enter your station, make good eye contact with the examiner that greets you and ask if you may sit down. Sit upright, smile, and be confident. Avoid crossing your arms and legs and if there are more than one examiner try and engage both of them even if only one talks to you. You will be given a minute or so to read the questions and understand the instructions before you start. Do not guess an answer if you do not know it. If the instruction allows you, start with the question you understand best but know that you must answer all the questions. Answering one question incorrectly is not a disaster, but allowing it to disrupt your concentration and ability to answer subsequent questions may well be. It is also worth remembering that you may have misjudged how you answered the question, and you may well have done better than you think.

As the bell goes, thank your examiners and leave the station promptly. The exam is over and no more marks can be gained.

References

1. Dhasmana DC, Bala S, Sharma R, et al. Introducing structured viva voce examination in medical undergraduate pharmacology: a pilot study. Indian J Pharmacol. 2016;48(1):S52–6.
2. Tutton PJM, Glasgow EF. Reliability and predictive capacity of examinations in anatomy and improvement in the reliability of viva voce (oral) examinations by the use of a structured rating system. Clin Anat. 1989;21:29–34.
3. Oakley B, Hencken C. Oral examination assessment practices: effectiveness and change with a first year undergraduate cohort. J Hosp Leis Sport Tour Educ. 2005;4:3–14.
4. Epstein RM. Assessment in medical education. N Engl J Med. 2007;356(4):387–96.
5. Rohini Bhadre A, Sathe MB, Mosamkar S. Comparison of objective structured viva voce with traditional viva voce. Int J Healthc Biomed Res. 2016;5(1):62–7.
6. Waseem N, Iqbal K. Importance of structured VIVA as an assessment tool in anatomy. J Univ Med Dent Coll. 2016;7(2):29–4.

7. Abuzied AIH, Nabag WOM. Structured viva validity, reliability and acceptability as an assessment tool in health professions education: a systematic review and meta-analysis. BMC Med Educ. 2023;23:531–9.
8. Madhukumar S, Pavithra MB, Amrita NS. Conventional viva and structured viva—comparison and perception of students. Indian J Public Health Res Dev. 2022;13(2):167–72.

Gynaecology Viva Voce 16

16.1 Basic Principles of Surgery

16.1.1 Question 1: Universal Precaution

- What is universal precaution?
- Explain the measures put in place as universal precaution in the operating room.

16.1.1.1 Answer Outline

Universal precaution is a set of recommendations aimed at reducing the risk of transmission of pathogens from patients to caregivers and vice versa. In universal precaution, all patients are considered potentially infected and therefore equally treated. Because health workers come in contact with all kinds of patients, all should be immunized against the common communicable diseases such as hepatitis B virus, tuberculosis, influenza, measles, rubella, and varicella and more recently COVID 19 virus.

In the operating room, the universal precautions that are observed to prevent infecting the patients and vice versa include:

1 All theatre workers should be immunized against communicable diseases, especially blood-borne infections like HBV.
2 Do not cross the red line with casual wears into the business area to prevent contamination of the theatre.
3 Anaesthetists and assistant nurses must wear their scrubs, face masks, and hand gloves to receive patients at the reception. This protects the health worker's mucous membranes from blood and body fluids while also protecting the surgical wounds from exhaled pathogens and droplets.
4 The perioperative nurses and surgeons enter the scrub room, scrub and gown before entering the operating suite:
   (a) Wear cap, face mask, eye goggles, boots, and waterproof apron
   (b) Hand washing to reduce the load of pathogens on the hands

C. Chama, *OSCE and VIVA VOCE in Obstetrics and Gynaecology*,
https://doi.org/10.1007/978-3-031-77262-7_16

(c) Wear sterile gowns and double sterile gloves

5 Patients cover from the wards or emergency room to be removed before scrubbing and draping.

6 Surgical instruments should be sterile or highly disinfected. Instrument handling should be such as to prevent accidental pricks and cuts.

7 In case of accidental cuts and pricks, post-exposure prophylaxis should be taken according to protocol; immediately remove surgical gloves and encourage bleeding by squeezing outwards, wash with soap and running water, and take blood samples from both patient and surgeon for screening before commencing prophylactic drugs.

Checklist for universal precautions

Task	Well done	Fairly done	Poorly done	Not done
Introduction – definition and importance of universal precaution	4	2	1	0
Primary prevention by all theatre workers through vaccinations	4	2	1	0
Theatre design to prevent contamination; reception, changing rooms, red lines at reception and operating suite area.	4	2	1	0
Handling of patients to prevent cross-infection; changing of trolleys, use of face masks etc.	4	2	1	0
Pre-operative preparations by surgeons and perioperative nurses – scrubbing and gowning: - Importance of cap, face mask and eye goggles - Importance of waterproof apron and sterile gowns - Importance of double gloving		2 2 2		0 0 0
Instrument handling - Proper capping of needles - Use instruments to pick sharps. - Passing sharps from scrub nurse to surgeon in a receiver - Proper disposal of sharps		2 2 2 2		0 0 0 0
Protocol for PEP following cuts or pricks: - Ungloves and washes hands under running water. - Take blood specimen from patient and surgeon for screening. - Inform physician to prescribe prophylactic drug. - Schedule follow-up with physician		2 2 2 2		0 0 0 0
Total scores	38			
Candidate's score ………/38				

Examiner's signature Date

16.1.2 Question 2: Informed Consent

- What is informed consent?
- Outline and explain the important issues when administering an informed consent to a patient to undergo an elective major gynaecological surgery.

16.1.2.1 Answer Outline

Introduction

With increasing medico-legal litigation, and the desire to provide patients with more say concerning their own treatment, it is important to obtain an informed consent before any major surgical procedure. Informed consent means the patient has been adequately informed about her medical condition and the options of treatment before she chose to have a particular procedure. Informed consent guides the patient to the right decision and dispel unrealistic expectations. It also creates trust between the patient and the doctor. The important issues to be discussed when obtaining an informed consent include the following:

Outline of issues to be discussed.

- Who to obtain consent
- When to obtain consent
- Explaining the procedure
- Explaining the benefits and risks of the procedure
- Explaining alternative treatment
- Explaining the possible outcome of not doing anything
- Special circumstances (vulnerable people)
- Who endorses the consent

Who Obtains the Consent?

- It is preferable that someone who can perform the procedure obtains the consent from the patient or the guardian of the patient; this means a senior medical personnel in the managing team.
- Someone who has been specially trained on advising patients about the procedure can also obtain an informed consent. Examples are nurse counsellors and medical social workers.

Timing of Obtaining Consent

- For an elective surgery, the best time to obtain an informed consent is in the clinic when decision has been taken that the patient requires a particular procedure. The patient can then be included on the operation list.
- The patient must be competent to decide.
- The patient must have received sufficient information concerning his/her medical condition.
- Patient should not be under duress; if the patient is in pain, it is better to admit the patient and stabilize him or her before obtaining the consent.

Explaining the Procedure

- Explain step by step the intended procedure to the patient including anaesthesia.
- Explain the risks and benefits of the procedure.
- Give alternative treatments (options) including their risks and benefits too.
- Explain the risks and benefits of not doing anything.

Explaining the Potential Risks

- How much information do you give?
  - Anything that poses substantial risk of grave consequences.
  - Mention risks that would affect the decision of a reasonable person.
  - Tell the truth if asked a direct question.
- Mention complications likely to occur more than 1% of the time.
- Too little information fails to inform; too much information may lead to confusion.
- Explain risks in proportions like 1 in 100, 1 in 1000 and not percentages quartiles, etc.
- Information regarding surgery has been shown to have positive/neutral effect.

Explaining the Potential Benefits

- Balance the frequency of success against the frequency of risks.

Explaining Alternative Treatments

- The pros and cons compared to the planned procedure.

Explaining the Outcome of NO Surgery

- Status quo:
  - Possible resolution—give proportion
  - Worsening condition—give proportion

Special Considerations

- Children under 18 years
- People with mental disability
- Procedure not requiring anaesthesia

Additional Materials

- Audiovisual aide
- Leaflets
- These materials only supplement and does not replace verbal consent

Finally, both the person obtaining the consent and the patient must sign the consent form. However, the signatures do not validate the consent; it is the discussion that took place that validates the consent. Sometimes, the presence of a witness gives credence to the consent that in fact it took place.

Checklist for informed consent

Task	Well done	Fairly done	Poorly done	Not done
Introduction				
- What is informed consent?		2	1	0
- Why is it important?		2	1	0
Outline of issues to be discussed:				
- Who to obtain consent,			1	0
- when to obtain consent,			1	0
- explaining the procedure,			1	0
- explaining benefits and risks,			1	0
- alternative treatment,			1	0
- not doing anything, vulnerable people,			1	0
- who signs the consent			1	0
Who obtains the consent:				
- Preferably someone who can perform the procedure.		2	1	0
- Trained counsellor		2	1	0
Timing of obtaining consent				
- In clinic for elective, in the ward for emergencies		2	1	0
- Not under duress, stabilize first or use consorts.		2	1	0
- Patient must be competent.		2	1	0
- After giving sufficient information		2	1	0
Explaining the procedure				
- Step by step from anaesthesia to recovery		2	1	0
- Risks and benefits of procedure		2	1	0
- Options including their risks and benefits.		2	1	0
- Risks of not doing anything		2	1	0
Explaining the potential risks				
- How much information do you give?		2	1	0
- Mention complications likely to occur >1% of the		2	1	0
time.		2	1	0
- Explain risks in proportions like 1 out of 100.		2	1	0
- Tell the truth if asked a direct question				
Explaining options				
- Explain only available options.		2	1	0
- The pros and cons compared to planned procedure		2	1	0
Explain outcome of NO surgery				
- Possible resolution-give proportion		2	1	0
- Possible worsening condition-give proportion		2	1	0
Special considerations				
- Vulnerable people		2	1	0
- Procedure not requiring anaesthesia		2	1	0
Who signs the consent – the doctor, patient and a witness	4	2	1	0
Additional materials –pamphlets, audiovisual, charts		2		0
TOTAL MARKS	57			
Candidate's score ....../57				

Examiner's signature Date

16.1.3 Question 3: Anterior Abdominal Wall Incisions

- List two types of anterior abdominal wall skin incisions used in gynaecological surgeries with two examples of each.
- Describe step by step how you would perform laparotomy using the Pfannenstiel skin incision.

16.1.3.1 Answer Outline

Types of anterior abdominal skin incisions

1 Transverse incisions
   (a) Pfannenstiel incision
   (b) Joel-Cohen incision
   (c) Kustner incision
   (d) Cherney incision
   (e) Maylard incision
2 Vertical incisions
   (a) Midline incision
   (b) Paramedian incision
3 Oblique incisions (Not popular in gynaecological surgery)
   (a) Gridiron (McBurney) incision
   (b) Rockey-Davis incision
   (c) J-shaped incision (for extra-peritoneal CS)

Pfannenstiel Incision

This is the most popular abdominal wall incision in gynaecological surgeries perhaps because of its numerous advantages.

Advantages

- Good cosmetic result
- Three times stronger than midline scar
- Less wound dehiscence; 3–5 times less than midline
- Less painful, requiring less analgesia
- Less interference with post-operative respiration

Disadvantages

- More time consuming
- Less exposure of abdominal cavity
- More haemorrhage intra-operatively
- More haematoma/seroma post-operatively

Procedure

- Patient in supine position under anaesthesia
- Cleaned and draped to expose anterior abdominal wall
- Slightly curved transverse skin incision 2–3 cm above the hair line

- 10–15 cm in length but can be extended
- Cut through skin and subcutaneous fat down to the rectus sheath
- Divide rectus sheath transversely on either side of linear alba
- Separate rectus sheath from underlying rectus muscle by inserting your finger on either side of the cut rectus sheath
- Cut the linear alba in the middle
- Separate rectus muscles manually in the midline
- Pick the peritoneum between two artery forceps and incise vertically
- The incision of the rectus sheath can be extended into the internal and external oblique muscles, taking care not to injure the iliohypogastric and ilioinguinal nerves
- Insert a self-retaining retractor and pack the intestines away with two moist abdominal packs
- After surgery the abdomen can be closed in layers or in mass.
- Closure in layers
  - Peritoneum and transversalis fascia with continuous or interrupted vicryl 2/0
  - Rectus sheath with continuous or interrupted vicryl 1
  - Skin with interrupted mattress nylon 2/0
- Mass closure with vicryl 2 to include all layers except skin which is closed with nylon 2/0

Checklist for Pfannenstiel incision

Task	Well done	Fairly done	Poorly done	Not done
Transverse abdominal wall incisions (4 marks)				
- Pfannenstiel incision		2		0
- Joel-Cohen incision		2		0
- Maylard incision		2		0
- Cherney incision		2		0
Longitudinal or vertical abdominal incisions (4 marks)				
- Midline subumbilical incision		2		0
- Paramedian incisions		2		0
- Rocky-Davies incision		2		0
Pfannenstiel incision				
- Most popular skin incision in gynaecological surgeries		2		0
- Advantages: cosmetic, good wound healing, less postop pain	4	2		0
- Disadvantages: haemorrhage, poor exposure, longer time	4	2		0
Skin incision				
- Crescenteric (curved upwards) 2-3cm above the hair line	4	2		0
- 10-15cm long but can be extended	4	2		0
- Cut through skin, subcutaneous tissue, down to rectus sheath	4	2		0
Rectus sheath and muscle				
- Divide rectus sheath transversely on either side of midline and manually separate from the muscle	4	2		0
- Cut linear alba vertically in the midline	4	2		0
- Separate the rectus muscles manually on either side	4	2		0
Entering the peritoneal cavity				
- Pick the peritoneum between 2 artery forceps and divide vertically	4	2		0
- The incision of the rectus sheath can be extended laterally to the internal and external oblique to create more room	4	2		0
- Insert a self- retaining retractor and pack intestines away	4	2		0
PERFORM THE SPECIFIC SURGERY		2		0
Closing the abdomen				
The abdomen can be closed in layers or en-mass		2		0
- In layers: peritoneum vicryl 2/0, rectus sheath vicryl 1, skin with vicryl 2/0 or nylon 2/0	4	2		0
- Mass closure with vicryl 2 (nylon 2) to include all layers except the skin; close skin with vicryl 2/0 (nylon 2/0)	4	2		0
Clean skin and apply dry dressing to the wound		2		0
Total marks		64		
Candidate's score .../64				

Examiner's signature Date

16.2 Paediatric and Adolescent Gynaecology

16.2.1 Question 1: Ambiguous Genitalia

- What is an ambiguous genitalia?
- How would you manage a term baby born with ambiguous genitalia?

16.2.1.1 Answer Outline

Definition

Ambiguous genitalia is a disorder of sexual development (DSD), formally called intersex, in which there is the presence of both male and female external characteristics, i.e. they are not clearly male or female. The DSD, though seen phenotypically as ambiguous genitalia, may involve the gonads, internal duct system, or external genitalia. The abnormalities present are usually hypospadias, undescended testes, micropenis, enlarged clitoris, labial fusion, labial mass, and a combination of these. Rates vary from 1 in 1000 to 4000 births.

Causes

- Sex chromosome DSD (gonadal dysgenesis)
  - 45X Turner
  - 47XXY Klinefelter
  - 45X/46XY mixed (mosaicism)
  - 46XX/46XY Ovotesticular
- 46XY DSD (undervirilization of 46XY individuals)
  - Testicular; gonadal dysgenesis
  - Androgen production abnormalities
- 46XX DSD (gonadal virilization)
  - Ovotesticular (true hermaphrodite)
  - Gonadal dysgenesis
  - Androgen excess—foetal, maternal, placental

The poorly developed testes are termed dysgenetic testes while the poorly developed ovary is termed streak gonads. The underdeveloped gonads ultimately fail as evidenced by elevated gonadotropins. Patients bearing the Y-chromosome are at risk of developing germ cell tumours.

Management Team
- Obstetrician and gynaecologist
- Endocrinologist
- Neonatologist
- Psychiatrist
- Urologist
- Geneticist

Brief History
- Past history of congenitally abnormal baby
- Drug history in this pregnancy
- Family history of congenital abnormality

Investigations
- Electrolytes and urea
- Hormonal assays to include FSH, LH, ACTH, TSH, etc
- Buccal smear or blood sample for Barr bodies
- Karyotyping
- Ultrasound
- Intravenous urogram
- MRI to rule out adrenal or ovarian tumours

Treatment
- Congenital adrenal hyperplasia may require electrolyte replacement and
- Corticosteroid to suppress the excessive ACTH
- Gender assignment based on appearance and future fertility
- Surgery
  - Clitoral amputation
  - Vaginoplasty
  - Gonadectomy
  - Urologic

Checklist for management of ambiguous genitalia

Task	Well done	Fairly done	Poorly done	Not done
Introduction: definition of ambiguous genitalia, its importance, prevalence	4	2	1	0
Causes at birth: congenital adrenal hyperplasia, in-utero exposure to androgens, chromosomal abnormalities	4	2	1	0
Management team: Obstetrician and Gynaecologist, Neonatologist, Endocrinologist, Psychologist, Geneticist and Urologist	4	2	1	0
Brief history: family history of congenital anomaly, history of congenitally abnormal baby from the mother, drug history in this pregnancy	4	2	1	0
Investigations:				
- Electrolytes and urea		2		0
- Hormonal assay; FSH, LH, TSH, ACTH		2		0
- Karyotyping or buccal smear or blood for Barr bodies		2		0
- Ultrasound		2		0
- MRI to rule out ovarian or adrenal tumors		2		0
- Intravenous urogram		2		0
Treatment:				
- Congenital adrenal hyperplasia may require electrolyte replacement		2		0
- Corticosteroids to suppress excessive ACTH also in congenital AH		2		0
- Gender assignment based on appearance and future fertility		2		0
- Surgery: clitoral amputation, gonadectomy, vaginoplasty, urologic		2		0
Follow-up: congenital adrenal hyperplasia is an emergency due to the electrolyte imbalance. The other causes may require gonadectomy at puberty and vaginoplasty	4	2	1	0
Total score	30			
Candidates score ……/30				

Examiner's signature Date

16.2.2 Question 2: Rape

- What is rape?
- Discuss the management of a 12-year-old pupil brought to the accident and emergency unit having been raped by her stepfather.

16.2.2.1 Answer Outline

Introduction

Child sexual abuse is becoming rampant and has recently gained attention in Nigeria. It comes in many dimensions, including sexual assault. Where parents/guardians are involved it poses a great challenge to health care workers, the sufferers, family members, and the populace in general. Handling of such cases has medical, psychological, and legal implications. Rape is defined as forceful vaginal or anal penetration in a woman or anal penetration in a man by another man's penis or object.

Management

Requires multidisciplinary approach; involving the gynaecologist, psychologist or psychiatrist, paediatrician, microbiologist, urologist, nurse counsellor, legal officers, and security agents.

History

History should be taken from the patient in the presence of an adult who should preferably be the guardian or mother, a senior nursing staff, and a psychologist/psychiatrist. Sometimes this may involve only the patient in the presence of a psychologist/psychiatrist or a social worker and a senior nursing staff. History should include focus on where, when, how, why, who:

- Details of alleged assault, description of assailant, meeting place, place of assault
- Since the assault when did she last eat, bath, shower, drink, douched, passed urine, opened her bowels, changed clothes, ingest any drug including alcohol
- Gynaecologic and obstetric history
- Previous history of assault
- Past medical history-handicaps; both physical and mental
- Social history-family circumstance, relationship with perpetrator

Physical Examination

- General-severity and type of distress; pain, anxiety, pallor, dehydration, bruises
- Injuries-body diagrams; distribution, dimensions in relation to body landmarks—petechial haemorrhages, bruises, lacerations, incisions
- Systemic examination-head, neck, CNS, chest CVS, abdomen, genitals, extremities
- Detailed vaginal and anal examination-perineum smeared with semen or blood, any bruises, tears, lacerations, active bleeding, look at hymenal remnants, take swab for MCS and DNA
- Oral-teeth, mucosal injury, tongue

Laboratory Investigations

- Consult infectious disease unit-FBC, HBV, HCV, HIV, VDRL
- Keep stained clothes, tampons/pads, condoms, etc. for forensic examination
- Forensic samples from fingernails, skin, lower abdomen, and other relevant areas
- Mouth swab and wash
- Vaginal HVS, ECS
- Anal swabs, proctoscopy-guided anal and rectal swabs

Treatment

- Immediate: IVL, TT, analgesics, antibiotics, PEP immunoprophylaxis, emergency contraception
- Treat physical injuries
- Follow-up refer to child psychologist
- Legal issues: inform hospital authority who may inform the police
- Document all findings and treatment offered

Checklist for rape

Task	Well done	Fairly done	Poorly done	Not done
Rape is:				
- Forceful,		2	1	0
- Vaginal or anal penetration in a woman,		2	1	0
- Or anal penetration in a man,		2	1	0
- By another man's penis or object.		2	1	0
Management team: Gynaecologist, Paediatrician, Psychologist/Psychiatrist, Religious leader, Police	4	2	1	0
History:				
- In the presence of mother or guardian and Psychologist		2	1	0
- Focus on when, where, who, why and how		2	1	0
Physical examination:				
- General; pain, anxiety, pallor		2	1	0
- Injuries; body diagram with distribution of bruises and lacerations		2	1	0
- Systemic; head, neck, CNS, CVS, abdomen, genitalia, extremities		2	1	0
- Detailed VE and anal exam with swabs taken		2	1	0
Investigations:				
- Keep stained clothes, pads, condoms if freshly presented.		2	1	0
- Forensic samples from nails, skin, mouth, and any relevant area		2	1	0
- HVS, ECS, Anal swab under proctoscopy guidance		2	1	0
- FBC, RVS, VDRL, HBV		2	1	0
Treatment:				
- IVL, analgesics, antibiotics, blood transfusion as		2	1	0
necessary		2	1	0
- PEP according to protocol, emergency contraception		2	1	0
- Treat physical injuries		2	1	0
- Inform hospital authority to inform the police				
Follow-up:				
- Treat according to results of investigations		2	1	0
- Continue psychological counselling.		2	1	0
- Hospital authority to take up legal issues.		2	1	0
- Document everything; findings, treatment, complications etc.		2	1	0
Total marks	44			

Examiner's signature Date

16.2.3 Question 3: Imperforate Hymen

- What is imperforate hymen?
- Describe step by step, how you would perform hymenectomy in a patient with haematocolpos.

16.2.3.1 Answer Outline

By the seventh week of gestation, the cloaca is divided by the urorectal septum to form the urogenital sinus anteriorly and the hindgut posteriorly. By the twentieth week of gestation, the urogenital sinus (hymeneal membrane) degenerates to become continuous with the newly canalized vagina. Failure of this membrane to degenerate leads to imperforate hymen. Following menarche, menstrual blood accumulates behind this vaginal obstruction forming haematocolpos and if unrecognized and treated may progress to haematometra—collection of menstrual blood in the uterus.

In our environment, most patients are diagnosed in adolescence when they are symptomatic—primary amenorrhoea, cyclical abdominal pain, abdominal swelling, and urinary and defecation problems. Occasionally, asymptomatic imperforate hymen may be found in early childhood, with or without mucocoele. In severe cases, the mucocoele can cause ureteric obstruction and renal failure in the newborn.

Hymenectomy

Preoperative Preparation

- Consent
  - Depending on her age, may require parental consent only, parental consent plus child assent or child consent alone
- Investigations
  - Pelvic ultrasound scan
  - PCV
  - Urinalysis
  - Urine MCS if symptomatic

Surgical Steps

- Anaesthesia
  - GA preferable since it is a short (day case) procedure
  - Spinal anaesthesia can be given
- Positioning
  - In lithotomy position under anaesthesia
  - Cleaned and draped
  - The bladder is emptied
- Hymeneal incision
  - A cruciate incision at 10 to 4 o'clock and 2 to 8 o'clock into the hymeneal membrane
  - Allow menstrual blood to flow with suprapubic pressure

  - Trim hymeneal leaflets from the hymeneal ring with dissecting scissors
- Irrigation
  - Copious irrigation with warm normal saline
  - Can use bulb syringe or a 50 mL plastic syringe
- Suturing
  - Suture cut edges of the leaflet bases with interrupted vicryl 3–0 or 4–0
  - Alternatively, haemostats may be used to crush the bases of the leaflets for a minute and the leaflets cut with scissors or electrocautery

Post-operative Care

- Oral or topical analgesia
- Sitz bath twice a day
- Inform patient that menstrual blood may continue to flow for a few days
- See in 2 weeks and inspect for patency and assessment of healing

Checklist for hymenectomy

Task	Well done	Fairly done	Poorly done	Not done
What is imperforate hymen? Prevalence, pattern of presentation	4	2	1	0
Pre-operative preparations: signed informed consent, pelvic USS, PCV, urinalysis	4	2	1	0
Anaesthesia: GA preferable since it's a short procedure, spinal anaesthesia can be used		2	1	0
Positioning: in lithotomy position, cleaned and draped, bladder emptied		2	1	0
Hymeneal incision: cruciate incision at 10 to 4 o'clock and 2 to 8 o'clock, allow menstrual blood to flow with suprapubic pressure, trim hymeneal leaflets with scissors	4	2	1	0
Irrigation: with warm saline using bulb syringe or 50ml plastic syringe		2	1	0
Suturing: suture cut edges of hymeneal leaflets bases with vicryl 3/0. Alternatively, use haemostats to crush the bases of the leaflets and cut the free ends with scissors or electrocautery	4	2	1	0
Postoperative care: analgesia, antibiotics, sitz bath twice a day. Review patient in 2 weeks	4	2	1	0
Total score	26			
Candidates score .... /26				

Examiner's signature Date

16.3 General Gynaecology

16.3.1 Question 1: Cervical Incompetence

- What is cervical incompetence?
- Describe step by step how you would insert McDonald's cerclage at 14 weeks of gestation.

16.3.1.1 Answer Outline

Cervical incompetence is the inability of the cervix to retain pregnancy to term. The clinical condition complicates up to 1% of all pregnancies. Classically it presents with:

- Recurrent painless mid-trimester miscarriages
- Of decreasing gestation age
- Usually complete, with live foetus in an intact foetal membranes (Coul)
- Minimal vaginal bleeding

The risk factors for developing cervical incompetence include:

- Trauma
  - Excessive cervical dilatation during induced abortions
  - Instrumental vaginal deliveries especially forceps delivery
  - Cervical lacerations
  - Cervical conization
- Uterine anomalies
- Prenatal exposure to diethylstilbestrol
- Congenital cervical weakness-Ehlers-Danlos syndrome

Diagnosis

- Largely based on history of repeated painless mid-trimester abortions
- Some supporting tests
  - Retrograde cervical dilatation; easy passage of 8 mm Hegar's dilator
  - Traction test: easy pulling out of transcervical intrauterine 16F Foley's catheter inflated with 2 mL saline
  - HSG-funnelling of internal os
  - USS in pregnancy, preferably serial
    Funnelling of internal os on TVS (T-shape to Y-shape and then U-shape)
    Endocervical canal <2 cm in length
    Internal os diameter >2.5 cm at 10 weeks gestation

16.3.1.2 Insertion of McDonald's Cerclage

McDonald IA first used this type of cerclage in 1957 on 70 cases and obtained 43% neonatal survival even though most of the patients already had cervical dilatation more than 4 cm. When he later applied the cerclage at 14 weeks before the cervix began to dilate, neonatal survival improved to 80%.

Step 1: Preoperative Patient Preparation

- Establish the diagnosis
- Exclude genital sepsis with HVS, ECS
- USS to confirm foetal viability, dating, and cervical length (2 cm or more)
- Check PCV and urinalysis
- Obtain consent after explaining the procedure to the patient

Step 2: Anaesthesia

- Regional preferred (spinal or epidural)
- GA can be used
- Cervical block; least preferred

Step 3: Positioning Patient

- Patient in lithotomy or Trendelenburg position
- Cleaned and draped
- Bladder emptied
- EUA for cervical length and dilatation, uterine size and position, any adnexal pathology

Step 4: Applying the Cerclage

- Expose the cervix with Sims' speculum.
- Hold the anterior and posterior lips of the cervix with long Allis forceps or sponge holding forceps at 12 and 6 O'clock positions, respectively.
- With 5 mm Marceline or Nylon tape, take the first bite at 12 o'clock position at the cervico-vaginal junction and come out at 9:30 o'clock position. Take second bite at 9 o'clock and come out at 6:30 o'clock position, then at 6 o'clock and come out at 3:30 o'clock position. Finally take the last bite at 3 o'clock position and come out at 12 o'clock position.

- Adjust the suture to have adequate length either side and cut the needles off.
- With the assistant's little finger in the cervical os (if dilated) a surgeon's knot is tied at 12 o'clock position and tightened until the assistant feels a firm grip around his finger; he then removes his finger.
- Additional 4–5 throws are added in the knot and the ends trimmed 2–3 cm long for easy identification.
- Clean the vagina with wet and then dry gauze and apply sanitary pad.

Step 5: Post-operative Management

- Analgesia
- Tocolysis-optional
- Antibiotics-optional
- Bed rest + tranquilizer for a few days—5 days
- Inspect pad for bleeding or discharge (liquor)
- After discharge home, mother should report to hospital if:
  - Vaginal bleeding
  - Drainage of liquor
  - Lower abdominal cramps occur

Checklist for cervical incompetence

Task	Well done	Fairly done	Poorly done	Not done
What is cervical incompetence? - Definition and prevalence - Clinical features and causes - Diagnosis and treatment		 2 2 2	 1 1 1	 0 0 0
Pre-operative patient preparation: establish diagnosis, exclude genital sepsis, confirm viability, PCV, urinalysis, obtain informed consent	4	2	1	0
Anaesthesia: Regional preferred, GA can be used, cervical infiltration least preferred	4	2	1	0
Positioning patient: lithotomy or Trendelenburg position, clean and drape, empty bladder, EUA for cervical length, uterine size and position	4	2	1	0
Applying suture: - Expose cervix with Sims speculum - Hold lips of cervix with Allis forceps or sponge holding forceps - Make a purse-string suture with 5mm Marceline or nylon tape and tie at 12 o'clock position - Cut suture long, clean vagina, apply sanitary pad		2 2 2 2	1 1 1 1	0 0 0 0
Postoperative management: analgesia, antibiotics and Tocolysis are optional, inspect sanitary pads regularly for bleeding or discharge (liquor)	4	2	1	0
Follow-up: after discharge home, patient should report to hospital if there is bleeding, abnormal discharge, or lower abdominal cramps	4	2	1	0
Total score	34			
Candidates score ... /34				
Weighted score				

Examiner's signature Date

16.3.2 Question 2: Bartholin's Cyst

- What is Bartholin's cyst?
- Describe step by step how you would perform marsupialization of a Bartholin's cyst in a 26-year-old nullipara.

  How would you treat her if she were 58 years old?

16.3.2.1 Answer Outline

Introduction

- Bartholin's cyst is a common gynaecological problem in women below the age of 30 years.
- Bartholin's glands are pea-sized vulvovaginal gland situated in the labia minora at about 4 and 8 o'clock positions and lubricate the vulva during sexual intercourse.
- They open into the vestibule via 2.5 cm duct; the distal portion of which may be blocked to form the majority of Bartholin's cysts (Bartholin's duct cyst).
- Infected cysts may form abscess though primary infection of the gland may also form Bartholin's abscess.
- Bartholin's cysts are typically unilateral, asymptomatic, and discovered during routine pelvic examination; symptomatic cases may present with vulvar swelling or pain, dyspareunia, and pain during walking or exercise.
- In women over 40 years, malignancy, though rare (1/1000,000) should be excluded. Because it is rare, I&D and biopsy of the cyst wall is sufficient if suspicious excise.

Marsupialization

This is a second-line treatment for Bartholin's cysts if there is recurrence after the use of word catheter. Marsupialization is popular in our environment due to lack of availability of the word catheter.

Step One

- Anaesthesia
  - IV narcotics with sedation like diazepam and pethidine
  - Short GA using face mask like propofol with nitrous oxide and oxygen by face mask.
  - LA with 1% xylocaine infiltration but this is painful

Step Two

- Clean and drape in lithotomy position.

Step Three

- Procedure
  - Vertical elliptical incision 1–1.5 cm either inside or outside the hymeneal ring using No 11 or 15 blade.
  - An oval wedge of vulvar skin and cyst wall is excised to create a window.
  - Drain cyst, break loculations with artery forceps or finger, and take a swab for MCS.
  - Sew cyst wall to adjacent vestibular skin using interrupted vicryl 3–0.
  - Apply direct pressure or silver nitrate stick to control bleeding at the skin edges.
  - Clean and leave a wig of eusol for about 6 h.

Step Four

- Post-operative management
  - Oral analgesic
  - Oral antibiotics
  - Commence sitz bath from second day post-operatively

Prognosis

- Recurrence rate about 10% due to adhesion formation or septic complication
- Haemorrhage rare but massive haematoma possible
- Abscess formation following infection possible

If the patient is 68 years

- Bartholin's gland tumour is a variety of vulvar tumour and should be considered at this age.
- Biopsy the cyst wall or excise if suspicious and send specimen for histology.
- If malignant treat as appropriate.

Checklist for Bartholin's cyst

Task	Well done	Fairly done	Poorly done	Not done
Introduction: The Bartholin's gland, function, causes of cyst formation, prevalence and management	4	2	1	0
Anaesthesia: Short GA preferable, regional block with spinal possible, local infiltration least preferred	4	2	1	0
Positioning: In lithotomy position, clean and drape, empty bladder	4	2	1	0
Procedure:				
- Make 1-2cm elliptical incision inside or outside the hymeneal ring.		2	1	0
- Excise a wedge of vulvar skin and cyst wall to make a window.		2	1	0
- Drain cyst, break loculations with finger or artery forceps.		2	1	0
- Take a swab at the base of the wound for MCS.		2	1	0
- Sew cyst wall to adjacent vestibular skin with interrupted vicryl 3/0		2	1	0
- Secure haemostasis, clean and leave a wig of eusol for about 6 hours		2	1	0
Postoperative management: - Analgesia, antibiotics, sitz bath, remove pack after 6 hours	4	2	1	0
Follow-up: haemorrhage rare, abscess formation due to infection possible, recurrence rate with marsupialization about 10%	4	2	1	0
If the patient is 58 years: take biopsy for histology or excise the gland if it looks suspicious. Bartholin's tumor is a variety of vulvar tumor and should be suspected at this age.	4	2	1	0
Total score	36			
Candidate's score ....../36				
Weighted score				

Examiner's signature Date

16.3.3 Question 3: Ectopic Pregnancy

- What is ectopic pregnancy?
- Discuss the medical management of ectopic pregnancy.

16.3.3.1 Answer Outline

Ectopic pregnancy is the implantation of the fertilized ovum outside the normal endometrium. Ninety-five to ninety-seven percent occur in the fallopian tube and 3–5% in the peritoneal cavity, ovary, and the cervix. Ectopic pregnancy is an important cause of maternal mortality and morbidity; the second leading cause of maternal death in the first trimester after abortion.

Course

- Tubal abortion
  - Absorbed
  - Forms tubo-ovarian mass (TOM)
  - Grows into abdominal pregnancy
- Tubal mole (carneous mole)
- Tubal rupture
- Spontaneous resolution (rare)

Clinical Features

In our environment, ectopic pregnancy is usually diagnosed following rupture and therefore present with the triad of amenorrhoea, vaginal bleeding, and lower abdominal pain with or without signs of hypovolaemic shock. With increasing availability of ultrasound scan, asymptomatic unruptured ectopic pregnancies are increasingly being diagnosed.

Medical Management

Ectopic pregnancy can be medically managed in some selected cases, thus avoiding the morbidity and mortality associated with anaesthesia and surgery. Currently, medical treatment is by using methotrexate either orally or parenterally. However, trials are ongoing using:

- Potassium chloride
- Hyperosmolar glucose
- Mifepristone (RU 486)
- Prostaglandins

Prerequisites for Medical Treatment

- Patient must be haemodynamically stable, no signs of rupture.
- No co-existing intrauterine pregnancy.
- Mother not breastfeeding.
- No cardiac activity on TVS (relative contraindication).
- Serum B-hCG <5000 IU/L (relative contraindication).

- No underlying medical condition like pTB, HIV, DM, HD, RD, etc.
- Patient is motivated and reliable for follow-up.
- Patient agrees to use effective contraceptive for 3–4 months.
- Gestational sac diameter <3.5 cm (relative contraindication).

Investigations
- FBC, LFT, RFT, FBS
- ABO-Rh grouping and cross matching
- Serum B-hCG
- TVS with or without Doppler
- HT, WT; calculate BSA = square root of HT X WT/3600.

Protocols
- Single-dose methotrexate
  - Day 0, IM methotrexate 50 mg/m^2
  - Rhesus immunoglobulin 1500 IU IM if Rhesus negative
  - Day 4, baseline B-hCG
  - Day 7, B-hCG should drop by at least 15%; continue weekly till <5 IU/L or undetectable
- Multidose methotrexate
  - IM methotrexate 1 mg/kg day 1, 3, 5, and 7
  - IM folinic acid 0.1 mg/kg day 2, 4, 6, and
  - Serum B-hCG day 1, 3, 5, and 7; can stop treatment if decline >15%
  - Continue weekly B-hCG till <5 IU/L or undetectable.

Precautions
- No VE to avoid tubal rupture
- No sexual intercourse to avoid pregnancy or rupture
- No sunbath to avoid methotrexate dermatitis
- No multivitamins and folic acid to discourage trophoblastic growth
- No NSAIDs to avoid aplastic anaemia and complicated gastric ulcer
- No alcohol which can concurrently elevate liver enzymes

Single Versus Multidose Methotrexate
- No significant difference in success rate
- No significant difference in treatment duration
- No significant difference in regression rate of serum B-hCG.

Prognosis
- High success rate, up to 90%
- Post therapy sonography could be misleading when B-hCG has regressed to <15 mIU/mL; persistent mass may be resolving haematoma
- In the first few days of treatment, a few patients may develop abdominal pain due to tubal abortion or haematoma or both. Analgesics usually sufficient but assess for possible surgery.

Checklist for medical management of ectopic pregnancy

Task	**Well done**	**Fairly done**	**Poorly done**	**Not done**
Introduction				
- Definition		2	1	0
- Prevalence and importance		2	1	0
- Natural course: abortion, rupture, resolution		2	1	0
- Medical management in selected cases using methotrexate		2	1	0
Pre-requisites for medical treatment				
- Patient must be hemodynamically stable, no sign of rupture.		2		0
- No coexisting intrauterine pregnancy		2		0
- Mother not breastfeeding.		2		0
- Ectopic pregnancy sac<4cm in diameter		2		0
- No cardiac activity in embryo		2		0
- Serum B-hCG<5,000IU/ml		2		0
- No underlying medical condition; pTB, HIV, DM, renal dx		2		0
- Patient motivated, agrees contraception for 3 months				
Investigations				
- FBC, EUC, FBS, LFT		2	1	0
- Serum B-hCG		2	1	0
- TVS with or without doppler		2	1	0
- ABORh grouping and cross matching		2	1	0
- HT, WT, calculate BSA=square root of HTxWT/3600		2	1	0
Precautions				
- No VE to prevent rupture.		2	1	0
- No sexual intercourse for same reason		2	1	0
- No undue exposure to sun to prevent drug dermatitis.		2	1	0
- Avoid NSAIDs, multivitamins and folic acid		2	1	0
Protocol 1- single dose methotrexate (mark only one protocol)				
- Day 0, IM methotrexate 50mg/m2		2	1	0
- Rhogam 1500IU if Rhesus negative		2	1	0
- Day 4, baseline B-hCG		2	1	0
- Day 7, B-hCG should drop by at least 15%			1	0
- Continue serum B-hCG till <5IU/ml or undetectable			1	0
Protocol 2: Multidose methotrexate				
- IM methotrexate 1mg/Kg on day 1, 3, 5, and 7		2	1	0
- IM folinic acid 0.1mg/Kg on day 2, 4, and 8		2	1	0
- Serum B-hCG day 1, 3, 5, 7; can stop if decline >15%		2	1	0
- Continue B-hCG weekly till <5IU/ml or undetectable		2	1	0
Follow-up				
- Contraception for 3 months		2	1	0
- Serum B-hCG; monthly for 3 months		2	1	0
TOTAL MARKS		54		
Candidate's score .../54				

Examiner's signature Date

16.3.4 Question 4: Total Abdominal Hysterectomy for Uterine Fibroid

A 42-year-old P3+0 A3, all three deliveries by caesarean section through Pfannenstiel incision presents with abdominal swelling of 3 years duration. She was evaluated and found to have uterine fibroids of 24 weeks size. She weighed 110 kg and was counselled on treatment options. She chose to have total abdominal hysterectomy (TAH).

- What are the challenges you anticipate during the surgery?
- Describe step by step how you would perform the surgery.

16.3.4.1 Answer Outline

Total abdominal hysterectomy is a common procedure for benign gynaecological conditions in the West African sub-region. Indications include uterine fibroids as in this case, adenomyosis, endometrial hyperplasia, and pre-malignant conditions of the cervix.

Challenges anticipated in this patient:

- Due to obesity
  - Thromboembolism
  - Poor wound healing
  - Possible diabetes mellitus and/or hypertension
  - Wound sepsis
  - Wound breakdown
- Due to previous surgeries
  - Adhesions distorting normal anatomy
  - Haemorrhage
  - Injury to adjacent structures like bladder, ureters, and bowel
- Due to size of tumour
  - Going through the previous Pfannenstiel scar is not feasible
  - Blood transfusion

Surgical Steps

Preoperative Preparation
- FBC, blood chemistry, FBS or OGTT, grouping and cross matching
- Abdominal USS and IVU if indicated by findings on USS
- Pap smear if not on regular screening
- Obtain informed consent

Positioning and Anaesthesia
- In supine position, pubic hair clipped
- GA preferred but regional anaesthesia possible
- Antibiotic prophylaxis at induction of anaesthesia

Abdominal Entry

- Midline incision because of the size of the fibroid—despite previous Pfannenstiel
- Sharp dissection down to the peritoneum
- Insert self-retaining retractor like Balfour retractor
- Pack intestinal loops away using moist abdominal packs
- Adhesiolysis may be necessary to restore normal anatomy

Round Ligament Transection

- Double clamp the round ligament at its mid-portion with curved Kelly's clamps
- Divide the round ligament between the clamps and extend the incision on the anterior leaf of the broad ligament by 2 cm on either side
- Transfix the cut ends of the round ligament about 1 cm away from the clamps with vicryl 1 suture
- Hold the distal stitch end with artery forceps and remove the clamp; cut the proximal stitch short and remove the clamp

Adnexectomy

- With tension on the stitch on the distal end of the round ligament, and the uterus pushed medially, the index finger is used to bluntly dissect the areola tissue in the broad ligament to identify the ureter.
- A hole is now made on the posterior leaf of the broad ligament below the infundibulo-pelvic (IP) ligament.
- Because the uterine cornu is enlarged by the fibroid, separately double clamp the utero-ovarian ligament with curved Kelly's clamp, divide between the clamps and transfix the distal clamp with vicryl 1 to preserve the ovary.
- Double clamp the IP ligament, divide between the clamps, and transfix the distal portion with vicryl 1 suture.
- The procedures done on one adnexum are now carried out on the opposite side.

Bladder Flap

- The loose utero-vesical peritoneum is now incised medially on both sides and the bladder pushed downwards with a swab-on-stick till at least 1 cm below the lower margin of the cervix.
- This dissection is aided by pulling the uterus upwards on the Kelly's clamps holding the cornu of the uterus or by the assistant surgeon.

Uterine Arteries

- Using a swab-on-stick, the areola tissue parallel to the uterine vessels is gently pushed down to expose the uterine vessels (skeletonizing).
- The posterior leaf of the broad ligament is also cut close to the uterus and parallel to the uterine vessels.
- The uterine vessels are doubly clamped with curved Kelley's clamps taking part of cervical tissue and cut between the clamps.

- The lateral clamp is twisted gently to create a pedicle containing the uterine vessels, transfix with vicryl 1 and cut short.
- The same procedure is done on the opposite side.

Fundal Amputation

- Because the uterus is large, the fundus may be amputated from the cervix to allow space for the remaining steps of the surgery.

Cardinal and Uterosacral Ligaments Transection

- A straight Heaney's clamp or Kocher's clamp is placed across the cardinal ligament medial to the pedicle of the uterine artery and angled medially to hold part of upper vaginal wall.
- The portion of the cardinal ligament medial to the clamp is cut with a scalpel. The ligament is transfixed with vicryl 1.
- The uterus (or cervical stump) is pulled upwards, and the uterosacral ligament similarly clamped, cut and transfixed with vicryl 1.
- The same procedure is done on the opposite side.
- Palpate the most inferior level of the cervix through the vaginal walls and apply Heaney's clamp below the cervix on either side to meet in the midline.
- Cut above the clamps to remove the uterus (or cervical stump) free from the pelvis.

Vaginal Cuff Closure

- The vaginal angle is sutured to the cardinal and uterosacral ligaments using vicryl 1 on either side to prevent future vault prolapse.
- The anterior and posterior vaginal walls are closed with continuous vicryl 1 suture.

Closing the Abdominal Wall

- The abdomen is closed in layers and dry dressing applied.

Post-operative Care

- Vital signs are monitored closely until stable.
- Parenteral nutrition continued until oral feeding commenced usually after 24 h.
- Because this patient is obese, thromboprophylaxis with low-molecular-weight heparin should commence 6 h post-operatively.
- Prophylactic antibiotics should be continued.
- Early ambulation is encouraged, and compression stockings may be useful.
- Post-op PCV after 48 h.
- Inspect operation site 3 days post-op.
- Stitches are removed 7 days post-op.
- Sexual intercourse can resume 6 weeks post-op.

Checklist for TAH with huge uterine fibroid

Task	Well done	Fairly done	Poorly done	Not done
Introduction: peculiarities of this patient are obesity, previous CS through pfannenstiel incision, now presenting with huge uterine fibroid which is to be operated	4	2	1	0
Challenges anticipated in this patient: - Due to obesity; thromboembolism, poor wound healing, sepsis - Due to previous CS; adhesions, haemorrhage, injury to adjacent organs - Due to size of tumor; haemorrhage, new midline skin incision		2 2 2	1 1 1	0 0 0
Preoperative preparation: - FBC, EUC, OGTT, grouping and cross matching - Abdominal USS, IVU, pap smear if not regular on screening - Informed consent		2 2 2		0 0 0
Anaesthesia and positioning: GA preferred, cleaned and draped in supine positon, antibiotics at induction of anaesthesia	4	2	1	0
Abdominal entry: - Midline incision can be extended above the umbilicus. - Sharp dissection down to the peritoneum - Adhesiolysis to restore normal anatomy. - Insert self-retaining retractor. - Pack intestines away		2 2 2 2 2		0 0 0 0 0
Adnexectomy: - Double clamp the round ligament at its mid-portion with Kelly's forceps and divide between the clamps. - Divide the round ligament between the clamps and extend the incision on the anterior leave by 2cm on either side. - Because the uterine cornu is enlarged by the fibroids, separately double clamp the utero-ovarian and infundibulo-pelvic ligaments, divide and transfix with vicryl 1		2 2 2		0 0 0
The uterovesical peritoneum is incised medially on both sides and the bladder reflected downwards to the margin of the cervix	4	2	1	0
Uterine arteries - The areola tissue parallel to the uterine vessels are pushed down with swab-on-stick (skeletonizing) - The uterine vessels are doubly clamped with curved Kocher's forceps and divided between the clamps. - The lateral clamp is twisted gently to create a pedicle and transfixed with vicryl 1		2 2 2		0 0 0
Cardinal and uterosacral ligaments - The cardinal ligament is clamped with straight Kocher's forceps medial to the pedicle of uterine vessels, cut medially and transfixed with vicryl 1		2		0
- The uterosacral ligament is similarly clamped, cut, and transfixed. The same procedure is repeated on the other side		2		0
Vaginal cuff closure - The vaginal angle is sutured to the pedicles of the cardinal and uterosacral ligaments to prevent vault prolapse. - The anterior and posterior vaginal walls are sutured together with continuous vicryl 1		2 2		0 0
The abdomen is closed in layers and dry dressing applied	4	2	1	0
Postoperative care: IVF, antibiotics, analgesia, thromboprophylaxis with heparin, early ambulation, transfuse if necessary	4	2	1	0
Total marks	62			
Candidates score .../62				

Examiner's signature Date

16.4 Endocrinology and Infertility

16.4.1 Question 1: Laparoscopy

- What is laparoscopy?
- Describe step by step how you would perform a diagnostic laparoscopy for evaluation of infertility.

16.4.1.1 Answer Outline

Laparoscopy is the endoscopic visualization of the peritoneal cavity for the purpose of making a diagnosis and/or performing an operative procedure in the abdominal cavity. Laparoscopy has a role in nearly all gynaecological procedures as nearly all gynaecological procedures can now be done by laparoscopy.

Diagnostic laparoscopy for evaluation of infertility.

Preoperative Preparation

- Establish diagnosis from history and relevant investigations
- Control any comorbidity like diabetes, hypertension, etc
- Obtain written informed consent

Step 1 Positioning the Patient

- Patient in dorsal lithotomy position, buttocks at the end of the table, hips slightly extended and abducted with knees flexed under GA with endotracheal intubation
- Cleaned and draped to expose both anterior abdominal wall and the perineum
- Assistant to empty the bladder, do VE and fix the uterine manipulator

Step 2 Insertion of Veress Needle

- Through a vertical umbilical stab incision, insert the Veress needle at 45° in the midline after manually elevating the anterior abdominal wall
- Ensure correct placement:
  - Palmer's test
  - Pressure test
  - Loss of liver dullness
- Connect insufflation tubing and adjust CO_2 flow at 3–4 L/min till intra-abdominal pressure reaches 10–15 mmHg.

Step 3 Primary Trocar Insertion and the Scope

- Remove the Veress needle and insert the primary trocar in its sleeve, directing it towards the hollow of the sacrum (with a force of 4–5 kg)
- Reduce the IAP and insert the laparoscope through the sleeve of the trocar

Step 4 Examining the Peritoneal Cavity

- First perform a panoramic view; starting with the pelvic structures, move in a clockwise direction to inspect the caecum, appendix, ascending colon, liver, stomach, spleen (if enlarged), and the descending colon

- Insert a second trocar (or two) to insert a probe or grasper for proper inspection of the pelvic organs
- Again, in clockwise direction, examine the right tube and ovary, the POD, left tube and ovary and the utero-vesical pouch. Look out for:
  - Fibroids
  - Ovarian cysts
  - Endometriotic deposits
  - Pelvic adhesions
- Perform chromotubation using methylene blue dye to demonstrate tubal patency
- May instil 200 mL NS to demonstrate peritubal and periovarian adhesions (hydroflotation test).

Step 5 Removal of Instruments and Closure

- The assistant removes the uterine manipulator under direct vision and can take endometrial biopsy.
- The second trocar and cannula should be removed under direct vision.
- The laparoscope is then removed, and the gas allowed to escape maximally.
- The primary trocar is re-introduced and removed together with the cannula.
- The entry points are closed with absorbable sutures and cleaned with antiseptic.

Checklist for diagnostic laparoscopy

Task	Well done	Fairly done	Poorly done	Not done
Preoperative patient preparation: Establish diagnosis, treat any co-morbidity and obtain written informed consent	4	2	1	0
Anaesthesia: GA preferable, regional block can be used, infiltration least suitable	4	2	1	0
Positioning: Lithotomy position with hips extended and abducted, buttocks at the edge of the operation table. Assistant inserts cervical cannula and lock	4	2	1	0
Insertion of Veress needle: insert Veress needle at 5 degrees, ensure correct placement, connect insufflation tubing and adjust CO2 flow at 3-4L/min till intra—abdominal pressure reaches 10-15mmHg	4	2	1	0
Primary trocar insertion and the scope: Remove Veress needle and insert primary trocar in its sleeve, remove the trocar and introduce the telescope through the sleeve	4	2	1	0
Examining the peritoneal cavity: First perform a clockwise panoramic view before inserting a probe or grasper through a secondary port for detailed pelvic examination	4	2	1	0
Diagnosis: pathologies that can be seen include fibroids, ovarian cysts, endometriotic deposits and pelvic adhesions	4	2	1	0
Perform chromotubation using methylene blue dye for tubal patency	4	2	1	0
Removal of instruments and closure: probe and second trocar remove by assistant under direct vision. Remove laparoscope and allow gas to escape, re-insert primary trocar and remove with cannula. Close entry points with absorbable suture.	4	2	1	0
Postoperative care: laparoscopy can be a day case if done early. Oral analgesia is sufficient	4	2	1	0
Total score	40			
Candidate's score .../40				

Examiner's signature Date

16.4.2 Question 2: Hysteroscopy

- What is hysteroscopy?
- Describe step by step how you would perform a diagnostic hysteroscopy on a 25-year-old woman being evaluated for primary infertility.

16.4.2.1 Answer Outline

Introduction

Hysteroscopy is the examination of the distended uterine cavity using an endoscope. Diagnostic hysteroscopy is fast replacing dilatation and curettage in many gynaecological practices for the evaluation of the endometrial cavity and obtaining endometrial tissue for histology.

1 *Instruments*
   (a) Camera and monitor
   (b) Light source
   (c) Distension medium (N/S, Ringers, dextran, glycine, sorbitol)
   (d) Fluid pump and monitor
   (e) Hysteroscope (flexible or rigid)
2 *Anaesthesia*
   (a) NSAIDs
   (b) Sedation with pethidine or diazepam
   (c) General anaesthesia
3 *Positioning and VE*
   (a) Lithotomy position
   (b) VE to assess uterine size and position
   (c) Insert a Sims' speculum to expose cervix and hold the anterior lip with a tenaculum
4 *Procedure*
   (a) Set up fluid pump or ordinary N/S infusion on a stand under gravity.
   (b) Assemble the telescope in its sheath and connect light source and infusion.
   (c) Run the fluid through the tubing and hysteroscope to expel air.
   (d) Connect the camera and place the hysteroscope into the external os.
   (e) As the fluid is run, examine the endocervical canal, identify the internal os and gently advance into the endometrial cavity.
   (f) With 0–30 degrees telescope, the entire cavity may be visualized; the ostia, anterior wall, posterior wall.

5 *Diagnosis that could be made*
   (a) Endometrial polyps
   (b) Submucous fibroids
   (c) Intrauterine adhesions
   (d) Uterine septum
   (e) Foreign bodies—bone spicules, IUCD
6 *Conclusion*
   (a) Measure the fluid balance
   (b) Stop infusion
   (c) Withdraw hysteroscope under direct vision
   (d) Disassemble instruments and handover to the scrub nurse
   (e) Document findings and plan of action

Checklist for hysteroscopy

Task	Well done	Fairly done	Poorly done	Not done
Introduction: what is hysteroscope, its importance in gynaecological practice	4	2	1	0
Anaesthesia: NSAIDs, sedation with pethidine or diazepam, GA usually for operative hysteroscopy with or without laparoscopy	4	2	1	0
Positioning and VE: lithotomy position, assess uterine size and position, hold anterior lip of the cervix with tenaculum	4	2	1	0
Procedure:				
- Set up fluid pump or ordinary saline infusion.		2	1	0
- Assemble instrument and flush with distension fluid.		2	1	0
- Connect camera and place hysteroscope into the		2	1	0
external os.				
- As the fluid is run examine the endocervical canal,		2	1	0
internal os, and advance into the endometrial cavity.		2	1	0
- With 0–30-degree telescope, examine the entire uterine cavity				
Diagnosis that could be made:				
- Endometrial polyps		2	1	0
- Submucous fibroids		2	1	0
- Intrauterine adhesions		2	1	0
- Uterine septum		2	1	0
- Foreign bodies – bone spicules, IUCD etc.		2	1	0
Conclusion:				
- Withdraw hysteroscope under direct vision.		2	1	0
- Stop infusion.		2	1	0
- Measure the fluid balance.		2	1	0
- Disassemble instruments and handover to the scrub		2	1	0
nurse.		2	1	0
- Document findings and plan of action				
Total score	42			
Candidates score .../42				

Examiner's signature Date

16.4.3 Question 3: Ovulation Induction

- What is the mechanism of action of clomiphene citrate?
- What is clomiphene failure and how would you manage it?

16.4.3.1 Answer Outline

Introduction

- Clomiphene is an oestrogen receptor blocker (anti-oestrogen).
- Commonest ovulation induction drug in gynaecological practice in our environment.
- It acts by blocking oestrogen receptor in the hypothalamus and pituitary gland thereby preventing the negative feedback effect of circulating oestrogens; this causes increased GnRH secretion and therefore increased gonadotropin release.
- Normally given in a dose 50 mg/day for 5 days in a cycle but can be increased up to 150 mg/day.

Clomiphene Failure

- When a patient is not adequately stimulated with 50 mg/day of clomiphene, it can be increased to 100 mg/day the next cycle and if stimulation is still unsatisfactory, 150 mg/day the next cycle. This should be the maximum dosage.
- Patients who ovulate but fail to conceive on 150 mg/day of clomiphene citrate for three consecutive cycles are regarded as cases of clomiphene failure.
- Clomiphene failure may be due to cervical factors, intrauterine factors, pelvic adhesions, or luteinized unruptured follicle.
- Those who fail to ovulate on 150 mg/day of CC for three consecutive cycles are diagnosed to have clomiphene resistance.
- Clomiphene resistance may be due to some hormonal imbalances like in PCOS or idiopathic.

Investigations

- Diagnostic laparoscopy-significant pelvic pathology in 60% of cases
- Postcoital test
- Follicular tracking for luteinized unruptured follicle
- Repeat hormonal profile-LH/FSH/PRL/androgens
- BMI >27 kg/m^2 associated with less chance of ovulation

Treatment

- Exercise and weight loss
- Extended dose of CC for 7–10 days
- Tamoxifen improves cervical mucus and endometrial response
- Glucocorticoids-prednisolone 5 mg/day for 10 days from day 6 of cycle suppresses androgens and achieves ovulation in 80% of cases
- HCG 5000–10,000 IU in luteinized unruptured follicles
- Bromocriptine in cases of hyperprolactinaemia.
- Metformin 1500 mg/day in insulin resistance; may be combined with CC
- GnRH agonist or antagonist
- Surgical-laparoscopic drilling
- IUI for cervical factors
- Laparoscopic adhesiolysis.

Checklist for clomiphene failure

Task	Well done	Fairly done	Poorly done	Not done
Introduction: what is clomiphene citrate, its mechanism of action, usual dosage	4	2	1	0
Clomiphene failure: Explain how you arrive at the diagnosis of clomiphene failure	4	2	1	0
Relevant investigations following clomiphene failure: - Diagnostic laparoscopy for significant pelvic pathology - Postcoital test to rule out cervical factors. - TVS for follicular tracking to rule out luteinized unruptured follicle. - Repeat hormonal profile; FSH, LH, PRL, TSH, Androgens - BMI>27Kg/m2 associated with less chance of ovulation. - Insulin resistance test		2 2 2 2 2 2	1 1 1 1 1 1	0 0 0 0 0 0
Treatment: - Exercise and weight loss if overweight - Extended CC for 7-10 days if no obvious pathology found. - Tamoxifen improves cervical mucus and endometrial receptiveness. - HCG 5,000-10,000IU for luteinized unruptured follicle. - Treat PCOS when diagnosed. - Laparoscopic adhesiolysis		2 2 2 2 2 2	1 1 1 1 1 1	0 0 0 0 0 0
Follow-up: - If there is no obvious pathology, 80% conceive with extended CC. - Treating identified pathology results in 60-80% conception - Some will require assisted conception using ART		2 2 2	1 1 1	0 0 0
Total marks	38			
Candidates score .../38				

Examiner's signature

16.4.4 Question 4: Secondary Amenorrhoea

Mrs. CC is a 30-year-old P2+1 who presented at the gynaecology clinic with secondary amenorrhoea. The pelvic examination done was normal.

- Mention seven differential diagnosis of secondary amenorrhoea.
- Outline seven investigations, and their indications, you would carry out on her to establish a diagnosis.
- How would you treat her if the cause is found to be non-endocrinological?

Checklist for secondary amenorrhoea

Tasks	Well done	Fairly done	Poorly done	Not done
Differential diagnosis of secondary amenorrhea (Max 7):				
- Pregnancy			1	0
- Polycystic ovary syndrome PCOS			1	0
- Asherman's syndrome			1	0
- Thyroid dysfunction (hyper- or hypothyroidism)			1	0
- Adrenal disease (Cushing's syndrome)			1	0
- Pituitary causes (Hyperprolactinemia)			1	0
- Hypothalamic (stress-induced, anorexia nervosa)			1	0
- Iatrogenic (radiotherapy, oophorectomy)			1	0
- Genital TB			1	0
- Sheehan's syndrome			1	0
Investigations and their indications (Max 7):				
- Pregnancy test; to rule out pregnancy.		2	1	0
- Hormonal profile, FSH, LH, T2, PRL,SHBG; to confirm PCOS		2	1	0
- TSH, free T4, T3; to rule out thyroid dysfunction.		2	1	0
- Androstenedione, FSH, LH; to rule out Cushing's syndrome.		2	1	0
- Pelvic USS; to rule out pregnancy, conform PCO		2	1	0
- HSG; to confirm intrauterine adhesions.		2	1	0
- Hysteroscopy; to confirm and treat adhesions.		2	1	0
- CXR, Mantoux, AFB; to confirm genital TB.		2	1	0
- CT, MRI; for pituitary adenoma		2	1	0
Treatment of non-endocrinological causes				
Likely non-endocrinological causes: Asherman's syndrome, iatrogenic causes, genital TB	4	2	1	0
Asherman's syndrome: hysteroscopic or blind Adhesiolysis, insertion of Lippes loop or Foley's catheter, hormone therapy	4	2	1	0
Iatrogenic (oophorectomy, radiotherapy): ART if desirous of childbirth, treat complications medically including HRT	4	2	1	0
Genital TB; anti-TB drugs, poor prognosis		2	1	0
Total score	35			
Candidate's score .../35				

Examiner's signature Date

16.5 Gynaecological Oncology

16.5.1 Question 1: Human Papilloma Virus

The causative role of human papilloma virus (HPV) in almost all cervical cancers and in significant proportion of vulvar, vagina, and anal cancers is firmly established.

- How would you prevent HPV infection in your environment?
- What are the challenges you will encounter?

16.5.1.1 Answer Outline

Introduction

- HPV is a double-stranded DNA virus; there are two types: cutaneous (causing warts) and mucosal (causing CIN).
- Mucosal HPV infection is the commonest STI; found in 80% of sexually active women.
- Most infections (70%) are transient, clearing in 6–12 months; the remaining persisting.
- HPV attacks the basal cells in the transformation zone; the viral DNA is integrated into that of the basal cells in the TZ leading to immortalization of the basal cells causing CIN.
- Persistent infection may cause CIN in approximately 10 years. The risk factors for persistent infection are:
  - Viral load and viral type 16, 18, 31, 35
  - Host immune status (HIV infection)
  - Smoking
  - Parity
  - Use of oral contraceptives
  - Other STIs
  - Inflammation of the cervix

There are two important aspects of prevention of HPV infection in our environment; behaviour change and administration of vaccines.

1. *Behaviour change involves*:
   - Sexual abstinence
   - Delaying coitarche
   - Limiting number of sexual partners
   - The use of condoms
2. *Use of vaccines*

   Vaccines elicit the production of high levels of type-specific antibodies which block the entry of the virus into host cells. HPV vaccine has the potential to prevent malignancy of the cervix, vulva, vagina, penis, anal canal, and oropharynx.

The HPV vaccines are recombinant technologies for the synthesis of L1 capsid proteins of each HPV type included in the vaccine. L1 capsid proteins are highly immunogenic and seroconversion rates in excess of 99% are reported. There are currently three types of HPV vaccines:

- Gardasil 9
  - Nanovalent HPV vaccine (9vHPV).
  - Acts against HPV 6, 11, 16, 18, 31, 35, 45, 52, and 58.
  - HPV types 6 and 11 account for 90% of genital warts and recurrent laryngeal papillomas.
  - HPV types 16 and 18 account for 60–70% of cervical cancers and significant number of anal, vaginal, and vulvar cancers.
  - The other viral types account for 15–20% of cervical cancers.
  - Gardasil 9 protects against 96% of incident infections and their resultant neoplasia.
  - Recommended regimen ACOG 2019:

    Girls and boys 11–12 years; two doses, 6–12 months apart.

    Girls and boys 13–26 years (catch-up vaccination), three doses if started after age 15; at 0, 1, and 6 months.

    Recent evidence suggests that single dose of Gardasil 9 may be sufficient for protection against infection and neoplasia.

    Screening for cervical cancer should continue according to schedule as HPV vaccine prevents most but not all of HPV infections.
- Gardasil 4
  - Acts against HPV types 6, 11, 16, and 18.
  - Two dose regimen at 0 and 6 months.
  - Comes in 0.5 mL pre-filled syringe suspension.
  - Prevents against cervical and anal cancers and genital warts.
  - For adolescents older than 15 years, three doses are recommended at 0, 2, and 6 months.
  - Intramuscular injection over the deltoid or upper thigh.
- Cervarix
  - Protects against HPV types 16 and 18.
  - 0.5 mL at 0, 1, and 6 months.

General Note

- There is limited benefit for catch-up vaccination for people aged 27–45 years.
- No need for screening for HPV before vaccination.
- Vaccination started with cervarix or Gardasil 4 can be continued with Gardasil 9.
- After completing vaccination with cervarix or Gardasil 4, there is no need to take Gardasil 9.
- Vaccine is contraindicated in acute febrile illness and known allergy to previous dose or yeast.

Two Challenges

- Cost; a dose of cervarix costs about N15,000 and a dose of Gardasil 4 about N45,000 in Nigeria.
- Non-availability: the vaccines are found only in a few cities in Nigeria.
- Sociocultural reasons: some cultures view the administration of the vaccine as a licence for promiscuity.
- Lack of political will; the government is reluctant to provide the vaccine to the adolescents.

Checklist for prevention of HPV infection

Task	Well done	Fairly done	Poorly done	Not done
Introduction: brief virology of HPV including type, transmission and cause of CIN and VAIN	4	2	1	0
Prevention strategies: behaviour change and use of vaccines	4	2	1	0
Behaviour change:				
- Sexual abstinence		2		0
- Delay coitarche		2		0
- Faithfulness (limiting number of sexual partners)		2		0
- Barrier contraceptives (use of condoms, diaphragms, and cervical caps)		2		0
Use of vaccines: mechanism of action, types	4	2	1	0
Gardasil 9:				
- Nanovalent, against HPV 6, 11, 16, 18, 31, 35, 45, 52 and		2		0
58		2		0
- Protects against 96% incident infections		2		0
- 2 doses, 6-12 months apart for girls and boys 11-12 years old				
Gardasil 4:				
- Quadrivalent, against HPV 6, 11, 16, and 18		2		0
- 2 dose regimen at 0 and 6 months		2		0
- Additional dose after 6 months for adolescents older than 15 years		2		0
Cervarix:				
- Protects against HPV 16 and 18		2		0
- 3 doses at 0,1 and 6 months		2		0
General note:				
- There is limited use for catch-up vaccination after 27-45		2		0
years		2		0
- Those who started cervarix or Gardasil 4 can complete with Gardasil 9		2		0
- No need for taking Gardasil 9 after completing cervarix or Gardasil 4				
Challenges:				
- Cost: a dose of cervarix is N15,000 and Gardasil 4		2		0
N45,000 in Nigeria		2		0
- Availability; available only in a few cities in Nigeria		2		0
- Lack of political will; the government is not willing to provide the vaccine for adolescents.		2		0
- Sociocultural; the vaccine is viewed as a license for promiscuity				
Total score	50			
Candidates score ....../50				

Examiners signature Date

16.5.2 Question 2: Gestational Trophoblastic Neoplasia (GTN)

What is stage III gestational trophoblastic neoplasia (GTN)?

A 30-year-old P6+1 A6 presents with an irregular vaginal bleeding of 6 weeks duration associated with weakness, nausea, and vomiting. Her last pregnancy ended in a miscarriage 8 months ago at a gestational age of 8 weeks, no histology. On admission, pelvic ultrasound scan showed bulky but empty uterus with bilateral adnexal cysts. There were multiple metastatic nodules in the liver. Serum B-HCG was 120,000 miu/mL.

- What other investigations would you request?
- What chemotherapy regimen would you offer her and why?

16.5.2.1 Answer Outline

Stage III GTN: GTN with metastasis to the lungs with or without genital tract involvement.

From the information given, the WHO prognostic scoring for this patient is:

- Age = 0
- Antecedent pregnancy 8 months = 2
- Type of antecedent pregnancy, abortion = 1 (no histology)
- Liver metastasis = 4
- Urine B-HCG 120,000 miu/mL = 4

Total score based on available information alone is 13, which is high risk (high-risk score of 7 or more). There was no information on largest tumour size, number of metastasis, other metastatic sites, and previous use of chemotherapy. The presence of liver metastasis and the high level of B-HCG were sufficient to score the patient high risk.

Other investigations to be requested include:

- CXR
- FBC
- RFTs
- LFTs
- Where available: CT/MRI of brain, chest, liver, spleen, kidneys, pelvis.

The preferred chemotherapy regimen for high-risk GTN is:

- Etoposide, methotrexate, and actinomycin-D, alternating with cyclophosphamide and Oncovin (EMA/CO)
  - Well tolerated
  - Highly effective with complete remission in up to 78% cases
  - Overall survival rate of 86–92%
- For cases refractory to EMA/CO which occurs in up 25% cases
  - EMA/EP; replace the cyclophosphamide and Oncovin (vincristine) with Etoposide and cisplatin.
  - Paclitaxel (Taxol) plus cisplatin alternating with paclitaxel with Etoposide (TP/TE) has comparable efficacy but less toxic.
- Those with large burden disease are at risk of early death with standard EMA/CO due to haemorrhage from tumour lysis. Induction low-dose Etoposide-cisplatin (EP) reduces the mortality risk by ten-fold.

Checklist for gestational trophoblastic disease

Task	Well done	Fairly done	Poorly done	Not done
Gestational trophoblastic neoplasia: explain what GTN is, prevalence, importance, clinical features and treatment modalities	4	2	1	0
WHO staging of GTN; categorize into low and high risk	4	2	1	0
Case presented is high risk just by the presence of liver metastasis (4) and hCG of 120IU/ml (4) which give a score of 8	4	2	1	0
Other relevant investigations:				
- CXR		2		0
- FBC		2		0
- LFT		2		0
- RFT		2		0
- CT/MRI brain, liver, kidneys, spleen, pelvis		2		0
Preferred chemotherapy regimen for high risk GTN:				
- EMA/CO; highly effective, well tolerated, survival up to 90%		2	1	0
- EMA/EP for those refractive to EMA/CO; TP/TE less toxic		2	1	0
- Induction low dose EP for those with high burden disease		2	1	0
Follow-up				
- Serial hCG follow-up		2	1	0
- Survival rate up to 90%		2	1	0
- Lifetime follow-up		2	1	0
Total score	34			
Candidate's score ……/34				

Examiner's signature Date

16.5.3 Question 3: Endometrial Sampling

- List the indications for endometrial sampling.
- Describe step by step the procedure of endometrial sampling using the manual vacuum aspiration.
- What other procedures can be done to obtain endometrial sample?

16.5.3.1 Answer Outline

Introduction

Endometrial sampling is a surgical procedure that involves taking a tissue sample of the uterine inner lining for histopathological examination. Histologic examination of the endometrial sample remains the standard diagnostic procedure for uterine abnormalities. Abnormal uterine bleeding remains the commonest indication for endometrial sampling.

Indications

- Abnormal uterine bleeding
- Post-menopausal bleeding
- Diagnosis of endometrial hyperplasia
- Cancer screening
- Infertility evaluation
- Chronic endometritis
- Follow-up of patients on hormone replacement therapy
- Abnormal Papanicolaou smear with atypia

MVA Procedure

Out-patient Preparation

- PCV, grouping, and cross matching
- Urinalysis, chemistry if necessary
- Obtain informed consent
- Optimize patient if necessary
- Prime cervix with misoprostol if necessary

Anaesthesia

- Reassurance only
- Paracervical block
- Conscious sedation
- GA by face mask

Positioning

- Surgeon scrubs and gowns
- Patient in lithotomy position under anaesthesia
- Cleaned and draped
- Urinary bladder emptied
- Examination under anaesthesia done

Endometrial Sampling

- Use Cusco's speculum to expose the cervix
- Hold anterior lip of cervix with vulsellum forceps
- Dilate cervix to Hegar's size 6 and sharply curette the endocervix
- Insert size 4 or 6 Karman's cannula and a charged Karman's syringe
- By rotatory to and fro movement curette the endometrium
- Lock the valves, disconnect the syringe, and remove the cannula
- Fix the two specimens in separate bottles
- Clean and reposition the patient

Post-operative Period

- Analgesia
- Antibiotics if indicated
- Discharge patient to see with histology result

Other procedures that can be done

- Dilatation and curettage
- Pipelle aspiration
- Tao brush
- Vabra aspirator
- Hysteroscopy

Checklist for endometrial sampling

Task	Well done	Fairly done	Poorly done	Not done
Introduction: definition, indications	4	2	1	0
Indications: abnormal uterine bleeding, postmenopausal bleeding, infertility evaluation, abnormal Pap smear, follow-up of patients on HRT etc.	4	2	1	0
Preoperative preparation: PCV, urinalysis, informed consent, prime cervix with misoprostol	4	2	1	0
Anaesthesia: reassurance only, paracervical block, conscious sedation, GA by face mask	4	2	1	0
Positioning: lithotomy position, clean and drape, VE/EUA	4	2	1	0
Endometrial sampling:				
- expose cervix with Cusco's speculum, hold anterior lip with vulsellum forceps.		2	1	0
- dilate cervix to Hegar's size 6, curate endocervix.		2	1	0
- use MVA to curette endometrium using size 4 or 6		2	1	0
cannula.		2	1	0
- fix endocervical and endometrial curettings in separate containers		2	1	0
- clean and reposition patient				
Postoperative care: analgesia, antibiotics, see with histology report	4	2	1	0
Other procedures for endometrial sampling (max. 4 marks):				
- dilatation and curettage			1	0
- Pipelle sampling			1	0
- Tao brush			1	0
- Vabra aspirator			1	0
- Hysteroscopy			1	0
Total marks	39			
Candidates score .../39				

Examiner's signature Date

16.5.4 Question 4: Complication of Chemotherapy

A 45-year-old P4+0 4 alive diagnosed to have serous adenocarcinoma of the ovary following debulking surgery is on carboplatin infusion as part of the first course of chemotherapy. Ten minutes into the infusion, she developed difficulty in breathing and generalized urticarial rashes.

- What type of chemotherapy was being given?
- How would you manage her immediate condition?

16.5.4.1 Answer Outline

- Chemotherapy is the mainstay treatment of cancer of the ovary in our environment since most patients present with late-stage disease requiring debulking surgery followed by chemotherapy. This patient was receiving adjuvant chemotherapy—chemotherapy for microscopic tumour cells after debulking surgery. Other forms of chemotherapy for advanced ovarian cancer include:
  - Induction chemotherapy—primary chemotherapy for advanced disease
  - Neoadjuvant chemotherapy—preoperative treatment for advanced malignancy to decrease the extent of disease
  - Salvage/palliative chemotherapy—chemotherapy for recurrent or refractory malignancy just to maintain quality of life
- STOP the infusion.
  - CALL for help
  - Assess airways, breathing, and circulation
  - Oxygen by face mask
  - Rush normal saline if hypotensive
  - Give:

    IV promethazine 25 mg stat

    IV hydrocortisone 100 mg stat
  - If there is bronchospasm (wheezing), give nebulized salbutamol.
  - If there is no immediate improvement and there is persistent hypotension and/or bronchospasm, give adrenaline 0.1 mg IV.
  - Prepare for CPR if patient arrests.
  - Reassure patient when stable.
  - Change cytotoxic regimen.

Checklist for complication of chemotherapy

Task	Well done	Fairly done	Poorly done	Not done
Introduction: short statement on the management of ovarian cancer, highlighting the importance of chemotherapy	4	2	1	0
This patient was receiving adjuvant chemotherapy since she had debulking surgery before the chemotherapy	4	2	1	0
Other types of chemotherapy:				
- Induction chemotherapy- primary treatment for advanced disease		2	1	0
- Neoadjuvant chemotherapy- preoperative for advanced disease		2	1	0
- Salvage (Palliative) chemotherapy-to maintain quality of life in recurrent or refractory disease		2	1	0
Management of anaphylactic reaction:				
STOP the drug infusion		2		0
Call for help – nurse to bring oxygen prongs, adrenaline and promethazine, HO to set another line, inform anaesthetist etc.	4	2	1	0
Assess airways, breathing and circulation	4	2	1	0
Oxygen by face mask		2	1	0
Rush normal saline if hypotensive		2	1	0
Give IV promethazine 25mg and hydrocortisone 100mg	4	2	1	0
If there is bronchospasm (wheezing) give nebulized salbutamol		2	1	0
If no immediate improvement but persistent hypotension or bronchospasm, give IV adrenaline 0.1mg	4	2	1	0
Prepare for CPR if patient arrests		2	1	0
If patient becomes stable, reassure, and change cytotoxic regimen	4	2	1	0
Total marks	42			
Candidate's score .../42				

Examiner's signature Date

16.6 Contraception and Sterilization

16.6.1 Question 1: Missing IUCD Strings

List four top-tier contraceptive methods.

A 35-year-old grand multipara came to the family planning clinic 6 weeks after insertion of Copper T IUCD, complaining of inability to feel the threads.

- Discuss her management.
- Mention five absolute contraindications to insertion of this device.

16.6.1.1 Answer Outline

Introduction

Contraceptive methods are grouped according to their effectiveness. Top-tier or first-tier methods are those that are most effective and are characterized by their ease of use. These methods require minimal user motivation or intervention and have a typical-use pregnancy rate of <1 per 100 women during the first year of use. The first-tier methods provide the longest duration of contraception after initiation and the fewest number of return visits. Examples of top-tier contraceptive methods are:

- Intrauterine contraceptive devices
- Etonogestrel/levonorgestrel implants
- Female sterilization
- Male sterilization

CuT380A IUCD

- The IUCDs is classified among the most effective methods (first tier) of contraceptives with a pregnancy rate of <1/100WY.
- About 14% of contraceptive users globally use the IUCDs; being most popular in China where 40% of contraceptive users patronize it.
- IUCDs induce intense endometrial inflammation which results in production of lysosomes and other inflammatory proteins which is spermicidal and prevents the blastocyst from implantation.
- When the marker strings cannot be seen at the cervical os, the diagnosis is "missing IUCD string" but, when the device cannot be located inside the uterus, the diagnosis becomes "missing IUCD".
- Missing IUCD string is a cause for anxiety to both the client and the service provider. It may be due to expulsion which could be unnoticed, partial, or total uterine perforation, sommersaulting of the device or enlargement of the uterus due to pregnancy or fibroids.

Vaginal Examination

- Explain the steps you intend to take during the vaginal examination.
- Wash your hands, wear sterile gloves, clean and drape the perineum in lithotomy position.
- Expose the cervix with Cusco's speculum to diagnose missing IUD thread.
- Gently probe the uterine cavity with uterine sound or tubal hook to rule out translocation; ultrasound scan can also be used to rule out translocation of IUD.
- Absence of the device inside the uterine cavity confirms translocated IUD.

Treatment

- If the device is inside the uterus, it's still effective as contraceptive and can be left alone; the alligator forceps or a rod with hook may be used to draw the thread down but the device may be inadvertently removed in the process.
- Translocated IUD may require further investigations like plain abdominal X-ray and/or HSG or laparoscopy.
- Laparoscopy may be used to remove the device from the peritoneal cavity but sometimes laparotomy may be required if adhesions have been formed or the device is entangled in the omentum.
- Embedded IUD may be diagnosed and removed by hysteroscopy or D&C but sometimes may require hysterotomy if deeply embedded.
- If ultrasound shows intrauterine pregnancy, the abortion rate is >50% if the device is left in situ. The miscarriage rate is reduced to 25% if the device is removed promptly.

Contraindications to Insertion of IUD

- Active PID or within the last 3 months
- Suspected pregnancy
- Undiagnosed genital bleeding
- History of previous ectopic pregnancy
- Distorted uterine cavity due to fibroids or congenital anomaly
- Significant immunosuppression-AIDS
- Wilson's disease
- Suspected genital malignancy

Checklist for missing IUCD strings

Checklist for missing IUCD strings

Task	Well done	Fairly done	Poorly done	Not done
Top-tier contraceptive methods:				
- Intrauterine contraceptive devices			1	0
- Etonogestrell/levonorgestrel implants			1	0
- Female sterilization			1	0
- Male sterilization			1	0
Managing missing IUCD-strings:				
Explain the condition to the client and the steps you are going to take in managing the problem	4	2	1	0
Speculum examination: to confirm the diagnosis and do USS (preferably TVS)) to rule out pregnancy	4	2	1	0
If not pregnant and IUCD in-situ:				
- Use endocervical brush or hook to bring down the strings		2	1	0
- Reassure client and leave device as it is; its contraceptive		2	1	0
effect valid		2	1	0
- Use Alligator forceps to remove IUCD if not wanted				
If not pregnant and IUCD embedded:				
- D&C to remove device		2	1	0
- Hysteroscopy can remove device where available		2	1	0
- Hysterotomy required for deep embedment		2	1	0
If not pregnant and device partially or totally translocated:				
- USS, plain X-Ray, HSG, laparoscopy to locate the device		2	1	0
- Laparoscopy to remove device, laparotomy required with adhesions		2	1	0
If pregnant and device in-situ:				
- >50% miscarriage rate if device left in-situ		2	1	0
- 25% miscarriage rate if device removed promptly		2	1	0
If pregnant and device translocated:				
- Laparoscopy or laparotomy to remove device		2	1	0
- If left in peritoneum, can cause intestinal perforation or obstruction		2	1	0
Contraindications to insertion of CuT380A:				
- Suspected pregnancy			1	0
- Active PID within last 3 months			1	0
- Undiagnosed genital bleeding			1	0
- Suspected genital malignancy			1	0
- Distorted uterine cavity due to fibroids or congenital			1	0
anomaly			1	0
- Wilsons disease			1	0
- Significant immunosuppression like AIDS			1	0
- History of previous ectopic pregnancy				
Total marks	41			
Candidates score .../41				

Examiner's signature Date

16.6.2 Question 2: Emergency Contraception

- Define emergency contraception
- List five indications for its use
- What are the various methods available and their mode of action?

16.6.2.1 Answer Outline

Emergency contraception is the use of contraceptives to prevent pregnancy following unprotected sexual intercourse, or a known failure of contraceptive method like ruptured condom.

Principle

- Prevent or delay ovulation
- Prevent implantation where fertilization might have occurred

Indications

- When no contraceptive has been used
- Contraceptive failure
- Condom breakage, slippage, incorrect use
- Two or more consecutive missed COCP
- Late taking of minipills
- More than 2 weeks late for progestin-only injectable
- More than 7 days late for a combined oestrogen-progestin monthly injection
- Sexual assault

Methods Available

- *Hormonal*

  Levonorgestrel only regimen: 1.5 mg in a single dose or in two doses of 0.75 mg 12 h apart.

  Combined oestrogen-progestin (Yuzpe) regimen: two doses of 100 mcg ethinyl estradiol + 0.5 mg levonorgestrel taken 12 h apart.

  Hormonal methods prevent pregnancy largely by delaying ovulation and prevent ovulation in some cases. It takes about 3 days for cervical mucus to thicken after taking progestogens, during which time the spermatozoa would have entered the uterine cavity and the tubes.

  New research indicates that ECPs can prevent pregnancy up to 5 days after unprotected sexual intercourse against the previous 72 h timing.

  Selective progestin receptor modulator (Ulipristal) taken as a single dose 30 mg tablet up to 120 h (5 days) after unprotected sexual intercourse acts by delaying ovulation. It has been shown to be more effective than levonorgestrel. Its side effects include nausea and delay of subsequent menses.
- *IUCD*

  Copper T 380A inserted within 7 days of unprotected sexual intercourse.
  - Inserted within 7 days of unprotected sexual intercourse.
  - Inhibits both fertilization and implantation by creating sterile inflammation of the endometrium.
  - Reduces pregnancy rate from 8% at single coitus to 0.5%.
  - Can be left in situ as an effective long-term contraceptive.
  - Risk of PID at insertion is increased.
  - It is the most effective emergency contraceptive.

By mechanisms yet unknown CuT380 IUCD has been shown to prevent or delay ovulation and interfere with corpus luteum function.

Checklist for emergency contraception

Task	Well done	Fairly done	Poorly done	Not done
Definition of emergency contraception:				
- Use of a contraceptive method		2		0
- Following unprotected sexual intercourse		2		0
- To prevent fertilization or implantation		2		0
Indications for its use:				
- Unprotected sexual intercourse		2		0
- Condom rupture or slippage		2		0
- Sexual assault		2		0
- 2 or more missed COCP		2		0
- 2 or more weeks late for injectable progestin		2		0
- >7 days late for monthly oestrogen-progestin injection		2		0
Levonorgestrel (2); administration and mode of action (2)	4	2	1	0
COCP (2); administration and mode of action (2)	4	2	1	0
Ulipristal (2); administration and mode of action (2)	4	2	1	0
CuT30A (2); administration and mode of action (2)	4	2	1	0
Total marks	32			
Candidates score .../32				

Examiner's signature Date

16.6.3 Question 3: Contraception for the Elderly Woman

- List the various contraceptive methods used in West Africa.
- A 45-year-old multiparous woman comes to the family planning clinic for contraception. What special considerations would you counsel her on with regard to method choice?

16.6.3.1 Answer Outline

The various contraceptive methods readily available in West Africa are:

- Combined oral contraceptive pills
- Progestins; both injectables and implants
- Intrauterine devices
- Barrier methods, especially condoms
- Sterilization
- Emergency contraception
- Natural methods of family planning

The case presented:

- This client is perimenopausal
- Menopause usually occurs between 45 and 55 years (average 51 years)
- By itself, age is not a barrier to contraception but, the medical conditions that come with age may modify the choice of contraceptive.

Combined Hormonal Methods (Pills, Injectables, Patch, Vaginal Rings)

- Women 35 years or more who smoke should not use any of these.
- Women 35 years or more with migraine should also not use these.

Progestin-Only Methods (Pills, Injectables, Implants)

- Good for those who cannot use oestrogen.
- DMPA decreases bone mineral density slightly, consequences unknown.

Emergency Contraceptive Pills

- Can be used by all age groups.
- Should not be prescribed as regular contraceptive.

Sterilization (BTL)

- Good for completed families.
- Medical disorders must be ruled out or controlled before contraception.

Barrier Methods (Condoms, Diaphragms, Cervical caps)

- Cheap and convenient for occasional sex
- Highly effective in older women due to infrequent ovulation

IUCD (Copper Devices)

- Expulsion rate lowers after 40 years.
- Insertion may be more difficult due to tightening of cervical os.

Fertility Awareness Methods

- Difficult to use due to irregular cycles.

When can she stop contraception?

- 12 months after last menses.
- Those on hormonal methods should discontinue at the age of 50 and switch to another non-hormonal method.
- Copper T can be left till menopause and removed at least 6 months after last menses.

Health Advice

- Moderate physical exercise
- Eat foods rich in calcium—dairy, fish, beans
- Moisturizers or lubricants during sex if vaginal dryness a problem.

Checklist for contraception for the elderly woman

Task	Well done	Fairly done	Poorly done	Not done
Available contraceptive methods in West Africa (Max 5):				
- Combined oral contraceptives.			1	0
- Progestins; both injectables and implants.			1	0
- Intrauterine devices.			1	0
- Sterilization; both male and female.			1	0
- Barrier methods especially condoms.			1	0
- Emergency contraception.			1	0
- Natural methods of family planning.			1	0
Introduction: the elderly mother and the implications of using contraceptive methods	4	2	1	0
Combined hormonal methods; elderly mothers who smoke or have migraine not suitable	4	2	1	0
Progestin only; can be used. There is slight decrease in bone density but implication unknown	4	2	1	0
Emergency contraceptives; can be used by all age groups, not suitable for regular contraception		2	1	0
Sterilization (BTL); suitable if completed family. Control medical disorders before surgery	4	2	1	0
Barrier methods; highly effective at this age due to infrequent ovulation, also cheap	4	2	1	0
IUCD; difficult to insert due to cervical stenosis but expulsion rate is low	4	2	1	0
Fertility awareness (Natural methods); difficult to use due to irregular menses	4	2	1	0
When to stop contraceptive; 12 months after last menses, stop hormonal methods after 50 years, remove IUCD 6 months after last menses	4	2	1	0
Health advice; moderate exercise, calcium rich foods, moisturizers for sexual intercourse	4	2	1	0
Total score	43			
Candidates score .../43				

Examiner's signature Date

16.7 Urogynaecology

16.7.1 Question 1: Pelvic Organ Prolapse

1 What are the risk factors for pelvic organ prolapse (POP)?
2 List the components of POP.
3 When is POP considered a disease state in the woman?
4 What causes decubitus ulcer, and how would you manage it?

16.7.1.1 Answer Outline

Pelvic organ prolapse affects millions of women worldwide and can lead to urogenital tract dysfunction and diminished quality of life. The symptoms of pelvic organ prolapse (POP) include descent of anterior vaginal wall, posterior vaginal wall, uterus and cervix, vaginal apex in those who had hysterectomy, or the perineum. POP is considered a disease state only if surgical or non-surgical reduction relieves the symptoms, restores function, and improves quality of life. Because most women do not report the symptoms of POP, the condition is underestimated. If examination alone is used to describe POP, 30–65% of women presenting for routine gynaecological care have stage 2 prolapse as against 3–6% by those who present with symptoms.

Decubitus ulcer is a trophic ulcer always at the most dependent part of the prolapsed uterus outside the vaginal introitus.

Aetiology

Ischaemic necrosis due to

- Narrowing of uterine vessels due to stretching effect.
- Constriction of the prolapsed uterus by the vaginal opening.

Initially there is surface keratinization, followed by cracking and then sloughing and ulceration.

Management

- Confirm the diagnosis of uterovaginal prolapse and rule out cervical or endometrial polyp which may mimic procidentia.
- Take wound swab for MCS.
- Cervical cytology to exclude malignancy.
- Manual reduction to restore blood supply. Patient can be taught to reduce the uterus into the vagina by herself at home and review her weekly in the clinic.
- Vaginal pack with roller bandage soaked in antiseptic or oestrogen cream.
- Antibiotics if infected.
- Schedule her for surgery when the wound has healed; pessary may be used but ulceration is a complication of the use of pessaries.

Checklist for POP

Tasks	Well done	Fairly done	Poorly done	Not done
Risk factors for pelvic organ prolapse (POP):				
- Vaginal childbirth			1	0
- Age			1	0
- Race			1	0
- Connective tissue disorders			1	0
- Raised intraabdominal pressure.			1	0
- Genetic factors			1	0
The components of pelvic organ prolapse are:				
- Descent of anterior vaginal wall		2		0
- Descent of posterior vaginal wall		2		0
- Descent of uterus and cervix		2		0
- Descent of vaginal apex (post-hysterectomy)		2		0
- Descent of the perineum		2		0
		2		0
POP is considered a disease state in the woman only:				
- If surgical and nonsurgical reduction leads to,			1	0
- Relieve of symptoms,			1	0
- Restoration of functions,			1	0
- And improvement in quality of life.			1	0
Decubitus ulcer is caused by ischaemic necrosis due to:		2		0
- Kinking of uterine arteries and		2		0
- Constriction of uterus at the vaginal introitus.		2		0
Basic investigations include:				
- VE to rule out cervical or endometrial polyp.		2		0
- Wound swab for MCS		2		0
- Cervical smear to rule out malignancy		2		0
Supportive treatment involves:				
- Manual reduction; teach patient to do same at home.		2		0
- Vaginal pack with antiseptic or oestrogen gauze.		2		0
- Antibiotics where wound appears septic.		2		0
- Nutritional rehabilitation including haematinics.		2		0
Definitive treatment include:				
- Vaginal hysterectomy		2		0
- Use pessaries if unfit for surgery.			1	0
- Colpocleisis can be used			1	0
Total marks	46			
Candidate's score .../46				

Examiner's name and signature Date

16.7.2 Question 2: Urinary Fistula

- Describe the types of urinary fistulas seen in gynaecological practice in West Africa.
- Describe the method of making appropriate diagnosis of each type.
- What are the principles of achieving a successful VVF repair?

16.7.2.1 Answer Outline

Introduction

Urinary fistula is an abnormal communication between the urinary tract and any other epithelial lining usually the genital and alimentary tracts. In the developing countries, VVF remains an obstetrics calamity affecting thousands of women of low socioeconomic status where antenatal care is lacking. For every woman seen with VVF, a hundred others suffer lifelong disabilities due to complications of childbirth.

Types of Urinary Fistula

- Vaginal
  - Juxta-cervical
  - Juxta-urethral
  - Mid-vaginal
- Ureterovaginal fistula
- Vesicouterine fistula

Methods of Diagnosis

All cases of urinary fistulae present with urinary incontinence sometimes associated with faecal incontinence. The past medical history together with physical examination usually clinches the diagnosis without resorting to investigations. In our environment, obstetrics fistula accounts for over 90% of the urinary fistulae seen. This is in contrast to developing countries where gynaecological surgeries account for the majority of urinary fistulae seen.

Diagnosis of VVF

- History and physical examination
- EUA and dye test to assess site, number, and sometimes debridement

Diagnosis of Ureterovaginal Fistula

- History and physical examination
- IVU
- EUA and dye test (with IV indigo carmine dye)

Diagnosis of Vesicouterine Fistula

- History and physical examination (menohaematuria)
- Cystoscopy and hysteroscopy

Principles of Achieving a Successful VVF Repair

Preoperative: treat UTI, treat dermatitis, improve patient wellbeing and nutrition, and treat all underlying disease conditions and infections.

Intra-operative: appropriate positioning of patient, good operative lighting and visibility, appropriate anaesthesia, identify all fistulae, dissection of fistula edges free, and closure in layers without haematoma or tension. Continuous bladder drainage for days, antibiotics cover, adequate hydration.

Post-operative: monitor vital signs, input/output chart, at least 50 mL urine/h, low residue diet, analgesia, antibiotics, monitor wetness of bed, bladder retraining exercise.

On discharge: inform patient and her relation of the circumstances leading to the VVF. Couple to abstain from coitus for 3 months post discharge. Inform couple about the need for CS in subsequent pregnancies.

Checklist for urinary fistula

Task	Well done	Fairly done	Poorly done	Not done
Introduction: definition of urinary fistula, prevalence, importance	4	2	1	0
Types of urinary fistula in gynaecology:				
- Vesicovaginal fistula (VVF)		2		0
- Vesicouterine fistula (Youssef's syndrome)		2		0
- Ureterovaginal fistula		2		0
Method of diagnosis of each urinary fistula:				
- VVF; history, physical examination, EUA		2	1	0
- Vesicouterine; history, physical examination, EUA, cystoscopy, hysteroscopy		2	1	0
- Ureterovaginal; history, physical examination, EUA, IVU		2	1	0
Principles of achieving successful repair:				
- Preoperative: nutritional rehabilitation, treat comorbidities		2	1	0
- Intraoperative: good surgical technique; positioning, equipment, etc.		2	1	0
- Postoperative: close monitoring of input/output, antibiotics, etc.		2	1	0
- Follow-up: avoid early coitus, ANC subsequent pregnancies		2	1	0
Prevention of urinary fistula: prevent childhood pregnancy, good ANC	4	2	1	0
Total marks	28			
Candidates score .../28				

Examiner's signature Date

16.7.3 Question 3: Vaginal Hysterectomy

- What is second-degree uterovaginal prolapse?
- Describe step by step how you would perform vaginal hysterectomy for second-degree uterovaginal prolapse.

16.7.3.1 Answer Outline

In second-degree uterovaginal prolapse, the cervix protrudes beyond the vaginal introitus, but the uterine body remains inside the vagina.

Steps in Vaginal Hysterectomy
Preoperative Preparation

- Pap smear with or without colposcopy for all patients
- Endometrial biopsy for those with abnormal vaginal bleeding
- HVS/ECS; treat bacterial infection or vaginosis before surgery
- FBC, EUCr, grouping and cross matching of blood

Discuss the choice of the procedure with the patient.

- Relatively small uterus
- Extensive adhesions not anticipated
- No significant adnexal pathology
- Some degree of pelvic organ prolapse
- Compared to TAH: faster recovery, less pain, reduced hospital stay, less cost
- Obtain informed consent

Anaesthesia

- General anaesthesia
- Spinal anaesthesia

Position

- Lithotomy position
- Cleaned and draped
- Urinary bladder emptied
- Auvard speculum inserted to retract posterior vaginal wall
- Angled vaginal retractor placed anteriorly
- Anterior and posterior lips of cervix separately held with a pair of long Kocher's, Vulsellum, or Lahey-thyroid forceps

Vaginal Wall Incision

- Pull the cervix outwards by applying traction on the Kocher's forceps.
- Infiltrate cervical skin with 1:200,000 adrenaline solution to separate tissue planes and minimize bleeding.

- Make a circumferential incision at the junction of the cervical and vaginal skin, superficial to the cervical stroma.

Posterior Peritoneal Entry

- Lift the Kocher's forceps anteriorly to expose the posterior fornix.
- Hold the proximal edge of the circumcised vaginal skin with Allis forceps and bluntly dissect the vaginal skin off the cervix using peanut swab till the peritoneum of the POD is seen.
- The peritoneum is cut with Mayor's scissors and a stay-suture applied posteriorly.
- The Auvard speculum is now adjusted into the peritoneum.

Anterior Peritoneal Entry

- The traction on the cervix is now applied posteriorly to expose the vesicocervical space.
- The proximal lip of the circumcised vaginal skin on either side of the longitudinal incision is held with Allis forceps and bluntly dissected off the cervix till the vesicouterine peritoneum is reached.
- The peritoneum is grasped and divided between two artery forceps and the peritoneal cavity explored with the index finger.
- A vaginal retractor is inserted to elevate the bladder and anterior vaginal wall.

Transection of Uterosacral and Cardinal Ligaments

- Pull the clamps on the cervix to bring the uterosacral ligaments into view.
- Palpate the cardinal and uterosacral ligaments on one side and double clamp with curved Kocher's forceps, transect and tie with vicryl 1.
- Repeat the same procedure on the other side.
- If the cardinal ligaments are broad, similar clamping and cutting can be repeated cephalad.
- The sutures are cut long for identification.

Uterine Arteries

- As traction is applied on the clamps on the cervix to one side, the uterine artery on the exposed side is palpated, clamped with curved Kocher's forceps, transected and tied as the clamp is remover.
- The procedure is repeated on the other side; the sutures are cut short.

Cornua

- The round and ovarian ligaments with fallopian tubes are doubly clamped, divide and vicryl 1 suture applied distal to the lateral clamp.
- The same procedure is repeated on the other side.
- If adnexectomy is to be done, the uterine fundus is delivered either posteriorly or anteriorly, pulled down to visualize the ovaries, and the distal clamp applied lateral to the ovaries.

Vaginal Cuff Closure

- The peritoneum may be closed with purse-string vicryl 0 suture.
- A vicryl 1 suture is passed through the anterior vaginal wall on one side, the cardinal and uterosacral ligament pedicles, through posterior vaginal wall and tied. Same procedure is repeated on the other side.
- The rest of the vaginal vault can be closed with continuous vicryl 1 suture.

Post-operative Care

- Clean the vagina and apply dry sterile pack for 6 h
- Prescribe antibiotics and analgesia
- Leave Foley's catheter for 24 h
- Diet as tolerated from 6 h post-operatively
- Avoid sexual intercourse for 6 weeks to allow vault healing.

Checklist for vaginal hysterectomy

Tasks	Well done	Fairly done	Poorly done	Not done
Definition of second-degree utero-vaginal prolapse:				
- Cervix protrudes beyond vaginal introitus.		2		0
- Uterine body inside the vagina.		2		0
Steps of vaginal hysterectomy:				
Preoperative preparation:				
- Pap smear		2		0
- Endometrial biopsy		2		0
- HVS, ECS for MCS		2		0
- FBC, EUCr, group and cross match blood.		2		0
Anaesthesia and positioning:				
- General or Spinal anaesthesia.		2	1	0
- Cleaned and draped in lithotomy position.		2	1	0
- Bladder emptied and cervix exposed with Auvard speculum.		2	1	0
- Both lips of cervix held with long Allis forceps		2	1	0
Vaginal wall incisions:				
- Infiltrate cervix with N/Saline or 1:200,000 adrenaline		2	1	0
- Circumferential incision with anterior longitudinal one		2	1	0
Posterior entry:				
- Hold proximal lip of circumferential incision and dissect vaginal wall off the cervix till peritoneum is reached,		2	1	0
- Open peritoneum, apply stay suture, adjust Auvard		2	1	0
Anterior entry:				
- Dissect vaginal wall off cervix till Vesicouterine peritoneum reached.		2	1	0
- Open peritoneum, explore with finger, insert retractor.		2	1	0
Cardinal and uterosacral ligaments:				
- Pull cervix downwards, palpate ligaments, double clamp, transect and tie with vicryl 1, cut suture long.		2	1	0
- Repeat same on the other side		2	1	0
Uterine arteries:				
- Palpate uterine artery on one side, clamp with curved Kocher's, transect, tie as the clamp is removed.		2	1	0
- Repeat same on other side, cut sutures short.		2	1	0
Cornua:				
- Palpate infundibulo-pelvic ligament, double-clamp ovarian and round ligaments and fallopian tubes together with curved Kocher's forceps.		2	1	0
- Divide between clamps and tie distal to the lateral clamp with vicryl 1. Repeat same on the other side.		2	1	0
Vaginal cuff closure:				
- Close peritoneum with purse-string vicryl 0.		2	1	0
- Pass vicryl 1 through anterior vaginal wall, cardinal and uterosacral ligament pedicles, posterior vaginal wall and tie on one side.		2	1	0
- Repeat same on the other side; close the rest of the vault with continuous vicryl 1 suture.		2	1	0
Postoperative care:				
- Clean the vagina, apply dry sterile pack.		2	1	0
- Prescribe antibiotics and analgesics.		2	1	0
- Leave Foley's catheter for 24 hours.		2	1	0
- Diet as tolerated from 6 hours postoperatively.		2	1	0
- Avoid sexual intercourse for 6 weeks to allow vault healing.		2	1	0
Total marks	60			
Candidate's score .../60				

Examiner's signature Date

16.8 Ethics and Medico-Legal Issues

16.8.1 Question 1: Contraception for the Minor

A 16-year-old girl consults you to request for oral contraception. She is sexually active and goes out with an 18-year-old boyfriend. She does not want her parents to know about the consultation.

- What ethical considerations will influence your clinical decision and why?

16.8.1.1 Answer Outline

The main ethical issues here are:

- Competence
- Confidentiality
- Best interest

Competence

This patient is a minor and her consent should be assented by her parents or guardian. However, if the minor has the maturity to understand the benefits and risks of the proposed treatment, her decision should be respected. The doctor should of course try to persuade the patient to agree to parental involvement by explaining the value of parental support.

Confidentiality

Her autonomy and confidentiality should be respected if she refuses disclosure to her parents. Even if the doctor is unwilling to supply contraception on the grounds of the patient's immaturity, maintaining confidentiality is a general duty of the physician. Exceptions to the rule are where the treatment may cause harm to the patient.

Best Interest

Take into consideration whether this girl is likely to engage in sexual intercourse without contraception and whether physical and mental harm may come to her if she does not receive the treatment. Consider in her best interest if she would require the treatment even without parental consent. In some exceptional situations, like sexual exploitation, abuse and incest, the doctor may decide to disclose the information to the parents in the best interest of the girl.

Checklist for contraception to the minor

Tasks	Well done	Fairly done	Poorly done	Not done
Ethical consideration: - Competence, - Confidentiality, - Best interest.		2 2 2		0 0 0
Competence: - The patient is a minor and sexually active. - Her consent should be assented by her parents. - She understands the benefits and risks of the contraceptive. - Her autonomy and confidentiality should be respected.		2 2 2 2	1 1 1 1	0 0 0 0
Confidentiality: - Discuss the value of parental support for her. - Suggest to her to seek parental involvement. - Confidentiality should be maintained even if she refuses to involve her parents (respect her autonomy).		2 2 2	1 1 1	0 0 0
Best interest: - Take into account whether she is likely to have sexual intercourse without contraception. - Assess whether she may suffer physical or mental insult if she does not receive the contraceptive. - Consider in her best interest whether she requires the treatment without parental assent (or consent).		2 2 2	1 1 1	0 0 0
You may disclose the information to her parents against her wish if she is involved in sexual exploitation and other sexual abuse, or incest.	4	2	1	0
Total score	30			
Candidate's score .../30				

Examiner's signature Date

16.8.2 Question 2: Clinical Negligence

- What is clinical negligence?
- How would you prevent clinical negligence in obstetrics and gynaecology?

16.8.2.1 Answer Outline

Clinical negligence involves a "lack of care" in some aspect of treatment provision. Where there is a lack of care in some respect, and that lack of care causes an adverse outcome, then there has been clinical negligence.

An unwanted outcome which was predictable, or was a known risk factor, carefully guarded against, is not negligence. In other words, clinical negligence constitutes breach of duty as confirmed by an expert or group of experts, and the breach of duty must have caused a foreseeable injury. The breach of duty, together with the injury caused is called "liability" by lawyers.

In developed countries, dealing with actual or alleged clinical negligence costs the governments millions of dollars. More than 60% of these litigations in the UK are generated within obstetrics. The most expensive component of these costs is the claims made on behalf of brain-damaged babies.

Like the patients affected, doctors accused of negligence can go through long-term stress as they become the "second victim". Health organizations and professional bodies should adequately support health workers when errors occur because those involved can be distressed. A no-blame culture should be cultivated in which individuals are only blamed where:

- Breaches of the law have occurred.
- Incidents have not been reported.
- Problems are recurrent for the individual despite support and counsel.

Preventing Clinical Negligence

This will involve:

- Evidence-based practice
- Regular review and feedback of patients' condition
- Training and retraining
- Morbidity/mortality review:
  - Review and analyse mistakes
  - Perform root cause analysis
  - Apply lessons learnt to improve services (response)

Evidence-based medicine (EBM) is the judicious and conscientious use of current best evidence from medical care research for making medical decisions. This will involve:

- Finding the best available evidence
- Rating the quality of the evidence
- Judging the applicability of the result of the research

Health education in the community is also very important. The health seeking behaviour of women must change. In our environment, women wait for their husbands to come from work before reporting their health issues. Coming to hospital at odd hours will affect the quality of care received and promote clinical negligence. The inability of women to pay for health services will also delay rendering of treatment which in emergency situations can result in medical negligence.

Checklist for medical negligence

Tasks	Well done	Fairly done	Poorly done	Not done
What is medical negligence:				
- Lack of care in any aspect of treatment.		2		0
- Lack of care has led to adverse outcome or harm.		2		0
Most litigations concerning medical negligence are in obstetrics.		2		0
Preventing clinical negligence in obstetrics and gynaecology				
Evidence based medical practice:				
- Searching for best available evidence (study)		2		0
- Rating the quality of the evidence		2		0
- Judging its applicability in our environment		2		0
- Knowing medical ethics and the local laws		2		0
Regular review of patients' condition and feedback:				
- During follow-up in the clinic.		2		0
- During ward rounds		2		0
- Morning reviews and scientific meetings		2		0
Training and retraining of doctors and other health workers	4	2	1	0
Regular morbidity/mortality reviews:				
- Record and analyze mistakes.		2		0
- Perform root cause analysis.		2		0
- Apply lessons learned to improve services.		2		0
- Follow up on responses		2		0
Health education in the community (social media, churches etc.):				
- Women to come to hospital early.		2		0
- Break some cultural barriers affecting access to health care,		2		0
- Women empowerment to pay for health care		2		0
Communication skill: confident, systematic, audible etc.	4	2	1	0
Total marks	42			
Candidate's score .../42				

Examiner's signature Date

17 Obstetrics Viva Voce

17.1 Preconception Care

17.1.1 Question 1: Preconception Counselling

A 35-year-old female journalist is planning to get married for the first time. She has come to the preconception clinic to receive care. How would you counsel her during this first visit to the clinic?

17.1.2 Answers

17.1.2.1 Introduction

The purpose of preconception counselling is to improve the knowledge, attitude, and practice of men and women to preconception health. This is to ensure that all childbearing age women enter pregnancy in optimal health. Interconceptional interventions are also implemented to prevent recurrent adverse pregnancy outcomes.

17.1.2.2 Counselling Team

Although the obstetrician sees the women (and her partner) during the first visit, as may be necessary, the clients would subsequently be managed jointly with physician (Internist), paediatrician, psychiatrist, nutritionist, haematologist, and family physician as may be necessary.

17.1.2.3 Biodata

Name, age, address, religion/tribe, occupation, marital status. This is important when discussing sociocultural practices affecting pregnancy. The age of the mother (and to some extent that of the partner) also affects the outcome of pregnancy.

C. Chama, *OSCE and VIVA VOCE in Obstetrics and Gynaecology*,
https://doi.org/10.1007/978-3-031-77262-7_17

17.1.2.4 Medical History

Diabetes mellitus, hypertension, epilepsy, SLE, phospholipid syndrome, SCD, HIV, and other medical disorders can affect the pregnancy and be affected by the pregnancy. Live vaccines cannot be taken during pregnancy; examples are rubella, measles, varicella-zoster, polio, chicken pox, and yellow fever vaccines.

17.1.2.5 Reproductive History

Previous miscarriages, molar pregnancy, eclampsia, stillbirth, preterm delivery, placental abruption, and infertility should be enquired. These are likely to recur, and the causes should be sought for and managed accordingly.

17.1.2.6 Family History

Haemoglobinopathies, birth defects, phenylketonuria, mental retardation, infertility, etc. tend to run in families and should be screened for in populations at risk.

17.1.2.7 Social History

Use of recreational drugs and smoking and exposure to mercury and lead can adversely affect pregnancy. Poor nutrition including obesity should be optimized for good pregnancy outcome. Folic acid should be started before conception where necessary. Intimate partner violence and bisexuality should be managed before pregnancy for optimal outcome.

17.1.2.8 Physical Examination

A detailed physical examination including vaginal examination and a Pap smear should be carried out.

17.1.2.9 Investigations

Relevant investigations should be requested, and the results discussed during post-test counselling. Appropriate referral will then be made to the physician, psychiatrist, nutritionist, etc. as may be necessary.

Checklist for preconception counselling

Task	Well done	Fairly done	Poorly done	Not done
Greets patient, introduces self and obtains permission		2	1	0
Introduction: importance of preconception counselling and care		2	1	0
Informs client of the need to involve other specialists where necessary: Psychiatrist, Internist, Nutritionist etc.	4	2	1	0
Biodata: name, age, address, occupation, marital status, educational level	4	2	1	0
Medical history: DM, HT, SCD, SLE, explain relevance of knowing these information	4	2	1	0
Ask client (or couple) if they need any clarification on any matter discussed so far		2		0
Reproductive history: parity, miscarriage, molar pregnancy, preterm delivery, placental abruption. Explain importance of knowing these	4	2	1	0
Family history: SCD, DM, HT, multiple gestation, birth defects, infertility, mental retardation and why these are important	4	2	1	0
Social history: use of hard drugs, exposure to poisons, diet and exercise, intimate partner violence, bisexuality	4	2	1	0
Physical examination: general and systemic including pelvic examination and Pap smear	4	2	1	0
Explains findings to client and the need for certain investigations	4	2	1	0
Allows client to ask questions or seek for clarifications		2		0
Relevant investigations: to confirm certain diagnosis and rule out some abnormalities	4	2	1	0
Follow-up: give appointment to see with results of investigations		2		0
Total score	46			
Candidates score .../46				

Examiner's signature Date

17.1.3 Question 2: Prenatal Diagnosis

1 What is prenatal diagnosis?
2 Discuss the role of ultrasound scan in prenatal diagnosis.

17.1.4 Answers

17.1.4.1 Introduction

- Prenatal diagnosis is the identification of foetuses with serious structural, genetic, metabolic, and haematologic abnormalities to assist in making clinical decisions in the management of that pregnancy.
- About 2 per 100 pregnancies may have serious congenital anomaly.
- Prenatal diagnosis involves the application of screening and diagnostic tests.

17.1.5 Congenital Abnormalities to be Looked for

- Structural
  - Congenital heart disease
  - Neural tube defects
  - Cleft lip/palate
  - Talipes equinovarus
  - Sacrococcygeal tumour
  - Amelia
- Chromosomal
  - Trisomy 21 (Down's syndrome)
  - Monosomy X (Turner's syndrome)
  - Other trisomies (13, 18)
- Genetic
  - SCD
  - Cystic fibrosis
- Viral infections
  - Rubella
  - Cytomegalovirus
  - Toxoplasmosis

17.1.5.1 Screening Tests

- Maternal history
- Maternal biochemistry-AFP
- Maternal virology
- Maternal haemoglobin genotype
- Ultrasound scan

17.1.5.2 Diagnostic Tests

- Ultrasound scan
- Amniocentesis
- Chorionic villus sampling
- Cordocentesis

17.1.5.3 Role of Ultrasound

- Can be used as both screening and diagnostic test
- Anomaly scan usually at 18–20 weeks gestation but some anomalies may be detected in the first trimester
- Neural tube defects
  - Anencephaly
  - Hydrocephalus
  - Spina bifida
- Congenital heart disease
  - Septal defects
  - Atrio-ventricular defects
- GI abnormalities
  - Duodenal atresia
  - Omphalocele
  - Gastroschises
- Renal tract abnormalities
  - Renal agenesis
  - Hydronephrosis
  - Posterior urethral valve
- Others
  - Cleft lip/palate
  - Talipes equinovarus
- USS-assisted procedures
  - CVS
  - Amniocentesis
  - Cordocentesis

17.1.5.4 New Developments

- Foetal cells in maternal blood
- Pre-implantation genetic diagnosis
- 3D/4D ultrasound scan
- Foetal MRI
- Pap smear for foetal DNA

Checklist for prenatal diagnosis

Task	Well done	Fairly done	Poorly done	Not done
Introduction: definition, importance	4	2	1	0
Scope:				
- Structural abnormalities; congenital heart disease, neural tube defects		2		0
- Chromosomal abnormalities; Trisomy 21, Monosomy X		2		0
- Genetic abnormalities; SCD, cystic fibrosis		2		0
- Abnormalities due viral infections; rubella, cytomegalovirus		2		0
Screening tests:				
- Maternal history		2		0
- Maternal biochemistry		2		0
- Maternal virology		2		0
- Maternal Hb Genotype		2		0
- Ultrasound scan		2		0
Diagnostic tests:				
- Ultrasound scan		2		0
- Amniocentesis		2		0
- Chorionic villus sampling		2		0
- Cordocentesis		2		0
Role of ultrasound scan				
- Can be used for both screening and diagnosis.		2		0
- Anomaly scan done at 18-20 weeks gestation		2		0
Anomalies diagnosed by ultrasound scan:				
- Neural tube defects; anencephaly, hydrocephalus, Spina		2		0
bifida		2		0
- Congenital heart disease; septal defects, AV defects		2		0
- GI abnormalities; duodenal atresia, omphalocele		2		0
- Renal tract abnormalities; renal agenesis,		2		0
Hydronephrosis, PUV		2		0
- Others; cleft lip/palate, Talipes equinovarus				
- USS assisted procedures; CVS, amniocentesis, Cordocentesis				
New developments: 4D USS, fetal MRI, Pap smear for fetal cells, pre-implantation genetic diagnosis, fetal cells in maternal blood	4	2	1	0
Total score	50			
Candidates score .../50				

Examiner's signature Date

17.1.6 Question 3: Prevention of Mother-to-Child Transmission of HIV

1. How would you diagnose HIV in pregnancy?
2. What are the treatment options to prevent mother-to-child transmission of the virus?

17.1.7 Answers

17.1.7.1 Introduction

Globally there were about 37.9 million people living with HIV in 2018 and about 70% of them live in sub-Saharan Africa (3). Although there has been global decline in the incidence of HIV infection, in West Africa, the story is not the same, with HIV still accounting for 50% of infective morbidities among cases of maternal near-miss and 30% of maternal deaths. However, the availability of highly active antiretroviral therapy (HAART) and prophylaxis for opportunistic infections have drastically reduced the rate of mother-to-child transmission of HIV to less than 2% in some areas of sub-Saharan Africa.

17.1.7.2 Diagnosis

All pregnant women booking for antenatal care should be counselled and tested for HIV. This is the entry point for prevention of mother-to-child transmission (PMTCT) of HIV. Because of the high patient load in our environment, the provider-initiated counselling and testing is the preferred approach. HIV testing is recommended to all mothers booking for antenatal care and the mothers informed that each of them has the right to refuse the test—the "opt-out" method. In a meta-analysis of 44 studies, the opt-out method was shown to have 94% acceptance rate with 70% of those identified as HIV positive initiating ARV prophylaxis (11). In situations where the patient load is not much, like in some private facilities, individual counselling and testing can be carried out. The antenatal clinic can also be used to mobilize pregnant and non-pregnant women to access HIV testing and counselling in the hospital, community, and even home-based testing.

- Screening tests
  - Rapid antibody tests
  - ELISA
- Confirmatory tests

  The antibody test *Western Blot* is the gold standard for confirming HIV infection. It is a chromatography test using the patient's serum and the CDC criteria for interpretation are:
  - Positive: at least two of the following bands: p24, gp41, gp160/120
  - Negative: no bands present
  - Indeterminate: HIV band present but does not meet above criteria, for example, single band or weak bands

Another antibody assay, the Line Immunoassay (LIA) can also be used to confirm HIV-1 and HIV-2 infection. The other confirmatory tests are the polymerase chain reaction tests, either HIV RNA assay or HIV DNA assay. The HIV RNA assay is used to diagnose acute HIV infection prior to seroconversion and to establish baseline viral load before treatment. Together with CD4 count, the viral load is also used to monitor response to treatment and to estimate the risk for opportunistic infections.

- National guideline
  - Rapid tests only
  - Serial algorithm
    Determine (highly sensitive)
    Unigold (highly specific)
    Stat pak (used as tiebreaker)

17.1.7.3 Antenatal Care

Both obstetric and medical care in HIV-infected pregnant women need to be strengthened and modified. Post-test counselling should include information on the following:

- Disclosure, partner notification, and testing
- Benefits of PMTCT intervention
- Nutrition
- Delivery
- Infant feeding and testing
- ARV adherence and follow-up
- Specific tests for HIV-positive mothers
  - CD4 count—to assess degree of immunodeficiency
  - VL—assess risk of disease progression and perinatal transmission
  - Resistance testing—for choice of antiretroviral drugs
  - RFT, LFT, FBC, Lipid profile—as recommended by ART guideline
  - CXR to rule out pTB
  - HVS/ECS to rule out other STIs

17.1.7.4 Treatment Options

The 2016 WHO HIV treatment guidelines recommend that ART be initiated in all individuals living with HIV/AIDS irrespective of the clinical stage or CD4 count in order to preserve patient's immune systems, control HIV replication and reduce further transmission. This is more so in pregnancy which has a limited time to act and achieve viral suppression before delivery. Overall, the quality of life of the mother and her baby and consequently that of the entire family is improved.

Because not all investigation results may be available on time, in choosing ARV combination in pregnancy, one should cover for possible co-infection with HBV or HCV and the fact that majority of women have CD4 count above 250 cells/mL. Until recently, WHO recommended Tenofovir (TDF), lamivudine (3TC) and efavirenz (EFV) as first-line ART in pregnancy. However, WHO now recommends the use of the integrase inhibitor, Dolutegravir (DTG) with TDF + 3TC in people initiating ART and even in those doing well on first-line TDF + 3TC + EFV. DTG-based regimens are associated with more rapid viral suppression, less need to switch to other ARVs, and there is lower risk of development of drug resistance even when compared to boosted protease inhibitor combinations. Since access to viral load testing is difficult in our environment, this approach has the potential to bring greater public health benefits. Dolutegravir has been shown to increase the risk of neural tube defects in the newborn, but the benefits far outweigh the risk.

In low resource areas, the WHO 2010 recommendation gave three options:

- Option A (WHO 2010)
  - AZT alone during pregnancy (after 14 weeks)
- Option B– use of HAART during pregnancy and breastfeeding
- Option B+ continues HAART throughout reproductive life.

17.1.7.5 Labour

The usual obstetric guidelines for management of labour should be followed. Universal precautions should be practised, and the HIV-positive woman should not be isolated or treated differently. The risk of puerperal sepsis is three times in HIV-infected women than uninfected women, and this risk increases to six times if delivered by caesarean section. For this reason, a broad-spectrum antibiotic prophylaxis should be given in labour.

17.1.7.6 Postpartum Care

The mother should be continued on broad-spectrum antibiotics immediately postpartum and be encouraged to continue taking HARRT. Those diagnosed for the first time in labour should be completely evaluated and would have commenced HAART in labour. Those who refuse to commence HAART immediately should be counselled to have their babies started on nevirapine suspension. Counselling should be continued until the mother starts ART. The mother should be co-managed with physicians. Infant feeding counselling should be continued, and the mother assisted to choose the best method for her and her baby. Subsequent follow-up is as for non-pregnant adults on ARV.

All HIV-exposed babies should receive nevirapine suspension within 24 h of delivery and continued for 6 weeks. Those whose mothers are not on ARV should continue the nevirapine plus zidovudine suspension beyond 6 weeks until 12 weeks after their mother has started ART.

In our environment, exclusive breastfeeding should be advocated and supported to avoid the complexities of using infant feeding formulas. However, a mother who chooses not to breast feed should be supported to use the breast milk substitute appropriately. Exclusive breastfeeding should be for 6 months after which complementary feeding is introduced and breastfeeding continued for 1 year of life.

PCR for infant diagnosis is first done at 6 weeks and positive cases referred to the paediatrician for ART and cotrimoxazole prophylaxis. A repeat PCR for those that were negative at 6 weeks should be done 6 weeks after stopping breastfeeding. The final diagnosis of infant HIV status should be done by antibody testing at 18 months of life when the maternal antibodies would have burnt out.

17.1.7.7 Prognosis

- NVP alone 7% transmission rate
- AZT alone 3% transmission rate
- HAART less than 1% transmission rate
- Without treatment up to 40% transmission rate

Checklist for prevention of mother-to-child transmission of HIV

Task	Well done	Fairly done	Poorly done	Not done
Introduction: prevalence of HIV, mode of transmission	4	2	1	0
Diagnosis:				
- Screening through voluntary counselling and testing		2	1	0
- Confirmatory tests		2	1	0
- FBC, EUC, LFT, Urine MCS		2	1	0
Prevention of MTCT antenatally				
- HAART to mother or	4	2	1	0
- ZVD+3TC to mother or		2	1	0
- ZDV alone to mother or		2	1	0
- Modification of obstetric practice; no invasive		2	1	0
procedures, ECV,		2	1	0
- Elective CS if VL>1000copies/ml at term				
Intrapartum care				
- Universal precautions		2		0
- No ARM till delivery imminent		2		0
- Avoid instrumental deliveries and episiotomy.		2		0
- Broad spectrum antibiotics		2		0
Postpartum care				
- Exclusive breastfeeding		2		0
- NVP suspension to baby		2		0
- Mother to continue HAART		2		0
Prognosis: depends on type of intervention	4	2	1	0
Total score	40			
Candidates score .../40				

Examiner's signature Date

17.1.8 Question 4: Monozygotic Twins

1. What is monozygotic twining?
2. Explain the classification of monozygotic twins by time of splitting.
3. What are the types of abnormalities specific to monozygotic twins?

17.1.9 Answers

Monozygotic twins occur due to the splitting of a single fertilized ovum. Monozygotic twins account for about 30% of all twin gestations and its incidence is constant throughout the world. Monozygotic twins, although having the same genetic heritage, also are usually not identical. For example, the division of one zygote into two does not necessarily yield equal sharing of protoplasmic material. In addition, monozygotic twins may be discordant for genetic mutations because of a postzygotic mutation, or they may have the same genetic disease but marked difference in its expression. Recently, sesquizygosity, a rare event of dispermic fertilization that leads to monozygotic twins has been demonstrated, and some cases may have sex discordance (Gabbett 2019).

17.1.9.1 Types of Monozygotic Twins

- DCDA twins
  - Separate placenta and separate amniotic sacs
  - Embryo splits before 3 days of gestation
  - Accounts for 8% of all twin gestations
- MCDA twins
  - Single placenta but separate amniotic sacs
  - Cleavage after cell mass has formed; 4–8 days of gestation
  - Accounts for 20% of all twin gestations
- MCMA twins
  - The embryo splits from 9 to 12 days of gestation.
  - The chorion and the amnion have already differentiated.
  - Rare, accounts for 1% of all twins.
- Conjoined or Siamese twins
  - The embryo splits at or after 13 days of gestation.
  - Cleavage is only partial, and the twins share some parts of the body.
  - Very rare, thoracopagus (Rostral joining) being the commonest.

17.1.9.2 Abnormalities Specific to Monozygotic Twins

The abnormalities specific to monozygotic twins are mainly those arising from monoamniotic twins; these include:

Foetal Malformations

- Conjoined twins; thoracopagus is the commonest type occurring in 1.5/100,000 births.
- External parasitic twins: these are grossly defective twins or foetal parts attached to a relatively normal twin. A functional heart or brain is absent in the parasitic twin.

Vascular Anastomosis

This could be arterio-arterial (AA), arterio-venous (AV) or veno-venous (VV). Vascular anastomosis is clinically diagnosed based on two sonographic findings: first monochorionic pregnancy and second polyhydramnios in one twin sac and oligohydramnios in the other sac.

- TTTS; twin-twin transfusion syndrome
- TRAP; twin reversed arterial perfusion
- TAPS; twin anaemia-polycythemia sequence

Cord Entanglement

This frequently occurs in monoamniotic twins. The cause of cord vessel constriction is unknown and foetal death is unpredictable. Delivery is suggestive at 32–34 weeks of gestation.

Foetal Brain Damage

This could be cerebral palsy, microcephaly, porencephaly, or multicystic encephalomalacia. The brain damage is due to ischaemic necrosis which results from hypotension in the donor twin and blood pressure instability in the recipient twin.

Twin Embolization Syndrome

With in utero death of one twin, there may be passage of thromboplastic material to the surviving twin, resulting in ischaemic structural defects.

Checklist for monozygotic twins

Task	Well done	Fairly done	Poorly done	Not done
Introduction: mechanism of monozygotic twining, prevalence, and complications	4	2	1	0
Classification:				
- DCDA; embryo splits 1-3 days of gestation, 8% of all twins.		2	1	0
- MCDA; embryo splits 4-8 days of gestation, 20% of all twins.		2	1	0
- MCMA; embryo splits 9-12 days of gestation, 1% of all twins.		2	1	0
- Conjoined twins; embryo partially splits ±13 of gestation, rare, thoracopagus commonest.		2	1	0
Specific abnormalities				
- Fetal abnormalities; conjoined twins, external parasitic twins		2	1	0
- Vascular anastomosis; AA, AV, VV, resulting in TTTS, TRAP etc.		2	1	0
- Cord entanglement, frequent in monoamniotic twins		2	1	0
- Fetal brain damage; CP, microcephaly, porencephaly etc.		2	1	0
- Twin embolization syndrome, with death of one twin		2	1	0
Total score	22			
Candidates score .../22				

Examiner's signature Date

17.2 Labour

17.2.1 Question 1: Mechanism of Normal Labour

1. What is normal labour?
2. Describe step by step, the mechanism of normal labour.

17.2.2 Answers

Normal labour is the spontaneous onset of regular uterine contractions at term, leading to progressive cervical dilatation and subsequent expulsion of a live singleton foetus in cephalic presentation, with a birth weight of 2.5 kg or more. It is therefore a retrospective diagnosis.

- Low birth weight is not normal delivery.
- Preterm delivery is not normal delivery.
- Breech delivery is not normal delivery.
- Augmented or induced labour is not normal delivery.
- Twin delivery is not normal delivery.

Mechanism of labour is the series of changes in *position* and *attitude* that the foetus undergoes during its passage through the birth canal. The steps are:

1. Descent and engagement
   (a) Foetal head enters the pelvis in transverse position which is the widest diameter.
   (b) Engagement occurs when the foetal BPD reaches the ischial spines of the maternal pelvis.
2. Flexion
   (a) As the head descends into the midcavity, flexion occurs passively, aided by the surrounding structures.
   (b) This minimizes the presenting diameter.
3. Internal rotation
   (a) The occiput leads in a well-flexed attitude.
   (b) As the head reaches the slopping gutter of levator ani, the occiput is rotated anteriorly to OAP.
   (c) If the foetus engages in OPP, internal rotation can occur to OAP through 180 degrees, but the duration of labour is increased.
4. Extension
   (a) The well-flexed head extends and the occiput escapes from underneath the pubic symphysis and distends the vulva (crowning).
   (b) With further extension, the bregma, face, and chin appear over the perineal body posteriorly.

   (c) Extension movement minimizes soft tissue trauma by utilizing the smallest diameters of the head at each stage.

5. Restitution
   (a) As the foetal head escapes from the vulva, slight rotation of the occiput occurs through 1/8 of a circle so that the occiput aligns with the shoulders which entered the pelvis in the oblique position.
   (b) This is called restitution.
6. External rotation
   (a) As the shoulders descend through the midcavity, it rotates to the AP plane.
   (b) Accordingly, the occiput further rotates 1/8 of a circle to the OTP.
   (c) This is called external rotation.
7. Delivery of the shoulders and foetal body
   (a) The anterior shoulder escapes under the pubic symphysis followed by the posterior shoulder.
   (b) Although this movement occurs spontaneously, it can be assisted by pulling the foetal head downwards to help release the anterior shoulder from beneath the pubic symphysis.
   (c) The rest of the foetal body is delivered easily.

Checklist for mechanism of normal labour

Task	Well done	Fairly done	Poorly done	Not done
Introduction: definition of normal labour	4	2	1	0
What is mechanism of normal labour	4	2	1	0
Step 1: decent and engagement; fetal head enters through transverse diameter of the pelvis, engages when BPD reaches maternal ischial spines	4	2	1	0
Step 2: flexion; occurs passively, minimizes presenting diameter	4	2	1	0
Step 3: internal rotation; as the fetal head reaches the slopping gutter of levator ani, the occiput rotates to OAP	4	2	1	0
Step 4: extension; the flexed head extends for the occiput to escape under the pubic symphysis and distends the vulva (crowning)	4	2	1	0
Step 5: restitution; as the fetal head emerges from the vulva, the occiput slightly rotates to align with the shoulders which enter the pelvis obliquely	4	2	1	0
Step 6: external rotation; as the shoulders reach the midcavity it rotates to AP plane, accordingly the occiput rotates to OTP	4	2	1	0
Step 7: delivery of the shoulders and body; the anterior shoulder escapes under the pubic symphysis by lateral flexion.	4	2	1	0
Total score	36			
Candidates score ....../36				

Examiner's signature Date

17.2.3 Question 2: Obesity in Pregnancy

1. What is obesity?
2. A primigravida presents to the antenatal clinic for booking at a gestational age of 10 weeks with a body mass index (BMI) of 35 kg/m^2. Discuss her antenatal, intrapartum, and postpartum care.

17.2.4 Answers

Obesity simply means extreme overweight as determined by height and weight of an individual. It is measured by body mass index which is the ratio of the body weight in kilograms to the height in metres squared.

• BMI 18.5–24.9 kg/m^2	Normal
• BMI 25–29.9 kg/m^2	Overweight
• BMI 30 kg/m^2 or more	Obesity

17.2.4.1 Obesity is a Cause of Maternal and Perinatal Morbidity and Mortality

- Gestational hypertension
- Pre-eclampsia and eclampsia
- Post-term pregnancy
- Emergency and elective caesarean sections
- Postpartum haemorrhage
- Puerperal sepsis
- Urinary tract infections
- Wound sepsis
- Difficult epidural/spinal anaesthesia
- Thrombosis
- Foetal macrosomia
- Stillbirth
- Birth asphyxia

17.2.4.2 Antenatal Care

- Routine PCV, blood grouping, haemoglobin genotype, HIV, HBV, HCV, VDRL
- 75 g glucose test or OGTT
- Urine MCS
- USS for foetal dating in first trimester, anomaly scan in second trimester
- Serial USS for growth assessment
- Co-manage with physician and dietician
- Regular IPT and TT immunoprophylaxis

17.2.4.3 Labour

- Anaesthetic review in labour
- Inform neonatologist, may require USS to determine foetal lie and FHR
- Open partograph
- If to be delivered by CS
  - Do not cut through the panniculus; weigh vertical or transverse options
  - Close subcutaneous layer
  - Inform neonatologist and anaesthetist
  - Thromboprophylaxis
    Compression stockings
    Early ambulation
    Rarely low-dose heparin

17.2.4.4 Postpartum Care

- Adequate analgesia
- Prophylactic antibiotics
- Tail off insulin if taking one
- Baby to be reviewed by neonatologist; may require SCBU admission
- Routine immunization
- Weight reduction for mother; bariatric surgery an option

Checklist for obesity in pregnancy

Task	Well done	Fairly done	Poorly done	Not done
Obesity:				
- Simply means extreme overweight as determined by individual's weight and height.		2	1	0
- Measured by BMI = weight in Kg/height in meters^2		2	1	0
- Normal range 18.5-24.9Kg/m^2		2	1	0
Preconception care: dietary modification and exercise, control any co-morbidity before pregnancy	4	2	1	0
Antenatal care:				
- Routine antenatal investigations		2	1	0
- Continue dietary modification and exercise.		2	1	0
- 75g glucose test or OGTT		2	1	0
- USS for dating, anomaly scan, and serial scan for fetal growth		2	1	0
- Co-manage with physician and nutritionist.		2	1	0
- Regular IPT and immunoprophylaxis.		2	1	0
Intrapartum care:				
- Anesthesiologist and Neonatologist to review.		2	1	0
- Set IVL		2	1	0
- PCV, group and cross match blood		2	1	0
- USS for fetal lie and position		2	1	0
- Admitting CFG		2	1	0
- Open partograph		2	1	0
- If delivered by CS: do not cut through panniculus, give Thromboprophylaxis, ensure early ambulation,		2	1	0
Postpartum care:				
- Adequate analgesia		2	1	0
- Antibiotic prophylaxis		2	1	0
- Tail off insulin if taking one.		2	1	0
- Baby to be reviewed by neonatologist.		2	1	0
- Encourage breastfeeding.		2	1	0
- Continue weight reduction		2	1	0
Follow-up				
- Regular childhood immunization		2	1	0
- Continue weight reduction.		2	1	0
- Contraception		2	1	0
- Manage co-morbidities with physicians		2	1	0
Total score	54			
Candidate's score .../54				

Examiner's signature Date

17.2.5 Question 3: Cervical Ripening

1. What is cervical ripening?
2. Describe step by step how you would use misoprostol to ripen the cervix for induction of labour.

17.2.6 Answers

In quite a number of situations, the need arises to induce labour before its spontaneous onset. The more common indications are postdatism, severe pre-eclampsia and eclampsia, premature rupture of membranes at term, etc. In such circumstances, it is important to consider the favourability of the cervix to successful labour induction.

One popular quantifiable method of assessing the favourability of the cervix to predict outcomes of labour induction is the Bishop score (1964)

Modified Bishop score

Score	0	1	2	3
Cervical dilatation (cm)	0	1–2	3–4	5 or more
Cervical length (cm)	3	2	1	<1
Position of cervix	Posterior	Central	Anterior	
Consistency of the cervix	Firm	Medium	Soft	
Station of presenting part	−3	−2	0–1	+1 or more

Maximum score = 13
Favourable (or ripe) cervix = 7 or more. Unfavourable (or unripe) cervix = 6 or less

Some pharmacological agents like prostaglandins or mechanical means like Foley's catheter balloon or hygroscopic substances can be used to soften the cervix thus making it favourable for vaginal delivery if labour is induced. *The use of pharmacological agents or mechanical means to change the condition of the cervix to a favourable state for induction of labour is called cervical ripening.*

Misoprostol, a synthetic prostaglandin E2 analogue, is the most popular pharmacological agent for cervical ripening in our environment.

17.2.6.1 Mechanism of Action

- Breakdown of the cervical ground substance, proteoglycan, by increasing the concentration of glycosaminoglycan and dermatan sulphate
- Dispersal of collagen fibres by increasing the concentration of collagenase and elastase enzymes
- Relaxation of cervical smooth muscle therefore allowing cervical dilatation
- Myometrial contraction by increasing intracellular calcium

17.2.6.2 Protocol

- Counselling and obtaining informed consent.
- PCV, grouping, and cross matching of one pint of blood.

- Antenatal CTG should be normal.
- Admit patient a day before procedure.
- Cervical ripening should be commenced in the morning on a working day.
- Place 25 μg misoprostol tabs in the posterior fornix and patient should remain lying in left lateral position for 30 min.
- Palpate for contractions and foetal heart rate hourly; a continuous foetal heart monitoring should be used where available.
- Reassess and repeat 6 hourly till the Bishop score is 7 or more to a maximum of 4 doses.
- Induction of labour with oxytocin to commence at least 6 h after the last dose of misoprostol.

17.2.6.3 Side effects and Complications

- Uterine hyperstimulation
- Fever
- Nausea, vomiting, diarrhoea
- Antidote: SC terbutaline or IV salbutamol infusion

Checklist for cervical ripening

Task	Well done	Fairly done	Poorly done	Not done
The use of pharmacological agents or mechanical means to change the condition of the cervix to a favourable state for induction of labour is called cervical ripening	4	2	1	0
Indications for cervical ripening: postdatism, pre-eclampsia, PROM etc.	4	2	1	0
Briefly explain the Bishop score and differentiate ripe from unripe cervix.	4	2	1	0
Brief pharmacology of misoprostol: PGE2 analogue, increases collagenase, myometrial contraction etc.	4	2	1	0
Outpatient preparation for cervical ripening:				
- Confirm diagnosis e.g. postdatism, PROM		2		0
- Counsel and obtain informed consent.		2		0
- PCV, cross matching of one pint of blood		2		0
- Antenatal CTG should be normal.		2		0
- Admit patient a day before cervical ripening/induction of labour according to departmental protocol.		2		0
In labour ward:				
- Cervical ripening to commence in the morning on a working day according to protocol.		2		0
- Place 25ug misoprostol tablet in the posterior fornix		2		0
- Patient to remain in left lateral position for at least 30 minutes of insertion.		2		0
- Palpate for contractions and FHR hourly; continuous CTG if available.		2		0
- Reassess and repeat 6 hourly till Bishop's score of 7 or more.		2 2		0 0
- Maximum of 4 doses		2		0
- Start oxytocin infusion at least 6 hours after the last dose of misoprostol if not in labour				
Possible complications:				
- Nausea, vomiting, diarrhea; treat symptomatic.		2		
- Fever; treat symptomatic.		2		
- Uterine hyperstimulation; IV terbutaline or salbutamol antidote		2 2		
- Uterine rupture; laparotomy				
Subsequent management				
- Monitor labour closely for complications		2		
- Active management of third stage		2		
- Continue oxytocin infusion for 2 hours postpartum		2		
Total score	54			
Candidates score .../54				

Examiner's signature Date

17.2.7 Question 4: Management of SCD in Labour

1. What is sickle cell disease?
2. Discuss the management of a 25-year-old known HbSS primigravida who presents in established labour at 37 weeks gestation.

17.2.8 Answers

17.2.8.1 Introduction

Sickle cell disease is an autosomal recessive red blood cell disorder in which the sickling gene occurs in a homozygous state (HbSS), or in combination with haemoglobin C (HbSC) or B-thalassaemia (HbSB-thal). The sickling gene has valine replacing glutamine at position 6 of the B-chain of the haemoglobin molecule. The sickle haemoglobin crystalizes under low oxygen conditions causing the red blood cells to sickle. The prevalence in the black African population is about 1/200 to 1/500 with 8–25% of the population being carriers. Globally, about 400,000 HbSS infants are born annually with about 90% of them in sub-Saharan Africa.

The stress of pregnancy and infarction of the placental bed in SCD makes both maternal and perinatal morbidity and mortality to be increased.

The aim of management of this patient in established labour at term is to prevent crisis, ensure normal progress of labour, and the delivery of a healthy baby.

17.2.8.2 Brief History

- Booking parameters
- Any antenatal events like crisis, blood transfusion, and infections
- Foetal growth pattern
- Drugs—IPT, TT, folate, etc.

17.2.8.3 Physical Examination

- General physical examination-pallor, jaundice
- Liver and spleen
- Obstetric examination
  - Lie, presentation, position
  - Descent, foetal heart rate
- Admitting CTG
- Open partograph

17.2.8.4 Immediate Interventions

- Set IVL-Ringer's lactate or normal saline
- PCV, grouping, and cross matching of HbAA blood
- EUCr
- Analgesia—epidural or narcotics

17.2.8.5 Subsequently

- Monitor labour partographically
- Maintain adequate hydration, may allow oral sips on request
- PCV 4 hourly; transfuse if PCV<20%
- Assist second stage but avoid episiotomy as much as possible
- Active management of third stage
- CS for obstetric indications only

17.2.8.6 Postpartum

- Continue IVF for 24 h postpartum
- Continue analgesia with oral narcotics
- May give oxygen by face mask for the first 2 h postpartum
- Broad-spectrum antibiotics
- Early ambulation; give thromboprophylaxis if delivered by CS
- Encourage breastfeeding

17.2.8.7 Postnatal Clinic

- Immunize child according to protocol
- Progestin suitable for contraception

Checklist for management of SCD in labour

Task	Well done	Fairly done	Poorly done	Not done
Introduction: what is SCD, prevalence, effect on pregnancy and vice versa	4	2	1	0
Brief history:				
- Booking parameters		2		0
- Antenatal events e.g. crisis, blood transfusion, UTI, malaria, etc.		2		0
- Fetal growth pattern; IUGR, normal		2		0
- Drugs; IPT, folate, TT etc.		2		0
Physical examination:				
- General physical exam-pallor, jaundice		2		0
- Liver and spleen		2		0
- Obstetric examination		2		0
- Admitting CTG		2		0
Immediate intervention:				
- IVL; Ringer's lactate or normal saline		2		0
- PCV, grouping and cross matching of HbAA blood		2		0
- EUC, LFT		2		0
- Analgesia; epidural or narcotic		2		0
- Open partograph		2		0
- Haematologist, Neonatologist, Anaesthesiologist to review		2		0
Subsequent management:				
- Monitor labour closely; CTG, partograph,		2		0
- Maintain adequate hydration, allow oral sips.		2		0
- PCV 4-6 hourly; transfuse if PCV drops <20%		2		0
- Assist second stage but avoid episiotomy (Vacuum)		2		0
- Active management of third stage		2		0
- CS for obstetric indications only		2		0
Postpartum care:				
- Continue IVF for 24 hours.		2		0
- Continue narcotic analgesic.		2		0
- Broad spectrum antibiotics		2		0
- Early ambulation; thromboprophylaxis if delivered by CS.		2		0
- Encourage breastfeeding		2		0
Postnatal clinic				
- Immunize baby according to protocol.		2		0
- Progestin contraceptive beneficial		2		0
- Refer to haematologist for continuing care		2		0
Total score	60			
Candidates score .../60				

Examiner's signature Date

17.3 Delivery

17.3.1 Question 1: Performing an Episiotomy

1. What is episiotomy?
2. Describe step by step how you would perform episiotomy for the purpose of vacuum delivery.

17.3.2 Answers

Episiotomy (perineotomy) is a surgical incision on the perineum for the purpose of increasing the pelvic outlet for vaginal delivery.

Episiotomy is a useful procedure for selected difficult vaginal deliveries— shoulder dystocia, breech delivery, macrosomic foetus, operative vaginal deliveries, persistent OPP, and other situations where perineal tear is highly likely.

It should be noted that episiotomy does not protect the perineal body but increases the risk of third- and fourth-degree perineal extensions. The risk of faecal incontinence is tripled and flatal incontinence doubled following episiotomy with or without extension. When performed in primigravidas, it confers five times the risk of second or higher order laceration in the second delivery.

There are various types of episiotomy and the mediolateral episiotomy is the commonly used type in our environment; this type has a protective effect against higher order perineal lacerations.

17.3.2.1 Preoperative Preparation

- Anaesthesia
  - If the patient was under epidural analgesia, no further anaesthesia is required.
  - Otherwise, the perineum is infiltrated with 5–10 mL of 1% xylocaine in fanwise manner from the fourchette.
- Positioning
  - In our environment, patients are positioned in the dorsal position in second stage of labour.
  - For assisted or instrumental vaginal deliveries, the patient is positioned in lithotomy position.
  - The accoucheur would have scrubbed and gowned and gloved for receiving the delivery.
  - The patient is cleaned and draped, and the bladder emptied.

- Incision
  - The middle and index finger of the left hand is insinuated between the crowning head and the perineum.
  - Episiotomy scissors is positioned at 7 o'clock and the incision extended for 3–4 cm towards the ipsilateral ischial tuberosity.
  - The vacuum cup is then applied to deliver the baby.
  - The episiotomy is sutured immediately after delivery to minimize blood loss.
- Repair
  - Pac vagina with sterile gauze
  - Repair vaginal skin starting 1 cm above the apex with continuous vicryl 2/0
  - Repair muscle layer using interrupted vicryl 2/0; repair transverse perineal and puborectalis muscles separately.
  - Close the perineal skin and subcutaneous tissue using interrupted or subcuticular vicryl 2/0
  - Remove vaginal pack, do rectal examination, and clean the patient.
- Postoperative care
  - Patient is cleaned and repositioned normally on her bed.
  - Prophylactic oral antibiotics and analgesia are given.
  - Sitz bath twice a day from second day of delivery
  - Discharge when appropriate

Checklist for performing an episiotomy

Task	Well done	Fairly done	Poorly done	Not done
Introduction: what is episiotomy, prevalence, indications	4	2	1	0
Preoperative preparation: episiotomy pack, surgical gloves, sterile gown pack, 2% xylocaine, 10ml syringe and needles	4	2	1	0
Anaesthesia: if patient under epidural analgesia, no further anaesthesia is needed, if not infiltrate perineum with 5-10ml of 1% xylocaine in a fanwise manner.	4	2	1	0
Positioning: the accoucheur scrubs and gowns before cleaning and draping the patient in lithotomy position for the vacuum delivery	4	2	1	0
Incision: - The index and middle fingers of the left hand are insinuated between the crowning head and the perineum. - Episiotomy scissors is positioned at 7 o'clock and the perineum cut for 3-4cm towards the ipsilateral ischial tuberosity. - The vacuum cup is then applied to deliver the baby		2 2 2		0 0 0
Repair: - The episiotomy is sutured immediately after delivery. - Pac the vagina with sterile gauze - Suture the vaginal skin with continuous vicryl 2/0, starting 1cm above the apex of the wound. - Repair the muscle layer with interrupted vicryl 2/0 - The perineal skin is closed with either interrupted or subcuticular vicryl 2/0 - Remove vaginal pack		2 2 2 2 2 2	1 1 1 1 1 1	0 0 0 0 0 0
Postoperative care: - Clean and reposition the patient on the bed. - Oral analgesics - Prophylactic antibiotics - Sitz bath from the second day		2 2 2 2		0 0 0 0
Postnatal clinic: - Check for healing. - Enquire about perineal pain, dyspareunia, and anal incontinence		2 2		0 0
Total score	46			
Candidates score .../46				

Examiner's signature Date

17.3.3 Question 2: Application of the Vacuum Cup

In vacuum-assisted delivery, the first and most essential piece of information is the identification of the flexion point.

- What is flexion point?
- What are the possible applications of the vacuum cup in relation to the flexion point and what are the implications?

17.3.4 Answers

17.3.4.1 Introduction

In vacuum delivery, a suction is created within a cup placed on the foetal scalp such that traction on the cup aids foetal birth. It is preferred to the obstetric forceps because it is easier to apply on the foetal head and does not occupy space like the blades of the forceps. Vacuum cups are metal or plastic and differ in shape, size, and reusability. The rigid flattened mushroom-shaped metal cups generate significantly higher traction force and are preferred in OPP and asynclitism. In addition to the conditions that must be fulfilled for forceps delivery, vacuum delivery can also be conducted in advanced first stage of labour.

17.3.4.2 Flexion Point

Flexion point is an arbitrary point situated approximately 3 cm in front of the posterior fontanel in the midline (on the sagittal suture).

- A traction applied perpendicular to this point will flex the foetal head to the narrowest suboccipito-bregmatic diameter (9.5 cm).
- A 6 cm cup applied so that its rear edge is just at the posterior fontanel should be over the flexion point.
- In other words, the leading edge of a correctly applied vacuum cup will be 3 cm (two finger breadths) away from the anterior fontanel.
- A vacuum cup applied off the central sagittal suture will cause asynclitism during traction and increase the presenting diameter.

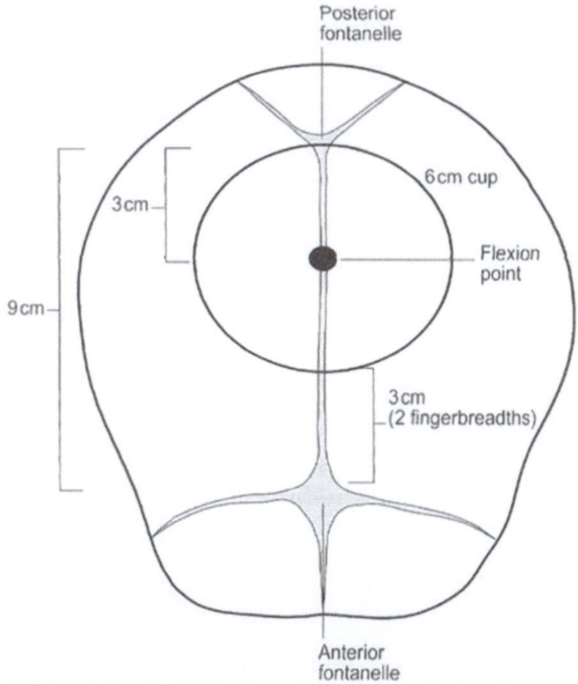

17.3.4.3 Possible Applications of the Vacuum Cup

- Flexing median—which provides the optimum and narrowest suboccipito-bregmatic and biparietal diameters
- Deflexing median—which produces the wider occipito-frontal diameter
- Flexing paramedian—which produces a wider paramedian diameter
- Deflexing paramedian—which provides the worst combination of wider diameters with the occipito-frontal and paramedian diameters

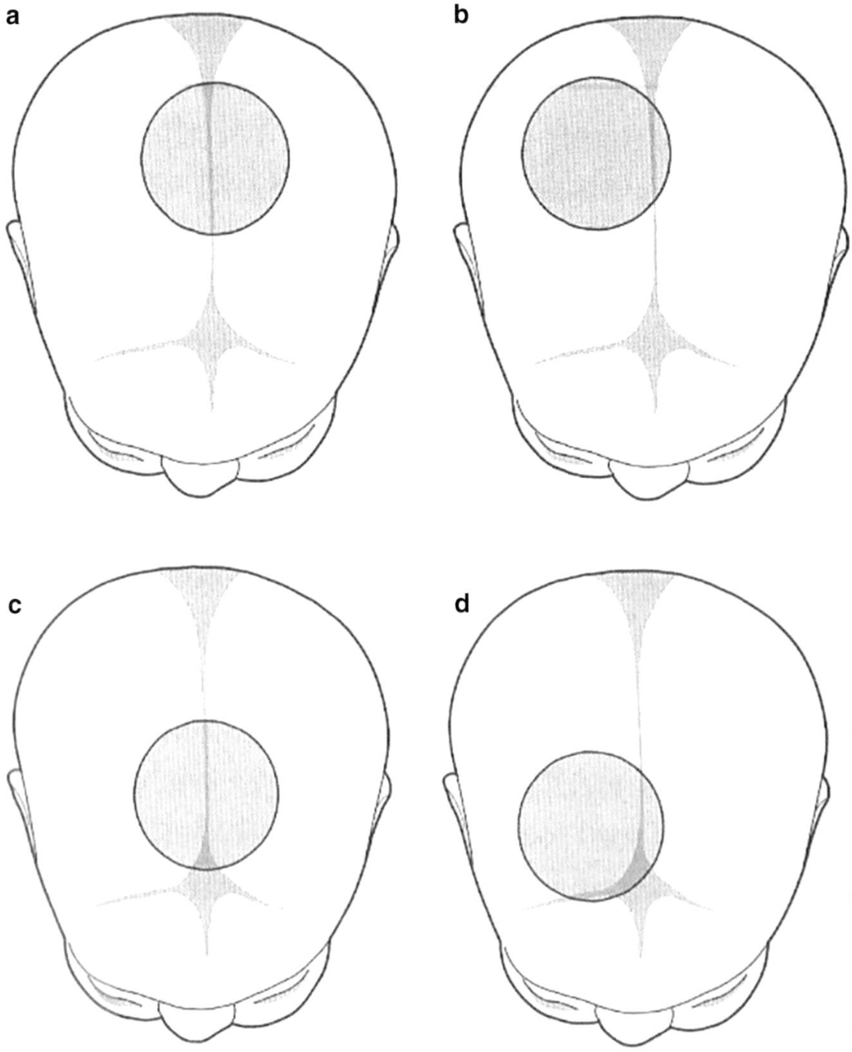

17.3.4.4 Importance of the Flexion Point

By applying the vacuum cup over the flexion point, the foetal neck is flexed and the smallest diameter (suboccipito-bregmatic diameter) is applied to the pelvic outlet. This maximizes traction and minimizes cup detachment. As a result, the success rate of vacuum delivery improves, foetal scalp injury is lessened, and perineal trauma lessened.

Checklist for application of vacuum cup

Task	Well done	Fairly done	Poorly done	Not done
Introduction: what is vacuum delivery, importance, advantages over forceps delivery	4	2	1	0
Explain flexion point; arbitrary, midline, 3cm in front of posterior fontanel	4	2	1	0
Properties of flexion point:				
- Traction at this point flexes the fetal head to suboccipito—bregmatic diameter		2		0
- A 6cm cup at the edge of the posterior fontanel will be over the flexion point.		2		0
- A vacuum cup applied off the central sagittal suture will cause asynclitism during traction		2		0
Possible application of the vacuum cup				
- Flexion median; optimal application		2		0
- Deflexing median; produces wider occiputo—frontal diameter.		2		0
- Flexing Paramedian; produces wider Paramedian diameter.		2 2		0 0
- Deflexing Paramedian; produces worst combination of wider diameters				
Importance of cup placement over the flexion point				
- Maximizes traction.		2		0
- Minimizes cup detachment.		2		0
- Flexes the neck of the fetus.		2		0
- Delivers the smallest diameter to the pelvic outlet		2		0
Total score	30			
Candidate's score .../30				

Examiner's signature Date

17.3.5 Question 3: Breech Delivery

A 26-year-old G2P1 + 0 A1 who had full-term spontaneous vaginal delivery in her last pregnancy presents to the antenatal clinic follow-up at 36 weeks gestation with breech presentation.

- What are the options of delivery of this patient?
- Describe how you would perform external cephalic version (ECV).

17.3.6 Answers

17.3.6.1 Introduction

Breech presentation is the commonest malpresentation accounting for 3% of all presentations at term. There are three types of breech presentation; frank (extended) breech, complete (flexed) breech, and footling breech. Breech delivery is associated with increased maternal, foetal, and neonatal morbidity and mortality.

17.3.6.2 Options for Delivery

To decide on the option of delivery for this patient who is currently at 36 weeks gestation, some factors will have to be put into consideration. These include:

- Foetal characteristics
- Pelvic dimensions
- Co-existing pregnancy complications
- Operator experience
- Patient preference
- Hospital capabilities

In this patient, a brief antenatal history to rule out comorbidities is important. Obstetric ultrasound to confirm the type of breech presentation, estimate foetal weight, localize the placenta, and rule out foetal anomalies is carried out. An antenatal cardiotocograph should be carried out. The results of these investigations are now used to counsel the patient on the following options of delivery:

- Await spontaneous labour at term for planned assisted breech delivery if the foetal weight is <3.5 kg and the antenatal CTG is reactive.
- External cephalic version (ECV) and spontaneous vertex delivery at term if successful.
- ELCS if the mother prefers or there are contraindications to vaginal delivery or ECV.

17.3.6.3 ECV

In general, ECV is attempted before labour at 36 weeks of gestation.

Contraindications to ECV Are
- Placenta previa
- Non-reassuring CTG
- Ruptured foetal membranes
- Scared uterus
- Uterine malformations
- Multifoetal gestation

The Success of ECV Is Improved In
- Multipara
- Foetal weight 2.5–3.0 kg
- Abundant liquor
- Unengaged presenting part
- Posterior placenta
- Non-obese mother

Conditions to Be Fulfilled Before Performing ECV
- Facility for CS available in the hospital
- Antenatal CTG reactive
- USS
  - Foetal weigh <3.5 kg
  - Placental localization
  - Non-vertex presentation
  - Amniotic fluid volume
  - Exclude foetal abnormality

Technique
- Mother in supine position.
- Each hand to grasp one foetal pole.
- Elevate foetal buttocks from maternal pelvis and push laterally.
- Gently guide the buttocks towards the fundus while guiding the head towards the pelvis.
- Discontinue if:
  - Excessive discomfort
  - Persistently abnormal foetal heart rate
  - Multiple failed attempts

- 7% failed attempts undergo spontaneous version to cephalic presentation (2% in nullipara and 13% in multipara).
- If version is successful, await spontaneous labour.
- Subcutaneous terbutaline 250 μg improves success rate (60% versus 30%).
- Spinal or epidural analgesia may improve success rate, but complications are increased (abnormal foetal heart rate tracings, vaginal bleeding × 10).

Complications of ECV (Rare)

- Abruption placentae
- Uterine rupture
- Foeto-maternal haemorrhage
- Preterm labour
- Foetal compromise—even IUFD
- Amniotic fluid embolism leading to maternal death reported in 1985

Checklist for breech presentation and ECV

Task	Well done	Fairly done	Poorly done	Not done
Introduction: prevalence, types and importance of breech presentation	4	2	1	0
Factors to be considered in deciding mode of delivery at 36 weeks: - Fetal characteristics - Pelvic dimensions - Maternal co-morbidities - Others-operator experience, hospital facility, pt. desire		2 2 2 2	1 1 1 1	0 0 0 0
Evaluation of this patient before taking decision - History and physical examination –rule out co-morbidities. - USS-type of breech, EFW, placental localization, anomalies. - Antenatal CTG		2 2 2	1 1 1	0 0 0
Options of delivery - Await spontaneous labour for assisted breech delivery. - ELCS if mother prefers or contraindications for VD. - ECV and possible spontaneous vertex delivery		2 2 2	1 1 1	0 0 1
ECV – to be attempted before labour at 36 weeks gestation		2	1	0
Contraindications to ECV: placenta praevia, non-reassuring CTG, congenital anomalies, ruptured membranes, twin gestation etc.	4	2	1	0
Factors improving success of ECV: multipara, fetal weight 2.5-3.0Kg, adequate liquor, unengaged breech, posterior placenta	4	2	1	0
Conditions to be fulfilled in this patient before ECV: facility for CS, reactive CTG, fetal anomaly ruled out, placenta praevia ruled out, fetal weight <3.5Kg	4	2	1	0
Procedure - Mother in supine position - With or without anaesthesia or tocolytics - Each hand to grasp fetal pole. - Elevate the breech from maternal pelvis, push laterally. - Gently guide the breech towards uterine fundus, head towards maternal pelvis - If version successful, observe and wait for spontaneous labour.		2 2 2 2 2 2	1 1 1 1 1 1	0 0 0 0 0 1
Discontinue procedure if: undue maternal discomfort, abnormal fetal heart rate, multiple failed attempts	4	2	1	0
Complications (rare): abruption, uterine rupture, fetal distress, Feto-maternal haemorrhage,	4	2	1	0
TOTAL MARKS	58			
Candidate's score .../58				

Examiner's signature Date

17.3.7 Question 4: Destructive Operations

1. List four common destructive operations
2. Describe step by step how you would conduct one of them on a primigravida presenting with prolonged obstructed labour, IUFD, cephalic presenting foetus at full cervical dilatation.

17.3.8 Answers

Common types of destructive operation:

1. Craniotomy
2. Decapitation
3. Evisceration
4. Cleidotomy

17.3.8.1 Craniotomy

For the patient presented, craniotomy is the ideal destructive operation to deliver her. Craniotomy is the perforation of the foetal head to evacuate brain tissue and collapse the head in order to extract the foetus through the vagina.

Indications

- Obstructed labour with IUFD in cephalic presentation
- Hydrocephalus—cephalic or breech
- Locked twins

Conditions to Be Fulfilled

- Cervix must be fully dilated.
- Cephalic presentation-except hydrocephalus.
- Foetus is dead.

Contraindications

- Severely contracted pelvis-true conjugate <7.5 cm
- Ruptured uterus

Preoperative Preparations

- Set IVL, rehydrate patient
- PCV, grouping, and cross matching
- Urinalysis, EUC
- Explain the procedure to patient and obtain informed consent

Preparation

- Under GA.
- In lithotomy position.
- With surgeon scrubbed, gowned with face mask and sterile gloves.Patient is cleaned and draped.
- Bladder emptied by catheterization.
- VE done to confirm findings.

Step 1: Insert the index and middle fingers of the non-dominant hand into the vagina to identify the point of perforation:

- Parietal bone in vertex
- Frontal bone in brow
- Orbit in face presentation

Step 2: With Simpson's (or Oldham's) perforator in the dominant hand, the closed blades are introduced under the surface of the fingers in the vagina to the point of perforation. You may incise the scalp between two Kocher's clamps to expose the skull bone.

Step 3: With an Assistant Steadying The Foetal Head per abdomen, the perforator is thrust into the foetal head up to the shoulders of the blades. The handles are compressed to open the blades. The blades are closed again, withdrawn to its tip, rotated at right angles, thrust in again and the blades opened. With rotatory movements, the brain tissue is churned, and the perforator carefully removed.

Step 4: The brain tissue is evacuated with the fingers of the dominant hand till the foetal skull is sufficiently collapsed.

Step 5: Two pairs of giant straight Vulsellum forceps are applied to the skin edges and skull of the foetus and traction applied along the pelvic axis to deliver the baby.

Step 6: The third stage is managed actively, and the utero-vaginal canal explored to rule out uterine rupture or vaginal tear.

Step 7: Anaesthesia is reversed, and indwelling Foley's catheter left in situ for 3–5 days. Give prophylactic antibiotics and treat anaemia if present.

Checklist for craniotomy

Task	Well done	Fairly done	Poorly done	Not done
Common destructive operations: - Craniotomy - Decapitation - Evisceration - Cleidotomy		 2 2 2 2		 0 0 0 0
The scenario given is suitable for Craniotomy: obstructed labour, cephalic presentation, cervix fully dilated.	4	2	1	0
Craniotomy: definition, indications, contraindications	4	2	1	0
Preoperative preparations: - Explain the procedure and obtain informed consent. - Set IVL and rehydrate patient. - PCV, grouping and cross matching of blood - Urinalysis, FBC, EUC		 2 2 2 2		 0 0 0 0
Anaesthesia and positioning: - GA preferable, spinal anaesthesia can be used. - In lithotomy position - Surgeon scrubbed and gowned, cleans and drapes patient. - Bladder emptied by catheterization. - EUA done to confirm findings		 2 2 2 2 2		 0 0 0 0 0
Insert the index and middle fingers of the non-dominant hand to the point of perforation; parietal bone for vertex		2	1	0
Hold the scalp over the point of perforation with 2 pairs of long artery forceps and incise to expose the skull bone		2	1	0
The closed blades of Simpson's perforator are introduced under the surface of the fingers in the vagina to the point of perforation		2	1	0
With an assistant steadying the fetal head per abdomen, the blades of the perforator are thrust into the fetal skull up to the shoulders of the blades	4	2	1	0
The handles are compressed to open the blades, closed again, withdrawn, rotated at right angles and thrust again	4	2	1	0
The blades are opened and rotated gently to evacuate the fetal brain; evacuation may be completed with the fingers of the dominant hand	4	2	1	0
Two pairs of giant straight vulsellum forceps are applied to the skin edges of the perforated skull and traction applied along the pelvic axis to deliver the baby	4	2	1	0
The third stage is managed actively, and lower genital explored for possible lacerations and uterine rupture		2	1	0
Anaesthesia is reversed and indwelling Foley's catheter left for 3-5 days. Give prophylactic antibiotics and analgesia		2	1	0
Total score	56			
Candidate's score .../56				

Examiner's signature Date

17.4 The Puerperium

17.4.1 Question 1: Neonatal Resuscitation

1. What is severe birth asphyxia?
2. How would you resuscitate a newborn with severe birth asphyxia following breech delivery?

17.4.2 Answers

Severe birth asphyxia is a condition in which a baby suffers profound hypoxaemia and hypercapnia leading to metabolic acidosis. It is usually assessed by a low Apgar score of <4 at 1 min or a blood pH <7.0. Clinically, the baby shows no effort to breath, is flaccid or comatose, and may have neonatal seizures.

Severe birth asphyxia is responsible for up to 50% of neonatal deaths. The causes of severe birth asphyxia may be intrauterine like abruptio placentae, intrapartum medications especially narcotics within 3 h of delivery, birth trauma as in breech delivery and postnatally due to congenital heart disease. A severely asphyxiated baby should be resuscitated as follows:

- Lie the baby on a resuscitaire with a head down tilt and under radiant warmer.
- Intubate and connect to IPPV machine with 100% oxygen.
- If there is no IPPV machine, do mouth-to-mouth ventilation and cardiac massage 1:3 and if after about 30 s of ventilation the HR < 60, give 0.1–0.3 mL epinephrine/kg of 1:10,000 solution.
- If there is hypotension, give 10 mL/kg of normal saline.
- For hypoglycaemia, give 60–80 mL/kg/day of 10% dextrose.
- Give 4 mL/kg of 4.2% solution of $NaHCO_3$ to correct metabolic acidosis.
- Transfer the baby to SCBU (NICU).

17.4.2.1 Prognosis

This depends on the maturity of the baby, the duration of hypoxia and facilities at the SCBU. The prognosis is poor when:

- Apgar score of <3 at 20 min
- Oliguria at 24 h of life
- Severe HIE
- Neonatal seizures

Because this baby was delivered by the breech, orthopaedic review will also be necessary to rule out musculoskeletal damage. Neuromuscular damage may require long-term treatment. Possible complications when the baby survives include:

- CVS; hypotension, cardiac failure
- Renal failure due to cortical necrosis
- Liver failure
- Necrotizing enterocolitis
- Seizures due to cerebral oedema; may progress to epilepsy
- Pulmonary hypertension
- Neuromuscular damage like Erb's palsy

Checklist for neonatal resuscitation

Task	Well done	Fairly done	Poorly done	Not done
Definition of severe birth asphyxia, its causes and neonatal outcome	4	2	1	0
Establish the diagnosis of severe birth asphyxia clinically	4	2	1	0
Step 1: lie the baby supine on a resuscitaire with head down tilt under radiant warmer	4	2	1	0
Step 2: intubate and connect to IPPV machine with 100% oxygen or mouth-to-mouth ventilation and cardiac massage (1:3=30+90) if no IPPV machine	4	2	1	0
If after 30 seconds of ventilation the HR<60bpm, give 0.1-0.3ml epinephrine/Kg of a 1:10,000 solution	4	2	1	0
If there is hypotension, give 10ml/Kg of normal saline		2	1	0
Take blood samples for RBS, EUC, FBC, lactate and if possible, blood gases		2	1	0
For hypoglycaemia give 60-80ml/Kg/day of 10% dextrose		2	1	0
For metabolic acidosis give 4ml/Kg of 4.2% NaHCO3		2	1	0
Transfer the baby to SCBU or NICU		2	1	0
Discontinue resuscitation if there is no heartbeat for 20 minutes		2	1	0
Prognosis: depends on baby's maturity, duration of hypoxia and facilities at SCBU. Poor prognosis with Apgar <3 at 20 min, seizures, oliguria at 24 hours	4	2	1	0
Because this baby was delivered by the breech, orthopaedic surgeon should review to rule out musculoskeletal injury	4	2	1	0
Possible complications when the baby survives include: - Hypotension and cardiac failure - Renal failure due to cortical necrosis - Liver failure - Seizure disorders - Necrotizing enterocolitis - Pulmonary hypertension			 1 1 1 1 1 1	 0 0 0 0 0 0
Total score	46			
Candidate's score .../46				

Examiner's signature Date

17.4.3 Question 2: Perineal Tear

1. What is fourth degree perineal tear?
2. Describe step by step how you would repair a fourth degree perineal tear.

17.4.4 Answers

A fourth degree perineal tear is an injury resulting in the disruption of the vaginal and perineal skin, internal and external anal sphincters, and the ano-rectal mucosa. The likely causes of perineal tears are poor conduct of delivery, precipitous labour, big baby, shoulder dystocia, and assisted vaginal deliveries.

Repair

- Place—delivery room (if patient on epidural analgesia in labour) or the theatre, with good lighting and facility for lithotomy position
- Team—experienced obstetrician, assistant, and anaesthetist
- Anaesthesia—spinal or epidural
- Surgical steps
  - Repair ano-rectal mucosa with continuous or interrupted vicryl 3/0
  - Identify and repair internal anal sphincter (thickened rectal wall) and repair with interrupted vicryl 3/0
  - Identify the external anal sphincter and grasp each end with Allis forceps. Mobilize the muscle ends by sharp dissection using scissors.
  - Repair the external sphincter in either of two ways:

    End-to-end technique using two or more figure of eight sutures of vicryl 1

    Overlapping technique by overlapping the mobilized ends by 1–2 cm and suturing with vicryl 1.
  - The remaining procedure is like repairing episiotomy

    Vaginal mucosa

    Perineal muscles

    Perineal skin
  - Post-operative management

    Broad-spectrum antibiotics

    Analgesia

    Stool softeners

    Sitz bath

It is important to advice elective episiotomy during subsequent deliveries, but if the patient is not well motivated, ELCS may be preferred.

Checklist for repair of fourth degree perineal tear

Task	Well done	Fairly done	Poorly done	Not done
Introduction: definition of 4th degree perineal tear, possible causes and how to prevent perineal tear	4	2	1	0
Preoperative preparation:				
- If fresh, do EUA to ascertain extent of injury and bleeding.		2		0
- PCV, grouping and cross matching of blood, resuscitate if necessary.		2		0
- If old wound, do bowel preparation to minimize infection and breakdown of repair.		2		0
- Book theatre and inform anaesthetist		2		0
Anaesthesia: epidural, spinal or GA		2		0
Positioning: clean and drape in lithotomy position, empty bladder	4	2	1	0
Step 1: repair anorectal mucosa with continuous or interrupted vicryl 3/0	4	2	1	0
Step 2: identify and repair IAS (thickened rectal wall) with interrupted vicryl 3/0	4	2	1	0
Step 3: Identify the EAS and grasp each end with Allis's forceps, mobilize the muscle ends by sharp dissection	4	2	1	0
Step 4: repair the EAS either end-to-end or by the overlapping method using vicryl 1	4	2	1	0
The remaining procedure is like repairing episiotomy:				
- Repair vaginal mucosa, then		2		0
- Repair the perineal muscles and finally.		2		0
- Repair the perineal skin		2		0
Postoperative care:				
- Analgesia		2		0
- Prophylactic antibiotics		2		0
- Stool softeners		2		0
- Sitz bath from second day		2		0
Future deliveries:				
- If patient is well motivated, vaginal delivery with episiotomy is preferred.		2		0
- If patient is not motivated, offer ELCS subsequently		2		0
Total scores	52			
Candidates score .../52				

Examiner's signature Date

17.4.5 Question 3: Exclusive Breastfeeding

1. What is exclusive breastfeeding?
2. How would you manage a primipara who presents 5 days postpartum with breast engorgement following an early neonatal death?

17.4.6 Answers

Exclusive breastfeeding means giving an infant breast milk alone, with no other food or drink, including water. The breast milk could be given directly or expressed. However, vitamins and mineral drops may be given when medically indicated.

The rate of exclusive breastfeeding in Nigeria is very low (17%) in the first 6 months of life. Even in the face of the HIV epidemic, exclusive breastfeeding has been shown to be superior to breast milk substitutes, even when the latter is given free in our environment. The policy of WHO, UNICEF, UNAIDS, and the FMOH is that breastfeeding be promoted, protected, and supported.

The advantages of breastfeeding include:

- Provides complete nutrients to the baby
- Cheaper than artificial milk
- Easily digested by the baby and efficiently used
- Protects against infections
- Helps bonding, growth, and development
- Delays a new pregnancy
- Reduces the risk of breast cancer and coronary heart disease in the mother

17.4.6.1 Breast Engorgement

Breast engorgement is excessive fullness of the lactating breast due to lack of emptying and associated with symptoms:

- Breast fullness
- Breast pain
- Milk leakage
- Transient fever, lasting 6–12 h in 10% of cases

Breast engorgement peaks 3–5 days postpartum and up to 10% of mothers experience it, especially primiparas and mothers who experience early neonatal death like in this case. The management of this case will entail relevant history and physical examination:

History

- Date of delivery
- Parity—primiparas are not experienced
- Gestational age (preterm babies have difficulty breastfeeding)
- Health of baby, sick, NND
- Difficulty with breastfeeding-especially attachment
- Social history—marital status, lack of support

Examination

- Symmetry of breasts (both breasts are always involved)
- Shiny skin, no induration, or excoriations
- Nipples for any cracks or soreness
- Full, tender, uniform, no fluctuant areas
- Milk ejection when expressed, may leak spontaneously
- No axillary lymphadenopathy—axillary tail may be enlarged too
- *(Observe the mother breastfeed her baby for positioning and attachment—if baby were alive)*

Treatment

- Well-fitting (sports) brassiere
- Oral analgesics-paracetamol, ibuprofen
- Ice packs
- *(If baby is alive and well, assist to establish regular breastfeeding.)*
- *(If baby is sick, express breast milk regularly—may use breast pump)*
- If baby died, as in this case, do not express breast milk.

Hormonal agents not recommended, may lead to rebound galactorrhoea except you treat for several weeks. The breast fullness itself reflexly inhibits production of prolactin thus stopping further milk production. Engorgement usually resolves within a week but may last up to 14 days in some cases.

Further Treatment

- Bereavement support
- Family planning counselling

Checklist for management of breast engorgement

Task	Well done	Fairly done	Poorly done	Not done
What is exclusive breastfeeding (max. 4 marks)				
- Definition		2	1	0
- Prevalence very low (17% in Nigeria)		2	1	0
- Advantages (complete nutrients, cheap, easy to give etc.)		2	1	0
Management of breast engorgement				
Introduction (max. 4 marks)				
- Breast engorgement is breast fullness due to lack of emptying.		2	1	0
- Symptoms are fullness, pain, milk discharge and sometimes fever.		2	1	0
- Affects 10% lactating mothers, primiparas commoner.				0
- Usually manifests 3-5 days postpartum		2	1	
		2	1	0
				0
History (max. 8 marks)				
- Date of delivery		2	1	0
- Parity; primiparas lack experience.		2	1	0
- Gestational age at delivery – preterm babies difficult to breastfeed.		2	1	0
- Health of baby – babies on admission, poor breastfeeding		2	1	0
- Social history – marital status, lack of support		2	1	0
Examination (max. 8 marks)				
- Symmetry of breasts – both breasts always involved.		2	1	0
- Nipples for cracks or soreness		2	1	0
- Shiny skin but no induration		2	1	0
- Full, tender, smooth, no fluctuant areas		2	1	0
- Milk ejection when expressed, may flow spontaneously.		2	1	0
- No axillary lymphadenopathy		2	1	0
Treatment (max. 6 marks)				
- Well fitting (sports) brassier.		2	1	0
- Oral analgesics		2	1	0
- Ice packs (physiotherapy)		2	1	0
- DO NOT express milk; breast fullness inhibits prolactin secretion		2	1	0
Supportive care				
- Bereavement support		2	1	0
- Family planning counselling		2	1	0
Total marks	34			
Candidate's score .../34				

Examiner's signature Date

17.4.7 Question 4: Postpartum Haemorrhage (PPH)

1. What is primary postpartum haemorrhage?
2. Describe step by step how you would manage a stable patient who presents to the labour ward with retained placenta for 12 h.

17.4.8 Answers

Primary postpartum haemorrhage is defined as blood loss from the genital tract, within 24 h of delivery, which causes a major physiological change such as hypotension, which threatens life. B-Lynch 2006

- Blood loss >500 mL following vaginal delivery
- Blood loss >1000 mL following caesarean section
- Most common cause of maternal mortality
- Accounts for 25% of maternal deaths worldwide

Management of Retained Placenta

- Brief history and physical examination
- Conduct of delivery
- Any intervention like augmentation
- Assess for pallor, BP, uterine contraction
- Set IVL with normal saline or Ringer's lactate
- PCV, grouping, and cross matching of two pints or more
- Vaginal examination
  - Cervical dilatation.
  - Can you feel the placenta?
  - Any active bleeding.
  - Attempt CCT if cervix is not closed.
  - If CCT fails, book patient for removal under GA.
- Procedure
  - In lithotomy position.
  - Empty bladder, repeat VE.
  - Follow the cord with the dominant hand as traction is applied using the other hand.
  - When insertion of cord is reached, identify upper edge of placenta.
  - Insinuate ulnar border of the hand between placenta and uterine wall.
  - With shearing motion, remove the placenta completely in the cup of your hand.
  - Inspect the placenta and membranes for completeness.
  - Clean the vagina and inspect the lower genital tract with speculum for any laceration.
  - Reverse GA and add 40 IU oxytocin to 1 L normal saline to run for at least 2 h.
  - Give antibiotics, ATS, TT

- Postoperative care
  - Continue antibiotics and haematinics
  - Postoperative PCV 2 days postoperatively
  - Transfuse required amount of blood if necessary
  - See postnatal clinic in weeks

Checklist for postpartum haemorrhage

Task	Well done	Fairly done	Poorly done	Not done
Introduction: definition of PPH, prevalence and its importance and prevention	4	2	1	0
Immediate intervention: set double IVL using wide bore cannula, take blood for PCV, grouping and cross matching, FBC, EUC	4	2	1	0
Brief history of conduct of delivery, interventions like augmentation or induction of labour	4	2	1	0
Physical examination: assess for pallor, BP, uterine involution and perform vaginal examination to assess bleeding, cervical dilatation and if placenta can be felt	4	2	1	0
Attempt controlled cord traction and if it fails book theatre for manual removal under anaesthesia.	4	2	1	0
Anaesthesia: GA preferred, spinal will do	4	2	1	0
Positioning: clean and drape in lithotomy position under anaesthesia, empty bladder if not previously catheterized	4	2	1	0
VE: follow the cord with the dominant hand till you reach the insertion of the cord	4	2	1	0
Insinuate the ulnar border of the hand between the upper edge of the placenta and the uterine wall	4	2	1	0
With shearing motion remove the placenta completely in the cup of your hand	4	2	1	0
Inspect the placenta and membranes for completeness		2	1	0
Clean the vagina and inspect the lower genital tract for any lacerations		2	1	0
Reverse GA and set 40IU oxytocin in 1L N/S to run for 2 hours		2	1	0
Postoperative: antibiotics, ATS, TT, transfuse if necessary		2	1	0
Total score	48			
Candidates score .../48				

Examiner's signature Date

17.5 Ethics and Medico-Legal Issues

17.5.1 Question 1: Managing APH in a Jehovah Witness Patient

A 34-year-old primigravida carrying triplet pregnancy following an in vitro fertilization and embryo transfer presents with mild vaginal bleeding at 32 weeks gestation. An abdominal ultrasound confirmed placenta previa. She is a Jehovah witness and refused any blood transfusion should the need arise.

- How would you manage her?

17.5.2 Answers

Since the bleeding is mild, this patient should be managed conservatively. Hoping to reach a gestational age of at least 34 weeks before delivery. With triplets and placenta previa, the delivery is going to be by caesarean section whether emergency or electively.

Immediate Intervention

- Admit patient into the antenatal ward.
- Inform anaesthetist, neonatologist, legal department, her pastor.
- Baseline FBC, EUCr.
- Give IM iron dextran 1 g alternate days for five doses if she is anaemic, if not anaemic give oral iron fumarate 150 mg three times a day with 5 mg folic acid daily.
- Give sulfadoxine-pyrimethamine tablets according to protocol.
- Give dexamethasone 12 mg 12 hourly for 24 h
- Magnesium sulphate 4 g IV, then 5 g deep IM 4 hourly for 24 h for neuroprotection in case of premature delivery.

17.5.2.1 Subsequent Management

If bleeding stops, counsel for autologous blood transfusion:

- Bleed one unit every week if her PCV is 35% or more
- Continue haematinics
- Schedule for ELCS at 34–36 weeks

  If bleeding becomes severe at any gestational age, deliver by EMCS:

- If she consented for autologous transfusion, use the blood already stored.
- If patient did not consent for autologous transfusion:
  - Use colloids intraoperatively; smaller infusion volume needed and has longer plasma expansion properties.
  - May contact legal department if her condition is critical to authorize blood transfusion.

Postoperatively

- Continue treating anaemia as is feasible
  - Autologous transfusion
  - Parenteral iron/oral iron
  - Colloids/crystalloids to maintain blood volume
- Antibiotics and analgesics
- Continue to counsel on options of management even at discharge if alive
- Treat complications as possible

Checklist for management of APH in Jehovah witness

Tasks	Well done	Fairly done	Poorly done	Not done
The issues that have to be managed in this patient are:				
- Antepartum haemorrhage		2		0
- Prematurity		2		0
- Refusal of blood transfusion		2		0
Immediate intervention:				
- Admit into antenatal ward.		2		0
- Set IVL and resuscitate as necessary.		2		0
- Start IM dexamethasone and		2		0
- IM magnesium sulfate		2		0
- Blood samples for FBC, EUCr.		2		0
Subsequently:				
- Haematinics; parenteral iron and folic acid.		2		0
- Monitor bleeding and PCV.		2		0
- Monitor fetuses with USS		2		0
- Inform anaesthetist, neonatologist, legal department.		2		0
- Counsel for autologous transfusion.		2		0
Delivery if bleeding becomes severe:				
- Book for EMCS.		2		0
- Inform anaesthetist and neonatologist.		2		0
- If agreed for autologous transfusion, use the stored blood.		2		0
- If not consented for autologous transfusion, use colloids, contact legal department if her condition is critical.		2		0
Delivery if bleeding stops:				
- Schedule ELCS at 34-36 weeks.		2		0
- Use stored blood if consented for autologous transfusion.		2		0
Postoperatively:				
- Continue managing anaemia as is feasible.		2		0
- Antibiotics and analgesics.		2		0
- Continue counseling even at discharge		2		0
Total marks	44			
Candidate's score .../44				

Examiner's signature Date

Suggested Reading

1. Haden RM, Stevenson M, Dawnie WW. Assessment of clinical competence using the objective structured clinical examination. BMJ. 1975;1:447–9.
2. Carpenter JL. Cost analysis of the objective structured clinical examination. Acad Med. 1995;70:828–33.
3. Webster dictionary, 10th ed. Merriam Webster Incorporated; 2020.
4. Ware J, El-Mardi A, Abdulghani H, Saddiqui I. Examination construction. In: OSCE manual. Saudi Commission for Health Specialties; 2014. pp. 24–31.
5. McCoy JA, Merrick HW. The role of the OSCE in the assessment of students' performance. In: OSCE manual. ASE Educational Clearinghouse; 2001. pp. 18–26.
6. American Educational Research Association. Standards for educational and psychological testing. Washington, DC; 1999.
7. Khan KZ, Ramachandran S, Gaunt K, Pushkar P. The objective structured clinical examination (OSCE). AMEE guide no 81. Part I: an historical and theoretical perspective. Med Teach. 2013;35(9):e1437–46.
8. Smee S. ABC of learning and teaching in medicine, "skill-based assessment". BMJ. 2003;326:707–6.
9. Van Der Vleutin CPM, Van Luyk SJ, Van Ballengooijen AMJ, Swansons DB. Training and experience of examiners. Med Educ. 1989;23:290–6.
10. Waren J, El-Mardi A. Relevant principles of assessment. In: OSCE manual. Saudi Commission for Health Specialties; 2014. pp. 1–9.
11. Boursicot K. Structured assessment of clinical competence. Br J Hosp Med. 2010;71:342–4.
12. Vargas AL, Boulet JR, Errichetti A, Zanten MV, Lopez MI, Reta AM. Developing performance-based medical school assessment programs in resource-limited environments. Med Teach. 2007;29:192–8.
13. Khan KZ, Ramachandran S, Gaunt K, Pushkar P. The objective structured clinical examination (OSCE). AMEE guide no 81. Part II: organization and administration. Med Teach. 2013;35(9):e1447–63.
14. Newble D. Techniques for measuring clinical competence. Objective structured clinical examination. Med Educ. 2004;38:199–203.
15. Pell G, Fuller R, Homer M, Roberts T. How to measure the quality of the OSCE: a review of metrics. AMEE guide no 49. Med Teach. 2010;32:802–11.
16. Epstein RM. Assessment in medical education. N Engl J Med. 2007;356:387–96.
17. Turner JL, Dankoski ME. Objective structured clinical examination: a critical review. Fam Med. 2008;40:574–8.
18. Dhasmana DC, Bala S, Sharma R, Sharma T, Kholi S, Aggarawal N, Kaira J. Introducing structured viva voce examination in medical undergraduate pharmacology: a pilot study. Indian J Pharmacol. 2016;48(1):S52–6.

C. Chama, *OSCE and VIVA VOCE in Obstetrics and Gynaecology*,
https://doi.org/10.1007/978-3-031-77262-7

19. Tutton PJM, Glasgow EF. Reliability and predictive capacity of examinations in anatomy and improvement in the reliability of viva voce (oral) examinations by the use of a structured rating system. Clin Anat. 1989;21:29–34.
20. Oakley B, Hencken C. Oral examination assessment practices: effectiveness and change with a first year undergraduate cohort. J Hosp Leis Sport Tour Educ. 2005;4:3–14.
21. Epstein RM. Assessment in medical education. N Engl J Med. 2007;356(4):387–96.
22. Rohini Bhadre A, Sathe MB, Mosamkar S. Comparison of objective structured viva voce with traditional viva voce. Int J Healthc Biomedical Res. 2016;5(1):62–7.
23. Waseem N, Iqbal K. Importance of structured viva as an assessment tool in anatomy. J Univ Med Dent Coll. 2016;7(2):29–4.
24. Abuzied AIH, Nabag WOM. Structured viva validity, reliability and acceptability as an assessment tool in health professions education: a systematic review and meta-analysis. BMC Med Educ. 2023;23:531–9.
25. Madhukumar, Suwarna MB, Pavithra NS, Amrita. Conventional viva and structured viva—comparison and perception of students. Indian J Public Health Res Dev. 2022;13(2):167–72.

Index

C. Chama, *OSCE and VIVA VOCE in Obstetrics and Gynaecology*,
https://doi.org/10.1007/978-3-031-77262-7

MIX
Papier aus verantwortungsvollen Quellen
Paper from responsible sources
FSC® C105338

If you have any concerns about our products,
you can contact us on
ProductSafety@springernature.com

In case Publisher is established outside the EU,
the EU authorized representative is:
Springer Nature Customer Service Center GmbH
Europaplatz 3, 69115 Heidelberg, Germany

Printed by Libri Plureos GmbH
in Hamburg, Germany